THE NEW MATERIA MEDICA
Volume II

By the same author

The Companion to Homoeopathy
The Practical Handbook of Homoeopathy
The New Materia Medica Volume I

Colin Griffith MCH, HMA is a highly respected and effective practitioner of homoeopathy. He studied at the College of Homoeopathy and, instead of writing a thesis, he set up a supervised drop-in clinic which continued for 11 years and became a teaching clinic where students under his supervision set up their own tables. He has always preferred to work in multi-disciplinary practice where other complementary therapies are offered: cranial osteopathy, reflexology, counselling, etc. He is a founder member of the Guild of Homoeopaths and lectures regularly at the Centre for Homoeopathic Education, Regent's College, London and has lectured in America, Canada, Japan and Greece. He is the author of the highly regarded *The Companion to Homoeopathy*, *The Practical Handbook of Homoeopathy* and *The New Materia Medica Volume I*.

To the memory of Martin Miles,
devoted disciple of Thomas Maughan,
inspirational homoeopath, inimitable teacher
and irreplaceable member of the circle

THE NEW MATERIA MEDICA

Volume II

FURTHER KEY REMEDIES FOR THE FUTURE OF HOMOEOPATHY

Colin Griffith, MCH, HMA

WATKINS PUBLISHING

LONDON

This edition first published in the UK and USA 2011 by
Watkins Publishing, Sixth Floor, Castle House,
75–76 Wells Street, London W1T 3QH

1 3 5 7 9 10 8 6 4 2

Designed by Jerry Goldie

Typeset by Dorchester Typesetting Group

Printed and bound in Great Britain

British Library Cataloguing-in-Publication Data Available

Library of Congress Cataloging-in-Publication Data Available

ISBN: 978-1-78028-022-6

www.watkinspublishing.co.uk

Distributed in the USA and Canada by Sterling Publishing Co., Inc.
387 Park Avenue South, New York, NY 10016-8810

For information about custom editions, special sales, premium and
corporate purchases, please contact Sterling Special Sales
Department at 800-805-5489 or specialsales@sterlingpub.com

CONTENTS

Part III

ACKNOWLEDGEMENTS

This second volume of new materia medica carries another 36 homoeopathic remedies proved through meditative practice. The protocol for the provings remained the same as for those in *Volume I* where a full description of it is to be found. The period of time during which the provings took place covered more than 15 years; in that time changes occurred among the participants of the circle. What has never changed is the quiet and unassuming presence of Janice Micallef who has led the meditations from the very beginning. Without her guidance and inspiration few of these remedies would have seen the light of day. The responsibility for the participants and the caring she has always shown us is humbling. Overseeing the well-being of each member of the circle of up to 10 people while guiding a 3-hour meditation and receiving information herself is draining work yet she has always maintained the same composure and gentle sense of humour throughout. We are all in her debt and can only wonder at how she also manages to run a practice that cares for over 250 families.

It is also important to mention Janice's contribution to the understanding of radiation remedies. Before she became a homoeopath she was a radiographer. Indeed, it was partly this profession that brought her into homoeopathy as her occupation contributed considerably to the reasons for seeking alternative medicine. She went to study at the College of Homoeopathy and became one of Martin Miles's patients. He found that no indicated remedies helped until **Radium Bromide**, repeated and given intercurrently over some two years, lifted the acquired radiation 'miasm'. With this background Janice has had a unique insight into the effects of the miasm and patients' reactions within it. Hence her cases on **Plutonium**, **MRPG3** and **Japanese White Oleander** are particularly valuable.

One of the original members of the circle is Jill Wright. She has been our indefatigable shorthand scribe for the 20 years these meditations have been running. She has been responsible for writing down verbatim reports to ensure that no information would be lost if the recording machinery broke down. To have typed up the notes for distribution must have taken quite literally hundreds of hours of out-of-clinic time. Without her undertaking this enormous task none of us would have been able to remember what had transpired during the meditations. The circle also has to thank her for hosting the most recent meditations in her home which provides such a tranquil setting. Personally I would like to thank her for her prompt and patient attention to my emails asking for yet more information that I have either lost or forgotten.

The present members of the circle are Jill Wright, Sylvia Treacher, Anita Garlick, Colin Griffith, Carole Baldie, Jennifer Maughan, Jerome Whitney, Maggie Gravells, Sue Baker, Lesley Suter, James Peel, Maureen Rose and Grahame Martin. Nick Griffith and Lisa and Edo Cossey have also been members of the circle when exigencies of family and study have allowed. The late Martin Miles was a regular member until his death in 2008 since when he has been very much missed. This has been the group that has proved the following remedies: **Sodium bicarbonate, Blackberry, Clear Quartz, Cardamom, Himalayan Crystal Salt, Hyacinthoides Non-scripta, Ivy Berry, Japanese White Oleander, Statice, Pomegranate, Rutilated Smoky Quartz, Turmeric** and **Viscum Album.** Apart from **Aquamarine, Dolphin Sonar, Rosebay Willowherb** and **Senecio + Tyria** which were proved by some of the above members with students at the Guild study weeks in Duncton Mill and Paros, Greece, the rest of the remedies were proved by the original circles.

In providing case studies to illustrate cases no one has been more assiduous and generous with time than Janice Micallef. She has spent hours talking me through her extraordinary cases. Jan Lewis, Helen Johnson and Linda Rogerson Heath have also been a tremendous support in their willingness to share their knowledge of the remedies. They spent their minimal spare time in collating the information and writing up cases. Sue Baker, Lesley Suter and Jan Taylor have all given their own personal experiences of the effects of the remedies in addition to their case histories. This is invaluable to a thorough understanding of the remedies. I cannot thank all these good friends enough. Carol Burroughs and Chris Braithwaite have not only provided their insights into the remedies but have positively bubbled with their infectious enthusiasm about using the new remedies in their practices.

Two people merit much more than thanks for the remedy made from the sounds that dolphins make: Maxine Harrison and Nick Sellick. When first I asked Maxine to obtain the remedy I had no real idea quite what would be involved. Though she was going to the Bahamas anyway, it was still a difficult task that also took in organization on an almost military scale, shepherding client-crew, skirting hurricanes and taking turns as cook and bottle washer. It took patience, speed, swimming skills, a deep pair of lungs and the ability to suspend scepticism that she was doing such a thing. Our good friend, Nick, an unwitting but enthusiastic prover of the remedy, made it possible through his enormous generosity and quiet but steely determination for us to find more dolphins to follow up on the first trip and then again on the second. All these expeditions were invaluable for getting first-hand knowledge of the behaviour and natural history of dolphins. Nicolas and Dragan Popov must be mentioned here too as they skippered with consummate seamanship the catamaran that took Maxine, Nick and the rest of us to the very place where Atlantic Spotted dolphins would be found. I believe that all four of these inveterate and intrepid travellers would be able to summon dolphins to them wherever they were in the world.

My sincere gratitude goes to the following people who, together, comprise the complete list of contributors:

AL	Alyson Larkworthy
AF	Ann Foster
CAB	Carol A Burroughs
CB	Chris Braithwaite
GM	Grahame Martin
HJ	Helen Johnson
JL	Jan Lewis
JT	Jan Taylor
JM	Janice Micallef
LE	Linda Eyre
LS	Lesley Suter
LRH	Linda Rogerson Heath
LR	Lizzie Rugman
ME	Margaret Ecclestone
MH	Maxine Harrison
PB	Pauline Black
RN	Rita Niehorster
SEB	Sue Baker
SB	Sara Bran
SP	Sue Palmer

ST   Sylvia Treacher
TH   Terry Hadoke
WW   Wanda Wright

Helios Pharmacy continues to give their support for the work that goes into these new remedies and their distribution. John Morgan and his team provide an exemplary service in keeping and preparing them and continue to show their faith and commitment in producing medicines, some of which undoubtedly stretch credulity despite the positive results that are accruing as evidence of their efficacy. I wonder, too, if we would ever have had the remedy, **Plutonium**, without John's intrepidity!

My daughter, Bella, has helped me enormously in understanding Chinese medical thought. She has spent lots of time guiding me to the right source material and with her explanations I have been able to see more clearly how the great oriental traditions might be adapted to homoeopathic usage. Peter Firebrace, acupuncturist extraordinary, has also been an inspiration. I learnt from him the basic techniques of 'listening' to pulses, an invaluable tool in practice that I cannot imagine being without. He has also been generous with his explanation of subtle meanings in Chinese traditional medicine.

Thanks once again to David Binns of The Stone Corner whose little shop of crystal wonder still delights me and provides us with many of the crystal remedies.

Fiona Spencer Thomas is a homoeopath's ideal agent; she is a homoeopath herself as well as being an expert pilot in the world of books. Her faith in homoeopathy, new remedies and alternative thinking in general is a good antidote to any of those doubts and anxieties I might have about writing such a book as this. Michael Mann is an author's ideal publisher; he only enquires when the job is done. This gives me great confidence as I know he has faith in the whole project for which I heartily thank him. My editor Annie Wilson deserves my thanks for her expertise and patience and my sympathy for having to trawl through such a mountain of arcane material. The late Penny Stopa, at Watkins, who must always have been one of those pillars on which companies rest assured, deserves the sincere gratitude of all the authors for whom she cared so well.

Part I

INTRODUCTION

The Remedies

As with *Volume I*, the 36 remedies in this book do not represent any consecutive flow of ideas. They are the collective inspiration of the individuals who make up the circle. Despite this random selection each one has proved to be of significance on a personal level. It is rare for the circle to prove a remedy that does not have a marked healing effect on more than one of the members or that does not become a standard remedy in the clinics of the participants. There are some that have not made it into these pages because there has been insufficient clinical evidence of their efficacy: **Neem**, **Green Beech**, **Banyan Tree** and **Black Tourmaline**[1] are just four such remedies. **Blackbird Song**, made by Martin Miles in the last few months of his life using a similar technique as was used for **Dolphin Sonar**, is also a remedy of significance but one that is extremely hard to qualify and, like the others, as yet has not enough corroborative evidence for the proving to be meaningful.

Within these 36 there are, however, remedies that form groups. The most obvious group is the colours. Inevitably they are chosen because of their association with the seven major chakras. So why are there only six of them? The colour range for the chakras used by the meditation circle differs from the traditional scale that follows the rainbow (see *Volume I*). **Blue** appears twice because it is the colour, albeit in paler and darker shades, of the sacral and throat chakras.

Another group is of culinary interest: **Blackberry**, **Brown Rice**, **Pomegranate**, **Cardamom** and **Turmeric**, though even a cursory look through the materia

---

1 **Green Beech** is a counterpart to **Copper Beech**; where the latter is dark in tone, the former is light. It is also a remedy that is best described as 'the wounded emotional warrior who needs respite from the battlefield' and when given in such a context does great work. **Black Tourmaline** is important in cases of constipation and toxicity of the bowel and is the remedy of choice when **Black Obsidian** is deemed too deep and uncompromising a remedy to use.

medica of each will show how diverse they are. **Sodium bicarbonate** and **Himalayan Crystal Salt** are both salts though quite different in application. Then, as in *Volume I*, there are several trees and plants and various crystals. Odd ones out are **Tunbridge Wells Water** and **Dolphin Sonar**. TWW is not like other spa waters in that it has distinctly passed its sell-by date; the material dose should no longer be sampled by anyone. **Dolphin Sonar** is a completely maverick remedy that is guaranteed to provide ammunition for anyone who finds homoeopathy anathema and has a wish to see it buried, yet it is proving its worth in the clinic. **Plutonium** and **Microwave Radiation PG3** are both radiation remedies and they have many features in common though their applications are quite different. Lastly there is **Senecio + Tyria**; unique in the history of homoeopathy in that it is a single remedy of a plant and the creature that lives off it. Some of the remedies have already been the subject of provings. **Himalayan Crystal Salt** was given a 'world proving', that is one conducted by various groups around the world simultaneously. They are usually, though there have not been many, dream provings when the provers are given the remedy at night and then record any dreams they have which are then shared. **Plutonium** has had two other separate provings, one of which was Hahnemannian in the strictest sense (Sherr). The proving of **Plutonium** presented here predates by a few years the other two and makes interesting comparative reading. The themes of the remedy are there in all three provings; the differences lie in the emphases and expression rather than the ground covered. Though we already have these published provings it was felt that the circle's results complemented and perhaps deepened what is in common knowledge. **Hyacinthoides Non-scripta** is already better known as **Agraphis Nutans**. **Bluebell** was chosen because it was felt that **Agraphis** was chiefly known for its affinity with some cases of adenoids and otherwise underestimated. It deserved a broader perspective.

The method of proving by meditation

In *Volume I* there is a full description of the protocol of meditative proving including the reasons for the choice of this unconventional method, the manner in which it is conducted and the means of producing the remedies before they are sent to the Helios Pharmacy for potentization beyond the 30th. It should be repeated here that meditative provings do not remove the need for Hahnemannian provings. Hahnemann's exacting method remains the most secure means of understanding the homoeopathic energy of our medicines. It is nevertheless true that there are quite a few remedies that have had skimpy provings and others that only have symptoms based on poisoning details and yet they appear in the mainstream materia medicas. If these or the remedies presented in this book prove to be significant additions to the common pharmacy of homoeopaths in general practice then the rigorous protocol of a Hahnemannian proving may well offer further enlightenment.

The common threads of the remedies

It was noted in *Volume I* that there were certain themes that kept appearing among the remedies. It is no different in this selection. We still find that there are remedies that cover these themes as they are expressed in individuals of varying susceptibilities. We still have radiation toxicity, vaccine damage, chronic injury patterns and biochemical toxicity. In these 36 remedies other themes have been identified in addition to the ones already mentioned:

- **Radiation toxicity** is represented by two remedies that are known to be extremely harmful to humanity despite their common usage. **Plutonium** is too well known from history books to mention it further here. Microwave radiation is still the subject of heated debate chiefly between scientists who want to use it and their financial backers, and those who suspect it of being an insidious negative influence on our health. **Ivy Berry, Japanese White Oleander, MRPG3, Orange, Plutonium, Statice, Turmeric** and **Turquoise** have affinity for the various effects of radiation (see Appendix I).
- **Vaccine damage** continues to occupy homoeopaths' minds and will do so for many years to come because clinical experience obliges us to take it into consideration in cases where inoculations appear to be the trigger for the wide range of pathology that has become associated with them. **Aquamarine, Dolphin Sonar, Hyacinthoides, Malus** and **Statice** have an affinity for the various effects of vaccination poisoning or damage. These and the others cited in *Volume I* may prove to be of value to practitioners who have studied and adopted the remarkable Tinus Smits' CEASE treatment of autism and the side effects of vaccination.
- **Chronic injury patterns** remain a constant theme because they are such important maintaining causes for patients not being able to

achieve positive change. The more we understand the way the body responds to chronic injuries and the reasons why they become a significant part of layers cases, the greater the facility we have in assisting patients to resolve their problems. **Clear Quartz, Green** and **Red** cover symptoms that may result from old injury.

- **Biochemical toxicity** remains another top maintaining cause. In this book there are several remedies that are noted for helping patients with blood cleansing, liver detoxing and improving lymphatic drainage. This aspect of practice, the prescribing of remedies to clean up the physical body, is a high priority especially among patients with a long history of suppression and drugging. The liver features strongly in this category. The following all have an affinity for patterns of reaction from biochemical toxicity: **Sodium Bicarbonate, Blackberry, Cardamom, Chalcancite, Clear Quartz, Green, Ivy Berry, Red, Senecio + Tyria, Turmeric** and **Yellow**.
- **Blood purifying** is covered by just a few new remedies: **Blackberry, Clear Quartz, Ivy Berry** and **Red**.
- **Glandular problems** such as those that affect the endocrine system are extremely common in practice and the following may be found useful: **Chalcancite, Cotton Wool, Jade, Japanese White Oleander, Orange, Plutonium, Rutilated Smoky Quartz, Statice** and **Yellow**.
- **Acid/alkali balance** in the body is a new theme and one that is addressed by the following remedies: **Sodium bicarbonate, Clear Quartz, Cardamom** and **Sequoia**. Hyperacidity of the system is a maintaining cause in that the state of an over-acidic system is usually characterized by too much 'heat' (even if the patient is a chilly mortal), too much adrenalin and too speedy a metabolism. This condition often means that the patient either 'burns up' the chosen prescription very quickly or it effects few changes.
- **Poor nutrition and absorption** are covered by **Organic Brown Rice, Pomegranate** and **Tunbridge Wells Water**.
- **Chronic fatigue** must be one of the most common serious conditions which we are asked to treat. It is not the same as ME though they are often treated as such. (CF may have any number of origins but is chiefly initiated by injury or emotional trauma and complicated by few or many other or minor complaints that appear in diverse parts. ME is more systemic and is usually characterized by blocked glandular

activity and a complete loss of real motivation.) Remedies to consider include: **Chalcancite, Cotton Wool, Japanese White Oleander, MRPG3, Plutonium** and **Tunbridge Wells Water.**
- **Shock** and its chronic sequelae may be covered by **Green, Japanese White Oleander** and **Plutonium.**

HOMOEOPATHY AND EASTERN MEDICAL PHILOSOPHY

In *Volume I* of this materia medica the preliminary chapter on the chakras suggested that remedies could be used to treat and support the areas of the body covered by the seven major energy centres: the base, sacral, solar plexus, heart, throat, brow and crown. The idea that remedial action can be taken on parts of the system that would threaten to destabilize the whole, even when that is being positively influenced by a constitutional remedy, is not by any means new. One only has to think of the common use of low potency drainage remedies for the support of specific organs to acknowledge the potential of this practice. Treatment of the chakras is an extension of this idea. Knowing when and how to prescribe a remedy (familiar or new) to support an afflicted chakra is dependent, as always, on observation of the individual and on how that individual's system behaves. It also depends on judging whether the chosen similimum on its own would be able to effect all the necessary changes or if it might need and benefit from the addition of a supporting remedy chosen for its good relations with the similimum and for its affinity for the identified problem chakra. One of the questions that arises amongst students most frequently is 'How do we know when a chakra is in need of support?' even if they have made a study of the chakras.

Apart from learning how to 'read' the chakras (which includes their associations with the miasms, their affinities for certain remedies, the type of pathology that might be associated with it, and the themes that characterize each one), it is very helpful to have a thorough understanding of the role played by the specific organs that belong to them. Unfortunately, Western medical thinking tends to restrict itself to the functional aspect of the kidneys, spleen, stomach and liver, etc., vital though that is. What can be of considerable help in assessing the state of individual organs within their sphere of individual chakras is a less material and more esoteric understanding. Such knowledge has long been available in Eastern medical philosophy.

The inferred integration into specifically homoeopathic thinking of the basic ideas of ancient Eastern medicine is another feature of these 72 new remedies.

Why do so many of us find Eastern medical philosophy so interesting? Perhaps it is because all holistic medical practices purport to be about body, mind and spirit and while Western medicine is pretty good at describing the body and the mind, it is hopeless at integrating the spirit into the scheme of things. So sovereign is materialistic medicine in the West that we need to go in search of what other cultures regard as the purpose for ultimate healing: the purification of the body and mind to achieve the unity of the spirit. By concentrating so strongly on the description of remedies and their roles as similima we may fail to see what lies beyond the curative effects they have. Cure becomes an end in itself and when it is evident it seems as if the job is done. We often forget to pay attention to the creative purpose that the spirit has in making use of the body and mind to manifest symptoms – the symptomatic metaphors it creates for its own ends and for perpetuating movement, be it positive or negative.

Reading cases cured by this or that remedy can create the delusion that people only need to find their 'own remedy' to achieve health – a limited concept to the Eastern mind. The truth of practice is usually far less clear-cut and far more fluid. The ever more precise practice of fitting patients into homoeopathic pictures rather than moulding prescriptions to patients is excessively demanding, largely impractical and dependent on perfect case-taking. Practice shows us that few patients remain wedded to one remedy (unless they have a hidden agenda in being 'stuck'); that we are all a complex tapestry of layers of emotional history (both our own and ancestral); that one of the functions of the physical body is to express through symptomatic simile and metaphor what the mind and emotions most need to resolve. Because of this complexity, there is so often an imbalance not only of the whole but between parts of the whole. It is here that we can usefully borrow from other models.

There are at least two streams of Eastern philosophy and these include the one from China and the one from India; it is from the latter that we have taken the concept of the chakras (though many other cultures have been aware of their significance). We may find ourselves more in sympathy with one than the other and if we look at both in terms of absorbing and adapting them into our homoeopathic traditions then it can seem like a goulash. Perhaps this is inevitable but we need to start somewhere in our search for the genuine holism of body, mind *and* spirit that is glaringly missing from occidental medicine. What should happen for each student is that a working philosophy evolves and whatever is not viable is forgotten. It is also of the utmost importance that each practitioner should find his or her own path and that the patients they treat should always remain individuals and never be subjected to the rule of the 'norm'. What follows is a much abbreviated description of the way Eastern medicine views the organs that make up the engine that keeps body and soul together. The purpose behind this is to help practitioners to appreciate, in a way their otherwise proper training in homoeopathy has not done, the extreme importance of being able to assess the role of the vital organs in the state of the patient.

Traditional Chinese medicine is based on the concept that the body/mind/spirit is a landscape infused with energies that circulate along well-worn routes. There are gates and pathways, important junctions and major roads. There are influences on this landscape much as weather changes the countryside and the internal weather of the body is subject to the constant flux of the elements of earth, water, fire, metal and wood.[2] The language of this philosophy is metaphorical and allusive. It is indirect because it describes what conditions within the body *are like* not what they actually *are* as Western medicine does. Before there is a prescription of herbs or needles there is the need to discover a sense of what the conditions are like. In ancient Hindu medical thinking there is a fundamental shift in perspective. We have an ascending ladder of at least seven energy centres, the chakras, each one linked with the rest through the subtle etheric or auric body with its seven (or more) levels. These stations represent not only hubs of vital force that maintain the integrity of the body's functions but also a progressive upward path that leads to spiritual enlightenment through the gradual purification of each centre. Ayurvedic practice further refines this by describing the doshas: constitutional types in all their variety of mixed conditions – hot, cold, damp, dry.

Chinese tradition sees water as the first of the elements. It is associated with winter, the north and cold. It can be fluid and subject to gravity or frozen and static, waiting for the warmth of spring sunshine (fire) to liquefy it once more. Its associated organs are the kidneys (yin) and the bladder (yang). It is from water that all other elements spring though they only do so when time, the etheric counterpart of water (and blood), carries the creative impulse in a particular direction with *purpose*. All movement requires this impregnating 'ignition', the equivalent of a nuclear reaction, a spark, an inspiration, an intention, a mini 'big bang'. An indicated homoeopathic remedy is an ignition.

2 Some other systems dispense with metal and wood and include air and ether in which the others are subsumed.

The kidneys

The organs that are most closely associated with water and its flow are the kidneys. They regulate not only the water balance in the body but also the earth element by controlling the retention of certain minerals, and fire by controlling the degree of fluidity in the fire-carrying blood vessels and the heart itself.

The kidneys are responsible for the upward flow of fluid energy to the heart. The heart controls the downward flow of heat (fire) to the kidneys. This relationship between the heart and the kidneys, between water and fire, is fundamental to the well-being of the body. In homoeopathic prescribing it is suggested that we pay attention to the state of the kidneys if the heart is involved in pathology and vice versa so, for example, a kidney drainage remedy supports the heart chakra and a heart support remedy underpins the emotions in a case of stricken kidneys.

The kidneys are subject to depletion from dehydration and lack of or compromised energy. Just as water is purified by evaporation (by the sun/yang) or by being filtered through rock (by earth/yin), so the kidneys perform similar yin and yang tasks for the body. Yet it is also seen that the stomach (an earth/yang organ) is the origin of fluid, as it is the appetite for food and drink that brings water into the system. This means that there is a vital relationship between the kidneys and the stomach – often upset by dehydration or flooding.

The kidneys carry what is known in Chinese medicine as 'essence'. Kidney essence or kidney energy, as homoeopaths might call it:

- describes a person's hereditary energy and determines the strength and vitality of the constitution as it was initiated and formed at conception and the quickening – it is also seen as the esoteric blue print of the soul's incarnated life journey;
- is responsible for the creation of bone marrow;
- is intimately connected (in conjunction with the spleen) with the physical process of absorption and assimilation of food *essence* into the system.

Kidney qi is subject to trauma, depletion and diminution. Like water, it can be easily dispersed or drained away. If kidney qi is deficient it becomes a priority of healing as weakened kidney qi affects every other aspect of the system. This means that we should find it helpful to know as much about kidney drainage and support remedies as possible. The second point above relates kidney energy to the spleen, the earth organ most associated with the creation of blood.

The third point above relates the kidneys to the stomach where the process of converting food into energy is begun. The spleen is also regarded as the organ which is responsible for deriving vital energy from food. The correct balance between kidney, stomach and spleen energy is partially maintained by a dietary balance of alkali and acid. Too much alkali will create too much yin/water in the system; too much acid will create too much yang/fire. Too much water in the system is bad for the spleen; too much fire in the system is bad for the stomach. Too much dampness causes water to rise and heat to fall; too much fire causes dehydration. If we are able to witness these events in the body then we will know better how to use remedies such as **Sodium Bicarbonate, Clear Quartz** and **Turmeric** as well as **Arsen-alb, Hydrastis** and **China** for example.

The relationship between the kidneys and the heart is direct. They must, so to speak, be able to communicate energetically at all times because of their influence on blood, the fluid that carries vital energy around the body. In these two organs the complementary nature of fire and water is illustrated perfectly: water cools ascending fire in the heart; fire warms cold water in the kidneys. For this reason it is useful to know that these actions would restore kidney energy to a state of balance:

- finding the correct amount of water for an individual to drink daily (not always 2 litres a day!)
- limiting the stimulants, such as tea and coffee, that interfere with kidney function and, to some extent, adrenal output
- eating foods that stimulate correct and balanced kidney function (green vegetables, nettle tea, cucumber, celery, etc.)
- discovering the remedies that will effect the most profound and subtle changes on them.

Familiar remedies are:

- **Arsen-alb, Benzoic Acid, Berberis Vulgaris, Calc-carb, Calc-arsenicum, Chimaphila, Equisetum, Helonias, Lycopodium, Nat-mur, Ocimum Canum, Phos, Pulsatilla, Sarsaparilla, Solidago, Squilla, Terebinth, Urtica Urens.**

New remedies are:

- Aquamarine, Blackberry, Blue, Organic Brown Rice, Cardamom, Chalcancite, Clear Quartz, Jade, Golden Beryl, Goldfish, Hazel, Hyacinthoides, Ilex Aquifolium, Malus, Moonstone, Oak, Orange, Red, Rhodochrosite, Salix Fragilis, Sandalwood, Sequoia, Silver Birch, Tunbridge Wells Water and White Chestnut Flower.

It is said that chronic disease will inevitably reach the kidneys because the kidneys are regarded as the root of all other organs. They provide the energetic impetus for their functioning because the kidneys are the storehouse of essence; they are the bank of spirit or qi with which we are invested on incarnation. The Chinese call the kidneys the 'root of pre-heaven qi' (energy that exists before conception and quickening). To find out about their parents' health and vitality is to discover a little of the quality of essence inherited by someone who is seeking treatment for a chronic condition that will inevitably reflect ancestry in some measure. In homoeopathy it is possible to prescribe not just for miasmatic inheritance but also for the effects of emotional and spirit inheritance.

The emotion that is most associated with the kidneys is fear. This may be slow fear that develops from accumulating anxiety or sudden, explosive fear that springs from shock. It can also be inherited fear from anxious or chronically shocked parents. Fear may cause qi to descend through the body; the result can be weakness of the bladder (especially at night in fearful children) and sometimes of the bowels. Or it can cause it to rise; there is a rush of adrenalin, a flushed face, dry mouth, restlessness and insomnia. (Remedies such as Ayahuasca, Aquamarine, Berlin Wall, Japanese White Oleander and Rose Quartz might come to mind in this context.)

One of the causes of anxiety that affects and depletes kidney energy is stress at work. Mental overwork combined with lack of relaxation, poor diet, late nights and a lack of physical exercise may lead to a depletion of yin energy – as the result of using too much yang/heat/adrenal energy and not allowing or inviting any 'giving and receiving'. This is too much 'doing' at the expense of 'being'. The long-term net result can be light-headedness, tinnitus, poor memory, reduced hearing, night sweats, thirst, a sore back, aching bones and constipation; the urine is likely to be darker coloured.

If anxiety or any other cause has created a condition of excessive compliance or victimhood (that is excessive yin, allowing or even inviting the loss of energy to others) then there is likely to be a deficiency of yang in the kidney energy. Here there is chilliness, weakness, lassitude, water retention, lack of thirst, poor appetite and loose motions. There is too much 'feeling' at the expense of 'thinking' or 'choosing'.

Sometimes the kidneys fail to receive qi themselves; they are unable to receive true qi[3] from above, usually because they are weakened by too much yang activity (after excessive mental or physical exertion) or from a chronic condition such as asthma which is characterized by lack of communication between lungs and kidneys. The lungs are part of this picture: rising qi accumulates in the lungs but there is not enough to be circulated back to the kidneys. This is partly because more of the true qi is being sent to the heart (raised pulse rate) and for defensive qi (night sweats) but also because the kidneys are weakened by the condition and its hereditary and miasmatic causes. The consequences include shortness of breath on any exertion, rapid, shallow breathing, difficulty inhaling, coughing, sweating, chilliness (especially of the extremities), emaciation, apathy and listlessness and soreness of the back. The urine is likely to be clearer and paler.

If kidney qi itself is depleted then the results are more like a general yin deficiency: in children there is poor development particularly of bone, poor nutritive condition, mental retardation, dullness. In an adult there will be softening of bone, weakness of the extremities (especially of the legs and knees), poor memory, loosening of teeth, premature greying of the hair and soreness of the back. All this can be due to ageing, excessive sexual activity (especially at puberty) or continually taking the wrong path that brings frequent disappointment and frustration and no resolution to life's lessons.

Kidney essence is also a fundamental attribute of mind; mind cannot function without it. Kidney qi must rise through the body for mind to be in harmony and to expand. If kidney qi is weak then the mind is dulled. If kidney qi does not rise due to weakness then the heart can become weak: there may be no collaboration between the two organs; the heart's fire does not warm the kidneys and the kidney's water does not cool the heart. This leads to palpitations, restlessness of the mind, lack of concentration, insomnia, poor memory, light-headedness, poor hearing, soreness of the lower back, night sweating and periods of feverish heat (mostly in the afternoon). When heart

3 True qi originates in the lungs and is the result of combining source qi from the kidneys, nutritive qi from the stomach and spleen, and heavenly qi inspired into the lungs. It is sent out to become defensive qi and to flow around the body in the blood vessels, any surplus being sent down to the kidneys.

and mind are affected by weak kidney energy the aetiology is often found in profound emotional problems, especially those to do with failed relationships or heart-shocks. Sometimes such issues may compound a hereditary link with heart pathology. Knowing the kidney support remedies means that we can support these vital organs when prescribing on the broader canvas of pathology in one of the other organs (i.e. the heart or the lungs) or the mind.

The following mini-repertory of remedies associated with kidney energy, when other organs or states are involved in the case, may prove useful in selecting for drainage or support:

- **spleen** and kidney: **Black Obsidian, Cardamom, Golden Beryl**
- **stomach** and kidney: **Clear Quartz, Sodium Bicarbonate**
- **heart** and kidney: **Cardamom**
- **liver** and kidney: **Clear Quartz, Hyacinthoides, Red**
- **blood** and kidney: **Blackberry, Red**
- **bowel** and kidney: **Black Obsidian, Sodium Bicarbonate**
- **nervous system** and kidney: **Chalcancite, Clear Quartz, Lotus, Orange**
- **poor nutrition** and kidney: **Organic Brown Rice, Tunbridge Wells Water**
- **emotions** and kidney: **Aquamarine, Goldfish, Hazel, Ilex Aquifolium, Jade, Lapis, Malus, Moonstone, Oak, Salix, Sequoia, Statice, White Chestnut Flower**

The Spleen

Spleen energy has several main roles to play in the body:

- transformation and transportation; of food and drink, of blood
- control of the quality and quantity of blood
- feeding muscles with nutrition energy in the limbs
- control of the raising of refined energy ensuring alignment of the vital organs and nourishment throughout
- fostering clarity of thought, concentration and facility of memory.

The vital energy of the spleen may be monitored by certain aspects of health.

- There is a connection with the mouth; when the spleen is weak, the sense of taste is impaired or distorted, the tongue shows indentation of the teeth around the edges, gums tend to bleed, the lips lose colour and become dry and pale. If the stomach is weak then there is redness and soreness and swelling on the external lips and around the mouth.

• There is weak musculature especially of the extremities.

• There is a tendency to haemorrhage or to anaemia.

• There is a lack of intellectual focus, poor concentration and poor motivation, a tendency to become ungrounded.

• There is a tendency to indigestion, stomach ulcers and conditions arising from female reproductive hormone difficulties. The knees and neck may manifest symptoms as they are associated through the meridians. If the stomach energy is poor then irritable bowel symptoms, hiatus hernia, mouth ulcers and problems with the eyes, sinuses, ankles, breast and female reproductive system will occur.

The spleen and pancreas are viewed, in traditional Chinese medicine, as being of the same energy. Yet the pancreas is also closely associated with digestion as it produces enzymes, a vital part of the digestive process, which are secreted directly into the small intestine. Problems arise in the pancreas when spleen energy and liver energy are both frustrated.

The stomach and spleen
The stomach and spleen are the central pivot on which most other physiological processes depend, not least as they are the organs that are most involved in receiving food. They are both earth organs and are opposite and complementary. As earth organs they require plenty of fluid if they are not to dry out. Both of them are susceptible to the emotional turmoil of the water element. Water is also vital to the digestive process; drinking an adequate amount of water[4] being one of the ways of maintaining the correct acid/alkali balance in the body.

---

4 Early signs of dementia may in fact be signs of dehydration in elderly people; an illustration of the connection between kidney and mind. It is also worth remembering there is no 'normal' amount of water for people to drink; they need to find their own level. Someone who has a lot of fire in their system is naturally going to need far more water than someone with less fire.

Stomach	Spleen
Yang	Yin
Descending energy to separate impure waste from food which is sent to the intestines for the assimilation of nutrients. Though yang, its mixing of food and fluids and provision of fluid energy are yin in nature.	Ascending energy to provide lungs and heart with essence of food. Though the organ is yin, its transporting activity is yang in nature.
+ & >> wet (damp); << dry If too dry, stomach energy cannot move downwards (stuckness/constipation). << excess	& >>dry; << damp & cold If too damp, energy can't move upwards leading to deficient motivational force. << deficiency
Prone to heat	Prone to cold
Familiar remedies: Arg-nit, Arsen-alb, Bry, Carbo-veg, China, Hydrastis, Lyc, Nat-phos, Nux-vom, Phos, Sulph	Familiar remedies: Arsen-alb, Bry, Ceanothus, China, Ignatia, Iod, Mur-ac, Nat-ars, Nat-mur, Sul-ac
New remedies: Black Obsidian, Cardamom, Okubaka, Organic Brown Rice, Pomegranate, Red, Rutilated Smoky Quartz, Sodium Bicarbonate, Tunbridge Wells Water.	New remedies: Berlin Wall, Blackberry, Black Obsidian, Cardamom, Golden Beryl, Hazel, Oak, Winchelsea Sea Salt

Ingested food arrives in the stomach where it is heated. The digestive process should already have started with the chewing and mixing of food with saliva that contains digestive enzymes. If food is too dry, stomach qi is <; if too cold, spleen qi is <. Whether food and drink are, by preference, ingested hot or cold becomes of significance as the information gives us clues about the constitution. The amount of water, juice, alcohol, tea or coffee which is drunk also becomes vital as each has an effect on the whole system and tells us about bad habits.

Food is best for us when it is of the right type, of the right consistency and with sufficient moisture for the individual. (No one would knowingly heat dry food in a saucepan or throw away sloppy waste food without draining it first.) There are no universally 'correct' diets; only the diet that suits the individual. In the following chart the liver and spleen are compared.

Liver	Spleen
Liver energy aids the process of transformation, separation and transportation initiated by the spleen.	Spleen energy helps the liver to maintain a healthy flow of blood-qi around the body while it is active, and to store healthy blood while at rest.
Governs the tendons and ligaments	Governs the muscles and the four limbs
Symptoms of disorder appear in the digestive tract, the mucosa, the eyes, the nails and the skin.	Symptoms of disorder appear in the muscles (weakness and atrophy), mouth and on the lips, as well as in problems of stamina and poor immunity.
Familiar remedies: Berberis Vulgaris, Card-mar, Chel, Chelone Glabra, China, Cholesterinum, Hydrastis, Iodum, Leptandra, Myrica Cerifera, Nat-Sulph, Nux Vomica, Podo, Zingeber	Familiar remedies: Arsen-alb, Arsen-iod, Asaf, Bell-per, Ceanothus, China, Ferrum, Ign, Iod, Nat-mur, Nux-vom, Phos, Plumbum, Sarsaparilla, Sul-ac, Urtica, Zinc

New remedies:	New remedies:
Bicarb-soda, Black Obsidian, Black Tourmaline, Cardamom, Clay, Ivy Berry, Okubaka, Organic Brown Rice, Turmeric, Yellow	Blackberry, Black Obsidian, Cardamom, Golden Beryl, Ivy Berry, Oak, Organic Brown Rice
Drainage combinations: • Chel + Card-mar + Tarax • Chel + Card-mar + Yellow • Golden Beryl + Hydrastis + Ivy Berry • Turmeric + Hydrastis + Ivy Berry	Drainage combinations: • Oak + Golden Beryl + Sulphur • Oak + Golden Beryl + Ignatia

The stomach is easily overwhelmed by negative energy from the liver when there is stress from overwork, poor dietary habits and emotional turmoil. When negative liver energy invades the stomach, irritability, distension, pain, fullness, heartburn, belching, nausea and vomiting can occur. In other words, stomach energy begins to bubble upwards, instead of maintaining its usual downward flow. This negative upward flow interferes with the lungs (breathlessness, shallow breathing, asthma, congestion) and with the heart (anxiety, discomfort, raised blood pressure). It can also lead to the formation of mucus in the airways, phlegm that will need to be expectorated upwards and outwards. Remedies such as **Clear Quartz**, **Sodium Bicarbonate**, **Turmeric** and **Ivy Berry** all help to support a struggling digestive system as they are complementary to so many of the polychrests. According to their indications they are capable of calming the energetic conflict between the stomach and the liver.

The small intestine receives food and drink from the stomach after the initial steps of digestion. The small intestine 'separates' clean food and drink from already putrefying waste products which are sent off to the large intestine and bladder for excretion. The large intestine further separates the waste from what is of benefit by siphoning off the excess water for recycling through the kidneys and the bladder. When there is pathology in the large intestine it is usually due to spleen trouble which may be direct or indirect. Supporting the spleen in bowel conditions becomes a reasonable prescribing strategy.

When an excess of dairy food, sugar or modified starch is ingested that causes negative chemical reactions in the intestines and an extra workload for the liver, the spleen is less able to raise energy to the heart and lungs. Spleen energy becomes stagnant. There is an excess of mucus and acidity in the system and a plethora of symptomatic changes in the digestive tract. The business of the patient's vital force is forced to remain below the diaphragm in a clearing operation instead of rising to assist the heart and lungs in their inspirational and creative processes. Fire may be drawn down into the digestive tract in order to cope with 'burning off' what is an excessive amount of waste instead of being used for purposeful creative activity or else excessive water is employed to flush out the system. The result may be inflammation, diarrhoea or oedema. However, if the chemical reactions to poor diet cause excessive and 'stuck' earth reactions, there may be a lack of water or fire to assist and this results in constipation and inertia.

When the stomach is replete with fluids, digestion is satisfactory and the sense of taste is normal. If there is a deficiency of water there will be poor digestion, a dry and cracked tongue, perversion of taste and a threat to the functional connection between the stomach and kidneys. One of the most common causes of stomach fluid becoming deficient is eating heavy meals late at night. The last meal of the day should be eaten no later than 7 or 7.30pm. (One might think of a well-rotting compost heap: when there is sufficient moisture the heap will rot the vegetation well and create little or no smell. If there is insufficient moisture there will be patches of foul-smelling matter and the rest will stagnate and become dusty and useless.) The kidneys, responsible for the overall governing of water in the system and of its filtration and purification, can be the underlying cause of stomach distress. If the kidneys are weak then the purification of water and retention of vital minerals is poor. The system may become dehydrated or waterlogged leading to insufficient fluids being available for digestion.

If the stomach is in a poor condition there will be a knock-on effect on the mind. If too much fire occurs in the stomach from excess acidity there will be agitation in the sensorium and irritability. Phlegm will be manufactured in the system and occur in the mucous membranes of the airways which will slow down the system as it tries to eliminate it. When the situation threatens to become chronic, excessive fire and stagnant water (thickening phlegm) can block up the channels of the lymphatic system.

The Small intestine

The small intestine (a fire organ) continues the separation and transformation process started by the stomach. The 'clean' water that is to be held back by the body is sent to the large intestine for later reabsorption while the waste water is sent directly to the bladder for excretion. The small intestine, separator of clean and waste material, also has an association with the mind. Just as it discerns the difference between what is required by the body and what is no longer of further use, so it has an influence over the decision-making processes of the mind. It has an influence over the clarity of discriminatory processes so that we are able to make decisions with confidence. Conditions of the small intestine give rise to loss of clarity in weighing up options and seizing opportunities. Remedies indicated by deficiency here support digestion in one who might need remedies for loss of mental acuity.

The Gall bladder

Physiologically close by is the gall bladder (with the common bile duct opening into the small intestine) which also has a connection with mind: it infuses us with courage to make decisions in the first place. It is also the organ associated with the capacity to deal with confrontations. The gall bladder provides us with the energy to galvanize ourselves to deal with challenges presented by liver energy and to deal swiftly and effectively with conflicts that arise from wrong choices. Remedies known to affect the gall bladder directly support the organ in one who lacks courage; this would certainly be true of **Lycopodium** and **Anacardium** though they often require support when prescribed constitutionally. **Ivy Berry** particularly comes to mind here.

The gall bladder, though part of the digestive system, holds no waste products. It should be clean though it is susceptible to being clogged up with a mixture of bile and cholesterol that forms the characteristic green 'stones' that can eventually cause cholecystitis. This is a condition that causes trouble in the stomach (nausea, belching and acidity), the intestines (pain and fermentation) and the spleen (discomfort, lowered immunity). The gall bladder has to be 'clean' because its connection with the heart and mind requires that it should foster clear decision-making as well as bolstering up a deficient heart. Anyone suffering from weak or deficient heart energy is aided by a boost of energy to the gall bladder. It is also very common for emotional trauma to be shifted from the heart centre and into the gall bladder to avoid the pain of grief. **Red** and **Ruby** are both remedies that cover this problem.

A sick gall bladder, making us unable to metabolize fats and holding too much bile, is one that has been unable to cope with challenges and conflicts in the past and has suffered from frustration and discouragement or timidity and indecision. One of the most common origins of gall bladder trouble is a history of boredom or frustration followed by the apportioning of blame on others for the lack of life movement.

The Large intestine

The large intestine continues the process begun by the stomach and the small intestine. It extracts the water from the waste in the body and recirculates it. It also excretes stools that are a combination of the waste from foodstuffs, broken-down blood cells and other waste products organized for expulsion by the liver and gall bladder. It is through the influence of the spleen that all this

Gall bladder	Small intestine	Large intestine
Familiar remedies: Baptisia, Bell, Berb-vul, Bry, Card-mar, Chel, Chin, Chionanthus, Cholesterinum, Coloc, Hydrastis, Iris, Lach, Lept, Lyc, Morgan, Morgan-Gaertner, Nat-sulph, Nux-vom, Phos, Ptelea, Sulph, Tarax, Verat-alb	Familiar remedies: Alum, Arg-nit, Arsen-alb, Baptisia, Bry, Carbo-veg, Chin, Clay, Colchicum, Coloc, Dulc, Dys-co, Gaertner, Hamamelis, Ipecac, Lyc, Mag-carb, Mag-mur, Merc-sol, Morgan-Gaertner, Merc-sol, Nux-vom, Phos, Podo, Puls, Silica, Sulph, Verat-alb	Familiar remedies: Abrot, Aloe, Alum, Amm-mur, Ant-crud, Arsen-alb, Bry, Chel, Chin, Coloc, Lyc, Morgan, Morgan-Gaertner, Nux-vom, Puls, Silica, Sulph, Thuja, Verat-alb, Zing
New remedies: Bicarb-soda, Black Obsidian, Cardamom, Ivy Berry, Red, Ruby, Yellow	New remedies: Bicarb-soda, Black Tourmaline, Lumbricus, Okubaka, Organic Brown Rice, Red, Ruby, Tunbridge Wells Water, Turmeric, Yellow	New remedies: Black Obsidian, Black Tourmaline, Clay, Okubaka, Organic Brown Rice, Turmeric, Yellow

happens. In considering the pathology of the large intestine we have to consider the role of the spleen and it would behove us to remember to support the spleen with low potency remedies in such situations.

The governing and conception vessels

There are 12 meridians, pathways of energy that traverse the entire landscape of the body. They take in every organ of the body and enable every function. A chart of the meridians can be invaluable to homoeopaths[5] but no description here could do them the smallest justice. Instead, it is worth noting the role of the governing and conception vessels. They are not counted among the 12 meridians but are extraordinary vessels with a less specific role; less specific because they travel through and even make use of points on one or more of the 12 meridians and because they cover a larger territory. They are to do with the midline (see **Clear Quartz** and **Sycamore Seed** in *Volume I*); the central axis of energy that carries the main body of circulating energy up and down the spine in a double helix.

The governing vessel is yang. It originates in the pelvic bowl; in the uterus in women and in the prostate in men. It emerges externally at the coccyx and rises up the spine along a parallel path to the bladder meridian. It then goes over the head and down across the forehead until it reaches the gum under the top lip. It is used to strengthen yang in the whole system and to strengthen and nourish the spine and the brain. It is indicated as in need of healing when the patient gives the impression that they need constant support, that there is a lack of grit in dealing with life's complications, when there is a weak and painful lower mid-back and general debility from weak kidney energy. (**Silica** is an obvious remedy here but so too are **Thuja**, **Lycopodium** and **Kali Carb**.)

The conception vessel is yin. It originates from the kidneys and flows into the uterus or prostate, down to the perineum and then rises up the front of the body taking in the abdomen, the thorax, the lungs, the throat and the lower jaw where it meets the descending part of the governing vessel. It is particularly associated with fertility (in both men and women), menstruation, conception, birth and menopause. It serves to nourish the tissues of the body with yin creative energy. It regulates the blood supply to the reproductive organs. It is used at the menopause to cool the embers of procreativity so that the fire

5 The best way to view the meridians is when they are displayed on separate charts as in *The Web That Has No Weaver* by Tom Kapchuk or *Meridians* by Tsao Hsueh-Lien and Bruce Thornton.

energy that was required in the uterus is able to rise to the heart. It is also useful to the lungs when they are unable to transfer true qi back down to the kidneys.

These two great channels are complementary and form a universal circuit which takes in other meridians in its path. Their integrity is essential to the vital force and to the etheric body as a whole. It is likely that all homoeopathic 'ignitions' are registered in their course. Some remedies have a very direct relation to them. This is partly due to the fact that the thymus gland lies within their orbit; in Chinese medicine this area of the chest has much to do with ancestral links. There are points here that are 'gateways' to connect with such energy. The thymus gland is the organ that has shown a marked degree of affinity for the body's memory of ancestral energy and the remedy, **Thymus Gland,** has profound effects on this esoteric aspect of one's being. So too have other new remedies. The main ones are **Aquamarine, Ayahuasca, Berlin Wall, Chalice Well, Clear Quartz, Goldfish, Hornbeam, Himalayan Crystal Salt, Jet, Olive, Rhodochrosite, Statice, Winchelsea Sea Salt.**

While the practice of homoeopathy certainly does not depend on knowledge of this kind, drawing on it may mean that difficult and complex cases become easier to understand. It means that we have a broader perspective and do not restrict ourselves to the expectations of a single prescription. It gives us greater flexibility and further means of ensuring that a patient with complex symptomatology is adequately supported in organs that would otherwise feel strain when attempting to eliminate to the advantage of the whole. It is opportune that so many of the new remedies appear to make it easier for us to adapt so many of the basic principles of oriental thought to homoeopathy. The use of support and drainage remedies is characteristic of those who would prescribe as if homoeopathy were a journey towards the purification of spirit rather than the pursuit of 'cure'.

A NOTE TO THE READER

The method and protocol of meditative proving that underlies these 36 remedies remains the same as it was for those in *Volume I*. For readers who are interested in it, a full description of the process of meditative proving is described in Part 1 of that book. Nothing has changed apart from some of the personnel of the group, as stated in the Acknowledgements, and the venue of the meetings. The symptom pictures of the remedies are still extrapolated from the transcripts of the meetings and added to from the clinical experience of both the attendees and, subsequently, practitioners who have attended lectures and who have felt encouraged to use these medicines.

As with the original 36, the greater part of each remedy is to be found in the general, mental and emotional symptoms. Though almost all the provers have become aware of physical symptoms at some time or another with some or all of the remedies, meditative provings tend to elicit emotional reactions and to concentrate thought patterns in particular directions peculiar to the remedy being proved. As with **Moldavite** and **Lotus** in *Volume I*, several of those presented here appear to suffer from a dearth of physical symptomatology: **Dolphin Sonar, Himalayan Crystal Salt, Lapis Lazuli** and **Orange**. It is only with more clinical experience that the characteristic physical symptoms of each will emerge.[6] However each one, no less than the other, fuller remedies, has been used successfully when chosen as a similimum appropriate to a particular stage of an individual's homoeopathic journey.

It will also be noted that there has been no attempt to weigh or qualify any of the symptoms by listing them with the numbers of provers who suffered this pain or felt that sensation, nor by the use of bold type. Such discrimination can be misleading and might encourage practitioners to prescribe according

6 For example, it was only clear that **Dolphin Sonar** was of value in the treatment of autistic children from the clinical experience of Sue Baker, Lesley Suter and Chris Braithwaite; nothing came up in the provings about this aspect of the remedy.

to statistics rather than the aggregate of a patient's unique symptom picture. If there has been an overwhelmingly universal reaction then it is referred to in the 'General symptoms' section.

It is easy to be carried away with enthusiasm for whatever is new. Much of the materia medica presented here would appear to make extravagant claims for these new remedies. It is worth remembering that it is only going to be years of observant practice that will establish the credentials of each remedy beyond doubt. It is also important to regard indications of healing for serious pathology only in the light of the *whole* picture of each remedy. Where it says that a remedy is useful in MS, AIDS or cancer, for example, it should be taken to mean that the remedy may arise as generally indicated in a case in which these conditions are extant; not that the condition will be cured by it. Healing, as we know, comes from the patient and not from the remedy.

So it is important to repeat the caveat that appeared in *Volume I* about basing a prescription solely on an aggregate of *seriously pathological physical symptoms*. It is always better to err on the side of caution when considering the use of one of these 36 remedies in such cases, just because of the need for a great deal more clinical experience. What has been reported here as having been physically experienced in meditation, may not be sufficient evidence to use a remedy in expectation of the elimination of physical symptoms. This is not at all to say that these remedies have not, at times, been of tremendous service in those who have suffered serious physical illness; a reading of some of the case studies shows how severe physical symptoms have succumbed to their healing energy and, in some examples, have been the only means of securing lasting healing. Nevertheless, the symptoms have been resolved as a result of the remedies being chosen as similima, not solely on their therapeutic indications.

As in *Volume I*, prescribing suggestions have been made which are based on the collective experience of practitioners already familiar with and employing the remedies. Where reference is made to using them for organ drainage and support, referral to 'Homoeopathy and Eastern Medical Philosophy' above, and to the chakra information in *Volume I* is suggested, to give a broader perspective of the potential of each remedy. Where combination remedies are suggested it is only for instances where there is no clear similimum though, as has been discovered by the use of specific combinations using **Thymus Gland** (see *Volume I*); a 'triad' remedy chosen for its combined similarity to a particular aspect of a complex case can attain the status of similimum, by virtue of its ability to shift a patient who otherwise lacks positive reaction to indicated remedies. It is hoped that every practitioner will use this materia medica as a book of inspiration and resource that might help to unlock difficult and many-layered cases which have thus far been hampered by maintaining causes that have not yet been resolved by any familiar indicated similimum.

The book is divided into three parts: the introductory material, the remedies and the appendices. The materia medica of each remedy is structured to give cohesion to the whole. Each remedy is examined under the following headings:

- The Background[7]
- Keynote effects
- General symptoms
- Miasms
- Mental and emotional symptoms
- Physical symptoms
- Considerations for the use of the remedy
- Esoteric therapeutics
- Chakras
- Case studies

'The Background' provides an introduction to the source of the remedy, looking at its history, its natural history, its mineralogy, its essence picture – whichever is applicable in each case. It is hoped that the material might suggest 'signatures' that might guide practitioners intuitively to fresh ways of seeing patients. In 'Keynote effects' the broad expectations of the remedy's prescription are covered. The 'Miasms' heading refers to the miasms with which the remedy has an affinity, suggesting that if a listed miasm appears strongly enough to influence a case then it might be considered as a contributing factor in prescribing the remedy. In the 'Considerations' section, comparisons are suggested not just between the remedies presented but also with old friends perennially in use. There is also further information based on collected experience from many of the practitioners already using the new remedies regularly. 'Esoteric therapeutics' and 'Chakras' are offered as an alternative way of looking at a remedy; they explore the more arcane aspects of the spirit of the remedy and describe the influence it has on the individual energy centres. The case studies given are from practising homoeopaths' casebooks. These cases

7 I am indebted to Frans Vermeulen and his exemplary publications, especially 'Prisma', for including this heading to introduce the remedies.

were either reported to me directly or sent by post or email. Apart from typos, spelling and punctuation, I have left them unaltered. Cases are accepted by readers as 'evidence', but by critics as anecdotal or hearsay. The cases here are offered as illustrations of empiricism at work.

NB I have used the conventional homoeopathic symbols throughout the book and I have listed below the abbreviations for dosage I have used:

o.d. = once each day; o.n. = once each night; b.d. = twice each day;
t.d.s. = three times each day; p.r.n. = as required.

PART II

1

AQUAMARINE

The remedy was first proved during a week's post graduate course run by the Guild of Homoeopaths on the island of Paros, Greece, in May 2005. It was chosen as one of two remedies to prove through meditation by two groups of students who took the remedy in the 30th potency. The students were unaware of the nature of the remedy though the leader of the groups, Janice Micallef, knew the name.

The Background

Aquamarine is a form of beryl, a hexagonal crystal form that has a hardness rate of $7^1/_2 - 8$. Its chemistry is complex: $Be_3Al_2Si_6O_{18}$ + iron. Other varieties of beryl include emerald (pale to dark green), heliodor (yellow) and morganite (pink). Beryl often appears in granite areas. The crystals are often short to long prismatic faces which are striated along their surfaces. There is a vitreous (glass-like) lustre to the surface. Aquamarine is of a pale blue-green colour and differs from emerald due to the presence of iron. It is found in the USA, Mexico, Russia, India, Brazil, Nigeria, Zambia, Zimbabwe, Madagascar, Mozambique, Afghanistan and Pakistan.

Traditionally, aquamarine is considered the birthstone for March. Legend tells us that many thought of this stone as the 'treasure of mermaids' and as such it was considered a powerful charm to keep sailors safe at sea. In the middle ages it was regarded as an antidote to poisons. As well as being the gemstone for the 19th wedding anniversary, it is also a stone for healing rifts between married couples; it is said to ensure long and happy marriages and is traditionally an anniversary gift between spouses. Rather more dramatically, it was claimed by some that aquamarine wards off the wiles of the Devil.

Keynote effects

Aquamarine soothes the heart that was wounded many years ago or that bears the scars of family (ancestral) trauma and grief. It fosters emotional enlightenment and helps patients to face uncomfortable and often buried truths. It can bring a sense of peace where there has been conflict within, even when that conflict is not acknowledged. It supports remedies chosen for their action on the physical heart (and will not interfere with chemical drugs that may be a necessary prescription at the same time). A common aggravation is a headache which should be left to resolve without further medication though Rescue Remedy may well speed up the process safely. Skin symptoms may also erupt and should be left alone except when infection threatens.

General symptoms

It works on the endocrine system, the nervous system, the heart and circulation and musculature. It is useful after a stroke (especially after remedies such as **Opium, Arnica** and **Calc-carb**); after seizures; with fainting especially when there is absent-mindedness, lack of self-awareness and shock anywhere on the system. It should be considered of use in Parkinsonism, MS and conditions marked by dystonia (impairment of muscle tone); also with asthmatic breathing particularly where the intercostal muscles and the diaphragm are held in spasm. The remedy has a bias for the left side of the body. It should be considered in those who have suffered vaccine damage that has gone beyond physical symptoms; in children who have been adversely affected in the mind, emotions or spirit by any vaccine. The remedy follows the isopathic vaccine remedies (**DPT, MMR** etc.), **Thuja** and **Silica** well, and works on the shock to the endocrine system that vaccines cause at the level of the pineal/pituitary connection. It appears to reset the body clock when that is put out of sync by artificial immunization. Swings of temperature; when the body's thermostat has no balance. Affects the five special senses: sight, hearing, taste, touch and smell; has great sensitivity to external impressions. Affects the thyroid gland and is especially useful in patients whose diagnosis is uncertain from blood tests or who appear to swing between hypo- and hyperthyroidism or who have a confusing mixture of symptoms of both. It is of use in patients affected by geopathic stress. It is a remedy to consider for children who carry mobile phones around with them all the time. It is protective against the auric influence of mobile phones held too close to the body and of the masts that emit electrodynamic radiation. For deep shock and trauma. NBWS (not been well since) a profoundly life-changing circumstance, physical, emotional or mental. Useful after **Arnica** and other physical trauma remedies when they have worked on the physical and mental bodies; the subtler etheric bodies also are often traumatized and the damage may not be susceptible to **Arnica** etc., a circumstance that may prevent thorough healing of the musculoskeletal system. **Aquamarine** is of use in healing the damaged aura and in helping to integrate body and vital force. It is said to be of great benefit to patients born after IVF treatment. It is thought to heal the inevitable disconnection that must result from the process of artificial insemination and other technical procedures required for mechanical conception. Can be used with safety by those who are on allopathic medicine; it will not interfere with the intended action of the chemical drugs.

Miasms

Psora, syphilis, cancer, tuberculosis and leprosy.

Mental and emotional symptoms

Shock and trauma to the psyche even to the point that the patient has been rendered unconscious. Sadness and grief: seems as if these came from a great distance and belonged to another time. Fearful of and haunted by the past. Fearfulness and unhappiness in those whose parents also felt fear and sadness; inherited tendency to sadness even in those whose lives are not especially marked by grief. A sense of the heaviness of years of emotional turmoil; wants to go out into the fresh air for relief from emotions but then broods and dwells on sad thoughts; a sense of loss that seems to stretch far into the past and to cast long shadows forward into the future. Deep feelings of grief connected to the diaspora. Particularly affected by the sea; being on the sea or the shore exaggerates the emotional gloom yet loves to be by the sea. A deep sense of being alone and loneliness yet often seeking solitude. Patients may feel the need to withdraw emotionally and even physically; may absent themselves for a while even without telling anyone of their whereabouts. A desperate feeling of needing space. Desolation; hopelessness; 'staring into the void'; foreboding; suicidal thoughts. A feeling that one cannot bear to hear of any more emotional traumas: useful for those who have reached beyond the limit of their endurance in the role of listener or 'confessor'. Wants to escape from psychic stress. Feels better and more secure when with close family or those who 'understand' and make few demands; wants to be held but finds it difficult to ask for it. Has been described as 'the **Arnica** of the soul'. Mental confusion: difficulty in discerning what is illusory from reality; finds it hard to tell whether another is speaking the truth or is spinning a delusion. Indecisive. Has difficulty with discriminating meaning in words. Absent-minded; mind wanders whenever the patient is not engaged in a present activity; finds it hard to stay in the present. This may be related to having taken hallucinatory drugs in the distant past. Daydreaming and tendency to go off at strange tangents in thought. Shyness and embarrassment especially when trying to cope with heavy emotional issues. May resort to telling lies especially about past events possibly to disguise a truth that is too emotionally painful to allow to continue unedited in their memory. Worry can cause overwrought adrenal activity. Forgetful of what one is doing; finds it hard to stay focused. Mind is full of clamouring thoughts; persistent unwanted thoughts. A tendency to drift off to sleep when stressed. Mental and psychic breakdown: for those who can no longer take the stresses of modern living and retreat into silence and confusion. The patient may appear eccentric due to the need to avoid what is distressing and painful to their sensibilities. The remedy helps to clarify what is muddled in the mind; it encourages discrimination and dispassionate appraisal of confusing emotions. It strengthens the intuition but not at the expense of the intellect. It strengthens self-confidence in those beaten down by years of emotional struggle. This is a remedy for those who feel (or give the impression) that they are in the emptiness of the emotional wilderness.

Physical symptoms

Head
Tendency to stress headaches; head feels heavy and clouded < noise and talking. Scalp feels tight; fainting or faint feelings with loss of coordination.

Eyes
Cataract < left eye. Eyes water < right. Possibly useful in exophthalmia especially < left eye.

Ears

Highly sensitive to noise; feel they must block out extraneous sounds < when emotionally stressed. Damage to the hearing apparatus and feel that ears will be damaged by noise pollution. Follows **Pulsatilla** and **Silica** well to consolidate their healing effects; a dose of **Aquamarine** can help prevent a return to the acute **Puls/Silica** state which so often happens in tubercular children after vaccination. 'None so deaf as those who won't hear,' (see **Green Jade**).

Nose

Watery < left nostril. (Right eye and left nostril watery simultaneously.) A feeling as if a cold would come on but it never develops fully. Sense of smell heightened but reduced by cold symptoms.

Throat

Sensation of swallowing across a lump. Globus hystericus. Helpful in young men whose voices are breaking. Thyroid pathology; myxoedema; goitre.

Chest

Heaviness and oppression of emotional origin in the middle of the chest. Sighing. Asthmatic breathing < tension held in the diaphragm. Tension felt in the heart (complementary to **Rose Quartz** which releases tension in the pericardium). Asthma > being outside in the fresh air; especially > by the sea.

Heart

Cardiac pathology. Symptoms can suggest angina which eventually develops when left unattended. A sense of anxiety held in the chest; disquiet felt in the heart. The remedy complements other heart remedies that may be indicated by physical pathology: **Aurum, Kalmia, Lachesis, Latrodectus, Naja** and **Rose Quartz**.

Kidneys

Sensation of being squeezed; pains felt in the kidneys < left. Frequent urging to urinate < lack of expression of emotions.

Skin

Dryness and a tendency to desquamation. After **Aquamarine** the skin may react by sloughing off: eczema, dermatitis, etc. Such reactions should be monitored but left alone unless the surface is broken and infection threatens (a rare occurrence).

Back

Shock and trauma from accidents; susceptibility to injury or pain symptoms in those who are overburdened by emotional issues.

Limbs

Lack of coordination of limbs due to muscular weakness and tension; muscles do not respond to intention. Cramp. Trembling and shaking in extremities. < left side of the body. Dystonia.

Sleep

Sleepy in the day; dozes off when stress increases. Daytime nap > sense of pressure and distress. Wakes at night with sense of unidentifiable disquiet. Cannot fall asleep easily for thinking of daytime stresses. Anxiety felt more strongly at night. Relieved to wake in the morning with a desire to get outside for air and light; to get away from dreams of disquiet.

Considerations for the use of the remedy

Aquamarine is a very psoric remedy. It covers the sense of inadequacy that is such a psoric manifestation, particularly emotional inadequacy. The quality of fearfulness is also psoric: of abandonment, of the past, of not being equal to tasks and burdens. However, the syphilitic and cancer miasms are also strongly evident in the later stages of the development of the **Aquamarine** picture. Nor is it difficult to see the tubercular state in the excessive sensitivity and the need to escape from being overwhelmed. The leprotic miasm should not be forgotten either; there is a similar sense of despair and abandonment in this miasm which is characterized by feelings of being outcast and beyond the reach of help from other people. The sense of the burden of years of unspoken grief and the weight of buried history are redolent of this state. It is not unusual for this remedy to be well supported by nat mur 6x, the tissue salt.

Aquamarine shares a number of symptoms with other well-known remedies:

- sense of grief, despair and desolation: **Aurum, Conium, Nat-mur, Phos-ac, Carcinosin, Helleborus**
- sense of dislocation and confusion: **Thuja**
- globus with feelings of grief: **Ignatia**
- < noise: **Aurum, Carcinosin, Helleborus, Ignatia, Latrodectus, Nat-mur**; especially of voices: **Aurum, Conium, Silica.**

Aquamarine works well before or after nosodes and is well supported by them; this is especially true of **Psorinum** and **Leprosinum**. Amongst new remedies:

- **Oak** (tension, the carrying of emotional burdens, the history of shelved traumas though **Oak** is unlikely to seek escape or solitude, rather, they just keep going);
- **Goldfish** (hypersensitivity, < left side, < stroke, loneliness, feeling disconnected and spaced out, the inability to focus on essentials of everyday life, sleepiness, musculoskeletal problems though **Goldfish** is much more fragile);
- **Hornbeam** (confusion and unfocused thoughts, poor discrimination, lying about the past to soften the pain of grief though the strong emotions here are remorse and regret);
- **Lumbricus** (pathology of the nervous system, dysfuntional body clock, vaccine damage, lack of self-confidence, introversion though **Lumb** can appear to be much more downtrodden, far more overtly fearful especially of change and would be unlikely to seek escape);
- **Buddleia** (history of devastating trauma – sometimes this remedy is for the immediate effects of the trauma and is followed well by **Aquamarine**).

Aquamarine is strongly related to various other remedies. It follows or precedes **Nat-mur** and **Aurum** very well. It can be mistaken for these remedies but actually is needed either to complement them (and deepen their work) or to take the patient to a deeper level of personal understanding about the past. It is complementary to **Ayahuasca** when that remedy is indicated by the similimum being deeply buried in the past history of family trauma (see

Ayahuasca in *Volume I* and how it has the ability to restore historical familial connections). **Thuja, Silica** and **Pulsatilla** are all complementary as are **Berlin Wall, Chalice Well, Green** and **Emerald** (another form of beryl). **Thymus Gland** is also related; **Aquamarine** is strongly associated with the thymus centre of energy. **Thymus Gland + Aquamarine + Syphilinum** make a combination triad remedy that has the capability of arresting the descent into self-destruction by encouraging the unearthing of buried syphilitic history. (As an LM potency it would complement and support the patient who is indicating **Aurum** as the similimum.)

Esoteric therapeutics

As a crystal essence Aquamarine is regarded as a stone to calm troubled waters, to encourage those in adversity to face their problems, to remain balanced and feel safe. It gives space to allow the intuition to reassert itself when the intellect is muddled and scared and overtaxed by adrenal energy. It works at the level of the throat to clear the voice; it works on the brow centre to clarify perception (of options, of the dynamics of a situation, of when to accept the inevitable without rancour). It is said to calm the mind of chuntering thoughts. Relieves the stress caused by phobias (see **Hyacinthoides**). It is a base chakra remedy, helping to maintain stability in the face of extraordinary pressures and the tendency to escape into unreality.

In various books on crystal remedies it is claimed that Aquamarine is beneficial for combating the effects of pollutants in the atmosphere, harmonizing the endocrine glands (specifically the pituitary and the thyroid glands) and is useful in the healing of the eyes. They concur as to Aquamarine's ability to clarify the mind in difficult circumstances; to calm the chattering mind and to assist the patient to find the way out of any thicket that may be causing particular stress.

In the meditative proving the remedy was reported to create a link between the pineal, pituitary, heart and base centres. It was noted that the damage to the higher energy centres from shock, trauma, grief, hallucinogens, some antidepressant drugs and vaccines can be beyond the reach of the well-tried and trusted remedies such as **Arnica, Opium** and **Thuja**. Essential though they are in dealing with such trauma, they need to be complemented by other remedies (**Aquamarine, Buddleia, Rainbow, Sandalwood** and **Ayahuasca**), homoeopathically indicated by the individual circumstance, in order to reach into the depths of the aura to which the trauma has gone. In working on the pineal, hypothalamus and pituitary the remedy helps to foster spiritual awareness. This is often initially manifest as a craving to be at one with Nature; to be out in the fresh air and feeling the energy of the elements and taking notice of things such as the flora and fauna. It is remarkable for its ability to allow the patient to leave the chaos behind and feel peaceful. It is said to be a remedy to lighten up the future; it relieves the pressure of impending difficulties so that the future seems less overwhelming. It was also said to be a remedy that would allow personal development or creative actions, that were begun in the past and left uncompleted, to be picked up and carried further to completion.

Aquamarine has influence on the elements of the body. As a crystal it is an earth remedy and excellent for establishing grounding. It has a strong affinity with water because of its association with emotion and the kidneys. It can encourage air to flow through the system better (for example in asthma) by the release of tension in muscles. The outcome of prescribing the remedy is often the regeneration of fire: inspired creativity or elimination of toxicity from the liver, both being aspects of this element. **Aquamarine** is seen as a remedy that galvanizes the base, sacral, solar plexus and heart chakras to eliminate better.

Chakras

Crown
Encourages awareness of spiritual energy that needs to come into consciousness. Sleep problems. NBWS taking hallucinogens or antidepressants. Feelings of disassociation; of being 'spaced out'. Wish to escape into other dimensions.

Brow
Fosters clarity of perception. Difficulty in seeing reality or telling the truth. Poor memory. Weakened intuition; too strong a reliance on the intellect leading to exhaustion and feeble motivation. Forgetful of past negative experience that should have taught one to avoid habitual negative behaviour patterns. Slackened or stultified growth of purpose. Clouded mind; restricted range of intention. Susceptible to being deluded.

Throat
Poor self-expression. Artistic endeavours fail to mature. Becomes susceptible to the effects of radiation.

Heart and thymus

Emotional imbalance; buried grief and trauma. Trauma to this centre often reflects past family history. Oppression of the chakra. Damage to the thymus gland from vaccination, childhood trauma or even unresolved ancestral trauma. Asthma from suppression of emotions.

Solar plexus

Frustration of creative impulses. Activity in this chakra is usually as a result of this remedy. The energy before it is given is often stagnant.

Sacral

Lack of kidney energy is an indication for the remedy. Pathology of (or damage to) the kidneys (especially the right) in a case of deeply held emotional trauma.

Base

Lack of grounding; fearfulness; insecurity; narrowing the bounds of one's limitations while at work but seeking escape into unreality to avoid more stress. (Beryl remedies are useful in assisting the penetration of other remedies deeply into the auric levels of the body when either physical or emotional trauma has infiltrated too far into them.)

Case studies

1 'While studying homoeopathy I was staying during those weekends with a very dear friend of mine from my schooldays. Her marriage had very recently collapsed with her husband leaving her for a younger woman, after 17 years of marriage. The effect on her was shattering, especially as they had no children and both her parents had died in the previous couple of years. She felt completely alone and abandoned. On returning to her house after a day at college I found her in darkness, curled up on the sofa in her lounge, unable to move and in a state of complete despair. She felt as if her life was over. She looked quite grey and totally lost. I had told my supervisor what had happened as my friend was one of the cases he was supervising, and we had discussed

the possibility that **Aquamarine** might be of use at some stage. I had been one of the provers of this remedy and so was aware of its potential. I only had **Aquamarine** 10M with me but felt so sure that this was the remedy she needed, and in a high dose. I gave her one dose and the effect was amazing. Within a few minutes she started to change visibly. She said that for her the effect was incredible. She felt this terrible despair start to lift and after a short while as I sat with her she was able to move and literally come back to life!

'We have never forgotten this experience, either of us, as it was so remarkable. She only needed the one dose and has never since experienced such a feeling of deep despair. Her recovery from this terribly painful time in her life continued and she has thankfully been able to move on.' **MH**

2   A colleague sent the following description after attending a seminar during which **Aquamarine** was presented as a new remedy.

'I was quite deeply affected by the mini proving of **Aquamarine** we did that day of the course. I felt like my lungs were burning and there was a sense of rage and grief all mixed up into one that I could not place. I felt strongly that it was ancestral and down the female line. I decided to stop off at a local park on the way home to feel the earth under my feet. I had an incredible need to be in nature and process my feelings before returning to my busy family life. As I parked my car, I sent a specific request to the Universe that I might be sent a symbol of clarity over what the **Aquamarine** had stirred up in order to release it.

'As I walked through the park gates, a friend and fellow homoeopath entered at the same time with her children. As this homoeopath is someone I am literally in the process of handing my practice over to and her daughter was one of my first patients, it felt very significant. We walked a while and settled down for a drink at the park cafe under a huge umbrella to shield us from the uncharacteristically intense early evening sun. All of a sudden the daughter (my patient) started skipping around us saying there was a rainbow above our heads. We humoured her thinking she was making it up; this particular girl has the most wonderful imagination and is always talking about fairies and butterflies. But she became quite insistent so we peered out from underneath our umbrella. And sure enough, hanging in the sky, directly above our heads, was a rainbow. But not an arc, just a strip of prism in the middle of the blue sky! What was strange was our reaction to the rainbow, which may logically have been a chemtrail or a strange result of the recent volcanic ash we'd had from Iceland, but this fellow homoeopath and I both felt completely, ridiculously joyous. We felt blessed, magical and peaceful. It felt like confirmation that we were doing the right thing, me in handing my practice over to this colleague and her in agreeing to take it on. But beyond this, it felt that something had been resolved on a very deep level just by being in the presence of the energy of **Aquamarine**. After seeing the rainbow I shared with my colleague my **Aquamarine** experience earlier in the day; she grinned and held up her wedding finger on which sat a perfectly cut aquamarine ring! We parted and as I got back in my car I looked up but saw no trace of the rainbow anywhere. It makes me wonder if the remedy **Aquamarine** has a connection to **Rainbow**. It also makes me wonder about the idea of **Aquamarine** pushing someone's fire upwards (that's what it felt like in my lungs; like the anger held in my liver got shoved up into my lung area) and I wonder if the rainbow dispersed it?' **SB**

3   'A woman of 45, a Piscean who was on dialysis, was waiting for a kidney transplant. She had done well on kidney support remedies such as **Berberis Vulgaris**. Nevertheless, she had been told that she would not be able to survive unless she had a transplant within three months. She had a difficult personality and was very fearful and had suffered a lot of trauma in her life. She often became deluded in the manner of someone turning senile in a way that suggested that her kidneys were failing seriously. She was given **Aquamarine** 10M o.d. for seven days. On day three after starting the remedy a donor organ was found for her and she went in for the operation. However, the remedy had already started to bring her personality back to normal. The patient continues to do well despite the negative prognosis and having to remain on rejection drugs.' **JM**

4   'Female, 45, Irish Catholic, mother of four, had joined my meditation groups but found it impossible to do the guided meditations. Felt restless and her mind would constantly wander to the household chores, etc. The reason for attending the meditation groups was with the aim of learning to give herself a little space, since her whole life

involved running around and caring very deeply and wonderfully for her family but at a huge cost to herself.

'After about three sessions of really gaining very little from the meditations I decided to give her **Aquamarine** 30 which she took twice a day for the two weeks. At the next meditation she was much more peaceful, could visualize much more clearly and realized she was keeping busy to suppress a "wild side" of her nature. She had fallen pregnant out of marriage and so had had to get married under pressure. Ever since, her guilt and fear of getting into any more trouble had kept her busy to the point of constant exhaustion. Since taking the remedy she has hugely relaxed, and finally started painting – although she had created a studio in her house about five years before.

'I was lucky enough to be in the proving circle of this remedy in Paros. My main experience was that it gave a deep feeling of stillness of mind.' HJ

5   'A girl of three was brought for eczema, sleep disturbances and problems settling at nursery school. She responded beautifully to homoeopathy and over the course of the next three years she was treated for a variety of childhood complaints such as molluscum contagiosum, impetigo, ear infections and so on. Part of the wider picture was that she was very shy in the company of strangers and would not talk to them. In fact, she never spoke directly to me during all that time and would only answer my questions by whispering to her mother who would relay the answers. This was despite sending me Christmas cards and drawings and her mother reporting that she felt a strong affection for me.

'When the child was six, I had a chance discussion with a colleague who suggested the possible diagnosis of selective mutism. I did my own research and discussed it with the child's mother who said that her GP had recently made the same diagnosis. (Selective mutism is a condition where a child speaks perfectly normally at home to their immediate family but cannot – rather than will not – speak to anyone outside a close inner circle. Conventional doctors class it as a social anxiety disorder.)

'Over the course of two years she was given a range of remedies such as **Lycopodium**, **Baryta-carb**, **Ambra Grisea**, **Ant-crudum**, **Ignatia**, **Carcinosin** and **Psorinum**. More therapeutic approaches were tried; there were remedies for anxiety in situations where she would be required to speak. There would always be some remedy reaction but no progress whatsoever was made with the selective mutism. There was no obvious aetiology in the case; no major grief or trauma. Her birth had been a joyous occasion at home and her loving family were child-centred and progressive in their parenting style. The child herself was intelligent, articulate beyond her years with her inner circle and an able pupil.

'Despite the lack of progress, I never gave up hope that homoeopathy could help but by the time the child was eight, I knew I needed to think outside the box. A triad combination of **Thymus Gland**, **Syphilinum** and **Ignatia** was given and although that remedy had no discernable effect on the child at all, at the next consultation with her something had definitely shifted for me in the way I perceived the case. The terror she felt at trying to talk to me was palpable. She seemed paralysed by fear.

'I asked her mother to come back and see me alone and I explored with her the history of the family in a much deeper way than just the diseases and causes of death I had taken initially. I had a sense that whatever ailed this child, it was not her own but ancestral in origin as though she were carrying a burden for others. The mother told me that her own father was Jewish (although she and the child were not) and that many of his family had died during the Holocaust in death camps. In addition, the child's paternal grandfather was English and her grandmother was German. Married just after the war, the grandmother was forbidden to speak German to her children. When coupled with the Jewish experience, the resonance between a woman unable to speak her mother tongue to her children and a child paralysed by anxiety when required to speak was so striking that it led me to prescribe **Berlin Wall** 10M.

Berlin Wall provided the breakthrough in the case. Within hours of taking it, the child felt overwhelmingly tired and had to go and lie down. She complained of earache in her left ear and pains in her lower legs but a day later all the physical symptoms had gone. Later that day I happened to meet the mother and child in a public place and was delighted that she made really good eye contact with me and we had our first little chat: only a few words but an extraordinary shift. The following day, remarkably I met them again, this time on a train with my own children. Much to the amazement of all the adults and the other children in the assembled group, the child joined in the convivial and excited conversation just like a normal eight-year-old.

'After a repeat dose of the **Berlin Wall** two weeks later, the child had a series of very vivid dreams. She has a strong love of horses and the most striking dream was one in which a stables was on fire. It was frightening and the horses were in terrible danger. She managed to rescue all 35 horses from the fire and when the stables were rebuilt she was given her own horse.

'Around the same time her mother also had a very vivid dream of the Holocaust. She was unable to recount the detail of the dream to me as she was too deeply moved and began to cry whenever she thought of it. Not long after the dream she developed shingles. Her doctor had given her antiviral medication which she did not wish to take and although the mother was not actually my patient, I suggested she try some **Nat-mur** from her kit as I felt the shingles were a physical manifestation of the grief that resulted from the dream. The shingles cleared really quickly with the **Nat-mur**.

'After the **Berlin Wall**, the child made further progress. She was better able to articulate what it felt like when she tried to speak to strangers. It remained a challenge for her and she still felt anxious but she was able to talk in more situations especially with her classmates. She was even elected form captain.

'Three months after the **Berlin Wall** I gave her a split dose of **Aquamarine** 1M. The intention was to further support the patient with a remedy that could lighten the burden of ancestral grief which the **Berlin Wall** had so clearly illuminated. In line with the remedy's reputation, she immediately got a return of her eczema and, although it was pretty nasty for a while, the mother did not treat it and it cleared up completely on its own. In the weeks that followed the child made big step changes in talking to complete strangers, even going out of her way to talk to strangers in shops, enjoying her new-found freedom. She still has some anxiety when talking to those people with whom she had always been silent but generally the selective mutism diagnosis is no longer applicable. A few days before writing this I had a long talk with her about her weekend activities.

'There is one further extraordinary event to report in the case. Shortly after the **Aquamarine**, the child was asked for a homework assignment, to write about something very scary. She told her mother her ideas before writing it. She described a "ship of horrors" and said that the scariest place on the ship was a room. People were locked in the room and poisonous gas was pumped into it to kill them. She described the room in detail. The mother was stunned to hear her child essentially describing a gas chamber. Although no one could be sure, she considered it highly unlikely that her eight-year-old daughter had ever heard about gas chambers especially as there was no TV in their home and reading material was carefully chosen. The mother then sat with her daughter and explained in an age-appropriate way what had happened during the Holocaust. She suggested that including the scary room in the homework assignment might upset someone unintentionally. The child was not fazed by any of this and simply said that she understood. After a further dose of **Aquamarine** the child also asked her father many questions about concentration camps (about which she now had some knowledge because of the conversation with her mother).

'The mother and I have talked about this at length and we are at a loss to understand the exact nature of what has gone on. The closest we get to it is that the child's selective mutism was a manifestation of ancestral energy and the remedies resonated with the depth of the ancient grief sufficiently to lift the burden carried by the child. After the **Aquamarine**, the child seemed impelled to talk about it as part of her healing process.' **CAB**

Author's note

Aquamarine was proved in May 2005 on the Greek island of Paros by two groups of students who had gathered for a week of study on new remedies and strategies of prescribing. The provings, for which I was not present, took place in an old converted farmhouse that overlooked the Aegean Sea with views towards Naxos, a place of outstanding natural beauty and considerable tranquillity. The following anecdote may be of interest. At the end of the week, when all the participants had left, I remained behind for a three-day break with my wife. We stayed on in the farmhouse. As soon as the ferry left carrying everyone back to the mainland, I was seized with an appalling sense of desolation. I was unable to enjoy any of the time we had left on the island. The grief seemed chiefly associated with our children, two of whom we had said goodbye to on the ferry; both hale and hearty and in no obvious danger. It was as if we might never see them again. The sense of desolation was overwhelming. So deep was the sense of tragedy that I had to get out of the farmhouse and travel round the very small island looking for distraction. When obliged to be at the house I attempted to read the time away in an effort to distract myself from the feelings that I was unable to find a cause for. Outside the house, where there was the spectacular view of the sea, was a threshing circle, disused but lately enjoyed by the group participants as a place for healing prayers and meditation. On the last morning, as I looked out to sea I suddenly became aware of the circle and all the 'gifts' left by the students in the centre: flowers mostly and attractive stones from the beach. I felt that I came to the sudden realization that I had been doing my own proving of the remedy. Intuitively I decided to attempt to antidote the effect of the energy of **Aquamarine** that seemed to have permeated the whole place by using **Ayahuasca** 10M, dissolved in a jug of water and dribbled anti-clockwise around the threshing circle. No sooner had I finished my impromptu ritual than I felt the burden of ancient grief lift entirely from me. I was able to enjoy the last hour of our stay though I vowed never to go back to the island.

2

BLUE

The materia medica for **Blue** is based on the remedy that was given two meditative provings by the Guild members, firstly on 7 November 1996 and secondly on 15 November 1996. A single dose of the 30th potency was taken by each participant.

The colour remedies, including **Blue**, were made by Katherine Boulderstone in association with the Helios Pharmacy of Tunbridge Wells in Kent in the UK. The remedy was made by capturing the essence of the blue part of the spectrum when sunlight was refracted through a prism. The following is quoted from Katherine's article in *Prometheus* on **Blue** (No 12: June 2000).

> I made the remedy **Blue** when I was ten weeks pregnant, two days after a partial eclipse of the sun. As I stared into the colours made by the prism I was aware how elusive the blue was, how it seemed to slip away into another colour like water disappearing. It also seemed to reflect other colours such as violet, yellow and green. It seemed gentle, fluid and diffuse, hard to focus on. I also found it hard to write about as I kept 'spacing out'. I felt that you have to be very still to hear it. It helps you to 'reach for the highest', to attune to the spiritual forces, to connect your physical condition to your spiritual potential and to overcome darkness with gentle healing. It is cleansing, purifying; makes you whole again, restores you.

The Background

Blue is one of the three primary colours; the others are red and yellow. Blue is mixed with yellow to make green and red to make purple. It is the fifth colour of the spectrum, coming after green and before indigo.

Colour meaning and symbolism has existed for millennia and blue has a rich history. It is particularly well known as the colour associated with the Virgin Mary's vestments. Byzantine painters used crushed lapis lazuli to create a deep blue pigment to clothe Christ's mother as this represented heavenly grace and spirituality. Throughout history blue has been associated with the sky and the sea, both seen as unfathomable aspects of Nature that give the impression of distance and separation from the turmoil of everyday life. Blue is used in both literature and art to represent certain values and meanings that help the reader and viewer to understand the subject matter. Variously blue has meant hope, loyalty, stability, confidence, faith, chastity, truth, trust and sincerity. It is regarded as the colour of pure inspiration, of good health, of friendship. It is also the colour of servitude; it represents the willingness to be of service to others. In Tudor times the sumptuary laws that governed aspects of social standing by stipulating a dress colour code, were updated and expanded by Henry VIII and both his daughters, Mary and Elizabeth, to ensure that royal blue was exclusive to aristocratic households while pale blue might be worn by servants. A blue iris, when given as a gift, represents true friendship. Traditionally, each day of the week is ascribed a colour and blue belongs to Wednesday or, as it was originally, Wodensday, the day sacred to Woden or Odin, the king of the Norse gods. Woad, *Isatis Tinctoria*, the plant that provides a deep blue dye, was the chosen warpaint of ancient British tribes.

Certain sayings and phrases also carry the meaning of blue:

- true blue: loyalty and unwavering support, though it has more recently come to have the further meaning of being politically Conservative
- once in a blue moon: a rare event based on the fact that there are very few months that have two full moons
- a blue study or mood: depressive
- the blues: music of a particularly soulful nature
- blue movies: pornographic films (though in other countries different colours are used to describe these)
- out of the blue: out of nowhere and usually suddenly
- the blue: the sea

It is worth noting that blue crystals also carry similar meanings and give out energies to match. Traditionally blue stones are a symbol of chastity. Most blue stones foster calmness and tranquillity. They have been worn as one might nowadays take a tonic. They are particularly associated with the communication of higher or deeper meaning; they would be useful for anyone on a diplomatic mission or for someone who wished to express anything deeply personal or anything of great significance. Blue tourmaline, for example, 'opens the way for service to others while encouraging those who constantly give also to receive'. It assists with 'living in harmony with the environment', it 'supports fidelity, ethical behaviour, tolerance and love of truth'. Similarly, blue lace agate is said to help those whose 'blocked self-expression settles in the throat chakra' where it 'may induce a feeling of suffocation'. The themes of the remedy's mental and emotional state are already inherent in the vibration of the colour itself and in most blue crystals as recorded historically and empirically by those who have used them.

Keynote effects

The remedy affords an opportunity to disconnect from those things that hold one back from positive change; allows one to look dispassionately at aspects of negativity in one's past that are influencing present patterns of response and behaviour to the point of causing depletion of energy and lowering of spirits. One of the usual responses to taking the remedy is calmness and cool dispassion; seeing things 'in the cold light of day'.

General symptoms

Has a strong connection with the water element of the body. Water retention with bloating and oedema. It encourages a general state of fluidity throughout the system thus helping to clear the lymphatic system. Purifies the blood by encouraging the elimination of toxins in the urine; it fosters kidney function by strengthening the tissues of the kidneys. Useful in conditions in which the blood carries toxins that are the root of inflammation and pain: rheumatoid conditions and autoimmune processes; especially when such states bring about a state of depression. It is markedly useful in conditions where congestion interferes with awareness and consciousness; useful in the detoxification of the blood in alcoholics. Has a profound effect on the venous blood and therefore has a relation to the liver and assists in its cleansing. Internal varicosity; diverticulitis; varicose veins (often painless but can be inflamed). It should be considered in poor circulation (often as a concomitant of congestion in the lungs) with cyanosis and cold extremities. Sinus problems (in any part) which cause slowness and sluggishness. Generally, the patient is chilly; cold in bed and unable to warm up. Reynaud's syndrome. Stiffness and aching of limbs which is > in warm weather. All symptoms are << in the evening. Dryness of the sensitive skin of the body: lips, anus, genitalia, fingertip, etc. Symptoms appear to move from right to left though the symptoms are < when they do appear on the left.

It has an affect, through the cleansing of the blood, on the central nervous system. In those with toxic waste in their bloodstreams there is often marked distress in the CNS causing such problems as trembling, tingling, numbness, neuralgia and pins and needles as well as poor conductivity and slowed hormonal activity. **Blue** improves the conduction of nerve impulses; it was felt that it works at the level of the synapses and the neural pathways. It especially seems to work on improving receptivity of external stimuli. Neuropathy: peripheral. Awkwardness and clumsiness; this may be due to congenital problems or thyroid trouble. Strongly associated with the thyroid gland and useful in thyrotoxicosis. Consider in exophthalmia; also in MS and ME. Marked weakness and torpor. Physical weakness of the muscles yet with a certain degree of restlessness from a 'buzzing' nervous system. Irresistible tiredness and sleepiness. Affinity for the left side.

Assists in processes of birth, rebirth and dying. Can calm babies in the final months of pregnancy or in the process of delivery when the waters have broken too soon. Has proved of value in calming dying patients who become agitated and unsettled. Can also be of use for those who go through rebirthing techniques and have trouble with breathing and tetany.

It has been noted that **Blue** can be very useful in the treatment of animals, especially dogs that are far too highly bred pedigree animals with weak constitutions.

Miasms

Psora, sycosis, syphilis and tuberculosis.

Mental and emotional symptoms

Depression. Lack any energy to express themselves. A feeling of oppression: 'as if covered by a blanket'. Expressionless and poker-faced. Seemingly dispassionate: not given to expressing personal views; if they say anything then it may be either critical (in an offhand manner) or world-weary. Uncertain about the immediate future especially when it leads to depression. Feels alone and isolated; wants to cry but cannot. Has a feeling that 'I just can't go on any more'. (Might be said in a flat, expressionless voice. May have wept so much in the past and without comfort or cure that they have no more energy left to weep.) Weeping over past mistakes: guilt and grief; self-criticism. Pessimistic: everything seems wrong. Wants to be left alone. Often say that they wants their own space or that they need to feel in control. Wants to speak out but is cautious about saying anything to hurt the other's feelings. Might attack others verbally especially when it is least expected. Post-natal depression. PMT: cyclic depression; PMT can be < after the period. Depression after hallucinogenic or allopathic mind-bending drugs. Aetiology might be < from loss of face or dignity; < loss of position (at work); < from recreational drugs or antidepressants; < from shock. The remedy tends to soothe the ego and softens the tendency to be critical either of the self or others. Nostalgia: selective memory for the good things that have happened; forgets and ignores the pain of all the bad things. (Appears to give off a negative vibration and live in a negative mindset but remembers and refers to positive things from the past even though they might, in reality, have been spoilt.) Loss of motivation; 'I can't see my way out!' Tends to make mistakes verbally. Poor sense of direction and spatial awareness. Can be on an emotional see-saw especially if there is a strong condition of the organs of the sacral centre (pelvic organs). Can develop sexual fixations that are expressed through pathology of the pelvic organs. Frigidity; aversion to sex; impotence; nympho-mania or satyriasis. Fixations with sex. Absence of libido.

Physical symptoms

Head

Severe congestive headaches. Migraines; period headaches of hormonal origin. Pain < right or < right to left.

Eyes
Difficult to focus; impaired vision. Left eye becomes watery, irritated and with stitching pains.

Ears
Earache: < right side. Hearing becomes more acute which = sensitivity. Shooting pains up into the left ear. It is thought to be helpful in children with impaired hearing or deafness who have not yet 'found a voice'.

Nose
Sneezing with right-sided obstruction of nose. Cold sore inside the right nostril.

Mouth
Dry lips. Cold sore on top lip (that might have spread from the nose).

Throat
Feels as if it is closing up. Aching and soreness. Feels scratchy. Throat and pharynx feel numb. Tonsillitis; pain can feel > talking. Pain < when on the left. Hay fever: palate feels itchy and sneezing. Voice deepens. Tension in the throat from not being able to express what one needs to say.

Respiration
Catarrh causing congestion of any of the airways; also causes coughing. Choking cough < lying down at night. Blue babies: > respiration in babies who have difficulty in breathing from mucous congestion.

Chest
Pains on the sternum with weakness 'as though pulling on the heart centre too much and I can't hold it together'. Ectopic heartbeats. High blood pressure with congestion of the lower extremities (poor drainage of the lower limbs due to liver congestion). (**Red** and **Ruby** have raised blood pressure with congestion of the solar plexus and tightness of the diaphragm.)

Stomach
Comfort eating; +++ chocolate and cheese. Nausea of pregnancy.

Abdomen

Severe pains that extend into the thighs. Bloating and wind < evening. After evening meal severe stitching in the lower abdomen. Soreness of the anus < haemorrhoids and constipation. Stools are hard to expel. (Marble-sized balls of faeces.) Herpetic eruptions that are recurrent. Sensation of weight pressing down onto the solar plexus.

Female

Infertility. Tender and swollen breasts < period. Very painful breasts with stinging and hot sensations even without touching: > the following period. Early menstruation. Single stabs of pain in the uterus. Congestion of the Fallopian tubes. Ovarian cysts or cancer. Uterine and ovarian cancer.

Male

Lack of libido. Congestion of the epididymis. Infertility as a result, it has been suggested, of being exposed to increased oestrogens in the environment.

Skin

Cold sores. Rash in the genital region, axillae, around the neck or around glands. Psoriasis on the scalp or in the pubic region. Hair falls out especially after grief or shock or after chemotherapy.

Extremities

Rheumatoid arthritis < autoimmune disease or autotoxicity. Stabbing pains in either hip (or both). Numbness. Swelling of the small joints. Varicose veins. Raynaud's. Great swelling of the left ankle, foot and leg.

Sleep

Insomnia from a busy, active mind. Waking for no apparent reason in the small hours. Sleepless until 2am. Gets up feeling exhausted. Dreams of witnessing horrors: murder, rape and pillage yet with curiously no emotion. Dreams of being excluded in family situations. Dreams of not having a voice. Dreams of sexual orgies. Dreams of running and of trying to win a race; of people trying to catch running horses.

Considerations for the use of the remedy

Blue bears comparison with several other remedies:

- **Amethyst:** also has a depression but it is marked by a deep sense of longing especially to do with 'home'. It is also more redolent of anxiety and tension than **Blue**.
- **Carbo-veg:** blueness of the complexion due to poor oxygenation of the blood, even incipient asphyxia; has more to do with lack of reaction or pathology of the lungs than **Blue** has though either or both may be called for to assist at a birth.
- **Crotalus Horridus:** blueness of parts or limbs with varicosities; chilblains though it is far more toxic and broken down in constitution than **Blue**.
- **Cuprum Metallicum:** has bluish skin but the temperament and particular pains of **Cuprum** differentiate it from **Blue** which is far more retiring and self-deprecating.
- **Digitalis:** blueness is usually limited to the tongue, lips and face and consequent on heart pathology while **Blue** is more associated with symptoms of the sacral area and the throat.
- **Lachesis:** is far more toxic either in terms of the physical body or in the emotions.
- **Laurocerasus:** has blueness of the face from cyanosis and asphyxia and may be called for in babies born with the cord round the neck. It is more associated with breathing difficulties (especially asthma < since being born with the cord round the neck) and bowel problems than **Blue**'s main areas of action.
- **Nat-mur:** can also be poker-faced and isolationist but they are more likely to be bitterly critical of others than of themselves.
- **Nux Moschata:** can be mistaken for **Blue** because it covers changeable moods, confusion and lack of spatial awareness, < from emotions and menstrual symptoms. There is also, as with many of the remedies that focus on the sacral centre, a sense of duality. However, **Nux Moschata** tends to be closer to wanting to shut out the world (they would rather fall asleep and avoid any crises), is far more lethargic and somnolent. **Blue** is less likely to feel faint and has no marked lack of thirst.

Blue is related to the sea remedies: **Sepia, Winchelsea Sea Salt, Aqua Marina, Squid, Sting Ray**, etc. Also associated with the water remedies: **Sanicula** and **Tunbridge Wells Water**. It is useful as a support after tree remedies especially those that have a sycotic tendency: **Silver Birch, Copper Beech** and **Sequoia**.

Can be very helpful as an organ support or drainage remedy when used in combination:

- **Blue + Thyroidinum + Spongia**: thyroid remedy in those who need a consistent support as they go through treatment that travels or even swings between differing constitutional states. This remedy has advocates among practitioners who have treated patients with either suspected thyroid conditions which have nevertheless been apparently contradicted by blood tests or those who have conflicting symptom pictures which have defied adequate repertorisation. It is usually used as a low maintaining dose in low 'x' potency such as 6x or 12x.
- **Blue + Arsen-alb + Carbo-veg**: used in low potency for varicose veins. The **Arsen-alb** can be replaced by **Pulsatilla** in cases where this is a more obviously similar remedy to the condition.
- **Blue + Arnica + Carbo-veg**: venous congestion in the pelvic area since the birthing process. The **Arnica** can be replaced by **Bellis Perennis** in subjects who are spare of flesh.
- **Blue + Arsen-alb + Oak**: enormous distress of difficult birth; this has also been given through a difficult pregnancy as a support when the mother experiences weakness, breathlessness and loss of fluids due to vomiting of pregnancy or dehydration from lack of thirst. This has been used successfully when given once weekly in the 30th potency as a supporting remedy.

Esoteric therapeutics

Affects the sacral, throat and brow centres principally. There is a difference of colour between the blue of the sacral centre (sky blue) and that of the throat (deep or royal blue). However, the remedy was made from the blue of the spectrum and results of its use seem to suggest that the patient's energy dictates at what level the prescription influences the body. It is said to link one into one's spiritual nature engendering awareness. As such **Blue** is considered a bridge remedy between the conscious and the subconscious. The throat centre is seen as the release point for the tension between the two when expression has been limited. **Blue** > clarity of vision; affects the brow by helping the patient to see beyond the everyday struggle for existence. As there is often a blockage between physical awareness (i.e. the pains, the swelling, the congestion, etc.) and the spiritual, it is necessary to forge a link between them for the patient to feel the value of lifting themselves out of their lowered state.

Chakras

Crown

This is properly the preserve of **Amethyst** and **Buddleia** and other remedies that are possessed of the colour of this chakra though **Blue**'s connection here is that it links with these remedies by preceding them well. This is especially the case when a patient wants to become more open to a spiritual path but finds that maintaining causes, especially held in the throat and sacral chakras, seem to prevent this.

Brow

The conscious mind usually holds sway in order that the subconscious does not get the chance to subvert a carefully managed facade. Emotional see-sawing, menstrual difficulties and a general sense of uncertainty contribute to confusion of this centre which makes the patient want to hold back. Not certain whether they want to move forward; the inwardness causes the lack of facial expression at times. The remedy tends to alter perception of things, changing negative experiences into positive memories in order for them to feel more comfortable.

Throat

Traditionally, this is the centre that is associated most closely with the deepest blue though, with this remedy, it is often needed as a result of problems stemming from the sacral centre for which the throat is the vehicle of expression as much as it is for the heart. The thyroid gland is most affected when the patient suffers emotional see-sawing which is nevertheless left inadequately expressed. Hears things differently from their reality; relays things in the same manner. (They are not liars like **Mercury** or **Thuja** because they are unaware of their trick of seeing negativity in a positive light.) Feel unable to carry on when negativity catches up and there is no further possibility of denying reality. This is when pessimism and criticism take over.

Heart

Sadness over the past especially of past mistakes. Grief may appear to belong to the past as so much weeping has been done but this is a delusion as the tears have left the heart centre exhausted. As weeping did not resolve the grief, there is now the tendency to deny its existence. (It is in this aspect that **Blue** supports the sea remedies so well.) The remedy also has a profound effect over breath and breathing and therefore the element of air. It is as if inspiration of air is what the physical and emotional bodies have been deprived of and are waiting for in order to find the means to recover.

Sacral

The roots of the need for **Blue** often lie in this centre. There is a profound difficulty in expanding awareness into this chakra; the patient is held back and held down by circumstances either of health, upbringing or miasmatic influence. Little joy emanates from here or, if it is experienced, it is furtive or clandestine; held in check by circumstance. The physical pathology of the organs of this centre is likely to reflect stagnation, blockage and lack of flow. There is weak kidney energy from the long struggle with diminishing energy following physical depletion or trauma.

Base

Blue is a remedy that has little concept of the base centre as they find present circumstances hard to deal with. They either deny them or see them as different from the way they truly are. They may appear to be well grounded (as all the colour remedies can do) but this is not the reality. They are out of sync with the Now and are therefore likely to suffer from conditions not just of the sacral centre but also structural weakness, circulatory disorder and endocrine imbalance.

Case studies

1 'I have used **Blue** a few times in newborn babies *as they have delivered.* Each of these babies and their mothers had been having homoeo- pathic remedies prior to birth. The first baby was full term but very reluctant actually to be delivered and was now going into distress. (I was

not meant to be at the birth but was called at the last minute as support – out of the blue!) The baby was cyanosed and not very responsive on delivery. The delivery process is when the change over from using the mother's oxygen in her blood supply to its own first breaths takes place. Though it is fairly common for the baby to look blue, the concern is if the baby does not breathe by itself straight away. So, prior to the baby being whisked away or the cord being cut I dropped some **Blue** 30 on to his skin. (The medicating liquid potency was used.) He seemed to respond instantly by taking some deep breaths.'

2 'In the second example I was the homoeopath in attendance at a home delivery. This was the third child and all had had natural births. For the delivery we used some of the basic remedies that come in a childbirth kit: **Puls, Carbo-veg, Kali-phos, Cimicifuga**. The baby delivered well; was blue for a while; had no difficulty in breathing but was just slow at turning pink. So I applied **Blue** 30 directly to the skin, a few drops and within 15 seconds he turned pink.

'The reason for giving these remedies was just the central state of being blue. I am also aware that this remedy has been said to be of use to help incarnate – well, what better time to do that? They are coming from that out-of-the-world state to be in the here and now and dealing with the shock that being born must cause. There cannot be a more clear interpretation for this remedy – the child is *blue in totality*. The blood is still in the deoxygenated state, hence the blueness from lack of oxygen. The skin tone and the colour of blood is blue, the nails are blue: typical cyanosis. They have just arrived from "out of the blue", almost from another realm! Certainly it is a new realm for them and often very much of a surprise. The baby responded to the remedy. The mother was given **Ignatia** 1M to help with the separation of the placenta.'

3 'The third time I was privileged enough to attend a birth was with a mother whose history is one of asthma; so there was a predisposing history of cyanosis in the mother herself. I treated her throughout her pregnancy to keep her asthma stable which worked well even under stressful conditions. Her last remedy prior to going into labour was **Aquamarine** as there were concerns regarding her own mother. She went into premature labour at 33 weeks. This is always a concerning time as

it is judged that the baby's lung capacity is not great enough for the baby to cope unaided. We managed to delay the delivery by almost one week just using **Arnica** 200. However it was felt by the medical profession that the mother should have two doses of steroids to help "the baby's lungs to toughen up prior to delivery". They really wanted the baby to wait at least 24 hours to help this to happen. The mother came out in a very fine red rash across her trunk and arms and had a slight temperature. A danger from the medical point of view is that infection may set in once the waters have broken. **Belladonna** was given with good affect on the mother. **Arnica** 200 was again used which slowed and stopped the contractions; as it was so premature, the longer the baby could be delayed without any contraindications, the better. However the waters had broken and the mother needed to be monitored to ensure no infection set in. The mother was warned that the baby would need to go into an incubator and would need assistance to breathe once born. However, though her contractions continued to develop strongly, the cervix was not dilating and **Aconite** 200 was given. The baby was delivered unassisted 20 minutes later. Due to the worry over the immaturity of lungs and the concern over oxygen exchange, **Blue** 30 was given onto the skin. He did breathe for himself and did not need to go into an incubator.' L R-H

4 'An 11-week-old baby was referred to me by an osteopath. She had had the cord around her neck but was born naturally by being dragged out. She was managing to feed and was putting on weight but was still in shock, very unsettled; sleeping in short bursts and was constipated. Initially I gave her **Buddleia** 1M three times in one day for the shock and trauma. After this she slept for eight hours straight and was more settled and her stools were more regular. We then had a joint session with the osteopath. The baby looked startled, wide-eyed and made little movement. The **Buddleia** had done its work, now the osteopath reported that her diaphragm was tight and held. So she was given **Stramonium** 1M which had the effect of releasing the tension in her face and diaphragm but the breath was not going any deeper. I thought of the next layer, the cord round the neck, the fear of this and around breathing. **Laurocerasus** did not seem to fit so I prescribed **Blue** 30c. The effect was immediate. The osteopath reported that "it just opened

up and had a whoosh about it"; the breath rushed into her body, deep into her belly and the CNS fluid also moved as it should. We left a gurgling, happy baby moving her arms and legs and exploring really being here in her body. Truly magical.

'Words from the osteopath when **Blue** was used on another patient who was recovering from glandular fever: "Immediately the body washed itself with fluid – like the sea washing into a rock pool and swirling around, lifting all the little fronds of seaweed and injecting life into what previously looked like dead detritus."' **AL**

3

CHALCANCITE

The remedy was proved on 20 November 1993 by 10 of the 13 original members of the Guild proving circle. Each participant took a single dose of the 30th potency. The only participant to know the name of the remedy was the leader of the group.

The Background

Chalcancite has only been known to science for a comparatively short time: less than two centuries. It is chiefly made of anhydrous copper sulphate and it is found in the vicinity of copper mines. The word 'anhydrous' means devoid of water and this suggests one of the keynotes of this remedy: friability, brittleness, dryness. On exposure to the air it absorbs condensed moisture very readily. It is extremely friable and will crumble on being handled. Chalcancite appears in clusters of wedge-shaped crystal points; it is poisonous and has corrosive properties. The colour of the tiny crystals is of the most extraordinary sharply bright deep blue.

In relation to this remedy, it is worth noting Dr Clarke's reference to **Cuprum Sulphuricum** in his great *Dictionary of Materia Medica*. This may give some possible insight into the physical aspect of a remedy that is, so far as the meditative proving is concerned, noteworthy for its psychic subtlety and mental and emotional frailty.

'Sulphate of Copper is a well-known emetic and caustic. It causes forcible vomiting and much nausea. Paleness of face; or jaundiced appearance; pale skin generally; a peculiar diarrhoea; enlarged liver . . . It is a well-known application in allopathic practice for stimulating flabby granulations and it has cured itching eruptions and manifestations of syphilis. Rest > pains.' He cites JD Tyrell's case of a woman who could not use **Cuprum-sulph** as it made her face hurt and swell so she could scarcely see and her lips became everted. He suggests a comparison with **Kali-bich** and **Merc-sol** and states that it is antidoted by milk and eggs.

Keynote effects

The remedy fosters the confidence to let go of negative, illusory beliefs and thought patterns so that one can move on from being completely fixed in the damaged ego; lifts one out of the mode of thinking 'I can't do it!' Encourages the system to become more flexible; the energy to be more fluid (particularly along the spinal column).

General symptoms

Frailty, vulnerability, fragility and brittleness yet often with a very polished, beautiful facade. It is particularly helpful in the treatment of individuals whose constitutions have been worn down or broken down by years of orthodox medical intervention (see also **Okubaka** in *Volume I*). For the easing of chronic destructive, incurable diseases which are usually treated allopathically so that the patient is 'propped up' but which mask the gradual and inevitable terminal decline. In this light it may be indicated in conditions such as MS, ataxia, AIDS and leukaemia. It has been suggested for the repair of the body after the excessive use of steroids. There is a great need for rest, quiet and sleep; overpowering sleepiness in the daytime. The patient may well appear to be very refined and delicate almost with the quality of glass or fine porcelain. Difficulty in maintaining the right body temperature. Osteoporosis; brittle bone disease. A profound sense of a lack of energy; absolute exhaustion. May be indicated in mothers who have poor milk supply or for their babies (who are slow to grow) because they cannot get enough milk. Consider this remedy in those children who are almost ethereal but who suffer from learning difficulties associated with reading and writing or from difficulty in interacting with others and lack of expression; these two states suggest dyslexia and autism. The remedy is generally right-sided.

Miasms

Cancer and psora.

Mental and emotional symptoms

A 'can't be bothered' attitude yet with an underlying sense that one should be getting up and getting on with something or going somewhere in order to do something. A feeling of being trapped though in a situation of one's own making; this is compounded by not wanting to let go of old attitudes. Not wanting to let go but knowing that one has to; a feeling of being in a no-man's-land between wanting peace, wanting to remain untroubled by change and knowing that one has to make an effort and that if one does not do so, there will be a terrible sense of failure. A historical feature may well be some form of physical or psychic abuse. The patient may have a marked concern about appearance while giving off the impression that there is not any strong substance to the personality. Mental clarity and acuity is poor; allows superficial, shallow thinking to dominate as it is easier and makes for a quiet life. Patient can be prejudiced or dogmatic in their effort to keep the status quo.

Physical symptoms

Head
Headaches that feel like a band around the head; < across the forehead. Sense of tightness or pressure in the head. Vertigo; sense of being tipped to the left. Sensation as if it is difficult to stay in the body.

Eyes
Blurred vision; floaters.

Ears
Destruction of the right auditory nerve. Tremendous buzzing in both ears; tinnitus.

Face
Heat in the cheeks and the face.

Respiration and chest

Heaviness in the right side of the rib cage. Pain in the base of the heart. Stabbing pain in the area of the thymus gland.

Stomach and abdomen

Pulsation felt in the stomach. Aching in the ileo-caecal region.

Extremities

Sharp pains in the right arm and neck. Irritating stabbing pains in the right foot.

Sleep

Great fatigue and sleepiness. Feeling cold and sleepy. A possible remedy for narcolepsy.

Considerations for the use of the remedy

Chalcancite is a carcinogenic remedy and it is very close to **Carcinosin**. These two remedies complement each other well. Delicate tubercular patients, including children, may well have a symptom picture that indicates **Chalcancite**. **Conium** may also turn out to be complementary.

- **Okubaka** is another remedy for the prolonged effects of orthodox drugs but there is far less sense of frailty than toxicity.
- **Thuja** is famed for its symptom of feeling fragile but while this can certainly be a physical symptom, it usually has its origin in the general insecurity and lack of trust in life to support one while **Chalcancite** is constitutionally fragile from years of gradual wearing down.
- **Silica** can look as delicate but is usually characterized by a determined or obstinate streak which can raise serious opposition to others while **Chalcancite**'s main concern is for a quiet existence.
- A tubercular or carcinogenic **Phosphorus** can also be as fragile as **Chalcancite** but has its characteristic modalities to help differentiate it.

Esoteric therapeutics

Chalcancite is a protective remedy for the aura in those whose life force has been worn to a ravelling. Pulse reading will often show that there is very little energy in the system altogether but it is particularly weak in the heart and the kidneys while most of the energy that is available is evident in the liver and lungs, both involved in attempting to maintain what little effort at elimination is possible. There is almost no evident fire or air; earth and water are both exercised in survival mode.

Chakras

Crown

It protects the spirit in a shattered body and mind. Of considerable value in those whose emotional and spirit bodies are fragmented by years on allopathic drugs. It may well be found to be of service in those who are addicted to sleeping pills. The patient is likely to be very psychically attuned. This faculty might be severely curtailed or distorted by allopathic drugs or be the cause of much sensitivity and even distress.

Brow

Unable to seize any opportunities as the mind is clouded and the damaged ego has little strength to make creative choices. 'Can't be bothered' attitude is more powerful than the certainty that turning thought into action is imperative. Thinking is easily overpowered by sleep. Fear born and held in the sacral centre (that has to do with expansiveness and development of awareness), tends to overshadow the perception of the third eye. Attempts to disguise any sign of distress or weaknesses by creating a polished, refined exterior.

Throat

Very little self-expression as events in the past may have convinced the patient that the effort was not worthwhile. The colour of the remedy is very much to do with this chakra and it may well be found to be a remedy of considerable benefit in thyroid cases.

Heart and thymus

The library of memory that is the thymus gland will sometimes call for this remedy, most particularly in those who are weakened by experience, medical intervention and family pressures. The patient will not necessarily immediately offer an emotional history that suggests trauma and grief. The main sense that comes across is the debility, fragility and lack of forward movement that are more to do with the base centre. However, there will be a deep history of suppressed physical pathology (either in the patient or in a forebear) that became necessary as a consequence of unresolved emotional trauma at some point in the past. It will be evident that sleepiness masks the despair held in the heart centre. There may well be a history of being subjected to bullying.

Solar plexus

Complete lack of any creative drive. All effort is expended on keeping the status quo or it is suspended in favour of using drugs to support the gradually declining physical body. Lack of motivation; very weak spleen energy.

Sacral

No expansion of worldly experience as there is often too much fear and anxiety held in this centre. The patient may well have chosen to be celibate as a way of stabilizing. Very little kidney qi; dangerously low in some cases. There may be no discernible kidney pulse.

Base

Very weak adrenal energy. Debility, weakness, fragility in every aspect of the structure of the body. Weak and fragile bones. Lack of any secure grounding often due to the overuse of allopathic drugs. Dependency on medication.

Case studies

1   'Female of 35. Arrived complaining of extreme debility and exhaustion which had been carrying on for 18 months. She was unable to drag herself about and was suffering from general aches and pains especially on the right side of her body. She suffered from headaches, one or two a week, which had not seemed to improve with painkillers. The headaches were like a band around her head. She suffered from a lack of clarity in the head. In her own words, "I feel fragile". She was sweaty and clammy the whole time. She wanted fizzy drinks and tea. Her

bowels were sluggish; she suffered from constipation. Otherwise there was no abnormality. She had had all the usual inoculations including two smallpox vaccinations. There was a family history of cancer, TB and arthritis. On the emotional front she wept without cause and seemed to be in a state of sheer hopelessness. She had no fears; she was too exhausted to be fearful. She was happily married with two children and there was no history of trauma. This patient had always had strong clairvoyant and healing powers but she had gradually lost her direction and these wonderful abilities. It was observed that she lost breath on talking too much; her voice was very weak. She also looked very pale and waxy, like a china doll. She seemed to be blocked as if she were not able to express her emotions properly. She had turned all her normally positive creative and healing powers against herself on all levels. She seemed in a fragile inert state. The first remedy she was given was **Carcinosin** 1M after which she showed a slight improvement for 10 days though this did not hold; she then got worse and felt terrible. The second remedy was **Phosphoric Acid** 1M which caused a slight amelioration for two weeks. Her bowel movements improved and her energy improved for about a month but did not hold. All else was the same. The third prescription was **Chalcancite** 30/200/1M in a day. There was a gradual amelioration over a period of two months of all her symptoms. The headaches eased off first then her general aches and pains. The debility and exhaustion gradually improved and her spirits improved at the same time. She no longer looked or felt fragile. Her appetite returned gradually. After four weeks an interesting aggravation occurred: she had a general anxiety about her state and oversensitivity which lasted 10 days then calmness returned. After six weeks her energy then surged and she became increasingly joyful. After eight weeks the remedy stopped working so she was prescribed **Chalcancite** LM1. Since then she has improved steadily and is still doing so.' JM (*Prometheus* Vol. 1 No. 1 June 1994)

2   'I gave **Chalcancite** 1M, once a week for four weeks on a Saturday night, to a retired woman who gave the distinct impression of not being at one with her family. The bullying she was subjected to during her marriage was something that she had never spoken about to anyone. She had put up with the judgemental comments of friends who felt that,

by leaving her husband, he was the wronged party even though he had neglected her. She gave off the feeling of vulnerability and sustained hurt on the inside that no one else would particularly have noticed as she hid it so well but which, because I knew her, she did not try to disguise in the appointment. She rang to say that after the first dose things were "not too bad but the second dose made me feel angry and impatient. When I took the third dose I became really angry and I felt that I could put my hands round anyone's throat and throttle them. I realize that it was because of the feeling that everyone criticized me for leaving my husband." She was clearly in a state that described **Staphysagria** which she took in the 200th potency. This remedy progression seemed entirely appropriate as the **Staphysagria** lifted her mood and spirits very well, suggesting that the **Chalcancite** had gone extremely deep and made her underlying unresolved feelings come to the surface for the **Staphysagria** to remove.' RN

4

CLEAR QUARTZ

The remedy was proved on 26 March 2010. Some of those present had also taken part in a proving some 12 to 15 years previously but had no memory of the remedy at all and none had used it in clinic in the intervening years. This second proving was undertaken without any in the group knowing what the remedy was, with the exception of the medium and the author who had made the remedy up to the 30th potency. It was felt beforehand that the remedy needed to be proved with some urgency. The 30th potency was taken.

The Background

Clear quartz is otherwise known as rock crystal. There is evidence that the ancient Egyptians and the Babylonians knew and used it not only in their art but for medical purposes. The Greeks named the clear quartz 'krystallos' (ice) as they believed it was ice that had been frozen permanently by extreme cold. Quartz is regarded as a gemstone even if an inexpensive and common one. It has often been and still is used to create cups, jugs and vases. Its market value is extremely low though antique examples of fashioned and cut ware can fetch relatively high prices. It is easily cut and resembles the diamond even though it cannot compete on any level.

Rock crystal is distinguished from lead crystal, a form of glass, by its birefringence, the quality of transmitting light unequally in different directions. Glass also commonly contains tiny bubbles of air. Rock crystal is 7 on Mohs' scale of hardness while glass is only at 5. The dynamic energy of the crystal is of note: the polarity of the point will change under pressure when subjected to heat; even the heat of a patient's hand. The tip of a point is usually positive and receiving but it changes to become negative and emitting; a negatively charged crystal will emit radiating energy from the tip and from the edges. Quartz can be used to dispel static electricity and can redirect and convert energy for beneficial purposes. It is used to amplify the body's own dynamic energy and to increase the power and direction of thought forms. This aspect of amplification is essential and of the greatest importance to anyone who would understand this crystal. (See the section below on experiences with the remedy.)

Modern crystal healers are familiar with a large variety of quartz forms, each with its own specific inherent use: transmitters, double-terminated crystals, ones for channelling, record keepers, generators, window crystals, wands, barnacles, sceptres and so on. There are also variations on the original theme: phantom quartz, smoky quartz and rutilated quartz being just three.

Clear quartz is found almost anywhere on earth though some of the largest quantities are in Brazil and Madagascar. Its chemical formula is SiO_2; silicon dioxide. It is formed hydrothermally in masses, grains or druses with prismatic hexagonal crystal points. It is of pure, silicic acid solution with no impurities. Crystal points that protrude out of the matrix rock crystal may be completely clear or they may appear cloudy; the former are reckoned to be yang in energy while the cloudy form is seen as yin. (The remedy was made from a yang quartz point.) Clear quartz features strongly in myths and legends; one of the most famous being the legend of Psyche, in love with and loved by Eros, who was challenged by Venus (his mother) to fill a crystal vase with the waters of forgetfulness, a perilous task that she only succeeded in accomplishing through the intervention of Jupiter himself. To the Japanese, the clear quartz is known as 'the jewel of perfection' or the 'breath of the white dragon' which they fashion into crystal balls into which they gaze as a source of spiritual guidance. The Chinese regard the stone with reverence as a talisman of concentration and perseverance. Many cultures have used clear quartz for crystal gazing; it is the original crystal ball. It has also been used in a form of surgery: light concentrated through a convex crystal to form a laser of sunlight has been used to excise lesions and tumours.

Clear quartz has been almost universally used as a healing crystal throughout history and by most cultures especially to enhance clarity, perception and understanding. It strengthens convictions hard won but held with imperfect confidence, and fosters self-development along the lines of one's true path. It brings into mind and focus memories that need to be brought into consciousness for full awareness associated with important experiences. It is a pathfinder when the seeker is unable to find the solution to a problem. It is a clearer of mental undergrowth when we have lost our way or need to remember how to use a skill once familiar but now long out of use. Physiological uses of the crystal include revitalizing parts of the body that have become numb, cold or paralysed. It is a crystal to equalize and balance the two halves of the brain and to strengthen the central nervous system. It has been used as a febrifuge and an analgesic.

Keynote effects

This is a remedy that allows us to look within ourselves and identify where the fault lines lie and where the problem areas are. It clarifies and amplifies our perception of ourselves in relation to others and to our personal world. It helps us to expand our conscious awareness that has been stultified by others and by circumstances, so that we are able to look beyond what is inhibiting and constraining us. One other effect that is worth noting is that the remedy can be used to enhance and amplify the positive effects of other indicated remedies that appear not to make any beneficial change despite being well selected.

General symptoms

The organs of the solar plexus are all influenced by the remedy: the liver and gall bladder are cleansed; the spleen and pancreas are revitalized; the stomach is calmed where there is too much acidity. It is another of the new remedies that can influence the acid/alkali balance positively (see especially **Sodium Bicarbonate**). The kidneys are also balanced and encouraged to drain properly. Blood and lymph are affected in the general drive to improve drainage of toxicity. Cerebrospinal fluid carries hormonal messages more efficiently as the pituitary is encouraged to take better control of the endocrine system (which it may have lost somewhat as the result of overdriving the adrenal glands for a long period or from torpor and stagnation). The spine is profoundly affected as the remedy influences the flow and circulation of energy up into the cranium; it realigns the spine and allows for greater flexibility. (Like **Sycamore Seed**, this remedy is useful when indicated if given during cranial osteopathic treatment.) Brittle bones; osteopenia. Sensations of internal trembling or shaking of the whole system. Sensation as if the whole body were slightly slewed round to the right; of being off-centre. It is also a remedy that can be used in patients who complain that all their remedies have caused them difficulty and aggravation; the patient seems to be not just over-sensitive but also to be intent on sabotaging their healing process. Eczema. Impairment of vision and visual acuity; should be considered for all conditions relating to the eyes.

Miasms

Psora and cancer.

Mental and emotional symptoms

Feelings of inadequacy, lack of self-esteem and self-confidence; self-doubt; a sense that one has become transparent and open to being judged for all one's shortcomings. Acute sense of vulnerability. A sense that one will be found out for being less than good enough; discovered to be a fraud. A terrible feeling that others will find out about one's deepest secrets; this even if one has not given any thought before to the fact that one might have any secrets. Feeling negative in a way that colours one's daily activity. Acute depression. Dismissive and cynical. Tends to judge things and people by appearances and too readily. There is a reluctance to participate because of prejudging. Resists change even when change is necessary or important. A reluctance to admit that change is needed or that clarification of difficult issues is overdue. The patient is held back by convention; by inherited or inculcated prejudices. There is a fear of appearing foolish; of being a nuisance; of being an outsider; or being unconventional; of being not politically correct. There is a tendency to do and say things that please others or that will illicit approval. There is the tendency to act or react without reference to what is good for the self; more according to what is perceived to be acceptable. There is an anticipation of what might be controversial with the feeling that it must be avoided. Parents may exhibit difficulties with their now adult children who have shown scant respect towards them and have taken them for granted; the parent has difficulty in saying exactly how they feel in case of offending their offspring.

This is a remedy that helps to restore one's faculty for critical thinking; one takes back initiative and self-respect so that what one has come to feel was 'correct' thinking may not necessarily be appropriate to oneself. The patient becomes easily drawn on for energy by others which leaves one feeling drained or scattered. Feelings of being constrained by others; by necessary routine; by time factors. It is for patients who become swept up by commonly held perceptions that influence decisions and attitudes; this causes them to lose their sense of self as the faculty most altered and blocked is the intuition. Time can feel distorted; it seems to flow either more quickly or more slowly than actually. Poor memory especially in the old. It is a remedy useful in men who have become confused about their role in relation to women; they find it difficult to tone down their masculinity and misjudge their approach. It may also be helpful in women who find machismo to be offensive; being unable to tolerate the priapic side of men they fail to wait for the softer side to emerge. There is a lack of awareness that symptoms have anything more than threat; the remedy can bring to consciousness the sense that symptoms have a meaning and purpose.

Physical symptoms

Head
Eczema on the forehead: burning sensation. Palpitations felt in the left side of the head. Congestion in the back of the head; constriction sensations felt in the middle of the head. Occipital headache < on waking.

Eyes
Black dots in front of the eyes. Glaucoma. Right eye becomes itchy; sensation as if it were expanding in the head. Bleeding behind the eye. Tension felt in the right eye that extends to the right jaw.

Face
Right side of the face feels enormously swollen that is connected with eye symptoms of pressure and swelling.

Throat
Palpitations felt in the throat. Catarrhal congestion in the throat. Pressure in the throat as if there were something that needed to be expressed.

Chest
Sensation of a weight on the chest in the thymus area. Discomfort in the right clavicle that can become quite intense.

Stomach
Acid indigestion; heartburn with gurgling.

Abdomen
Sensation of fullness in the abdomen particularly associated with bladder and kidney problems. Heaviness of the whole abdomen.

Male
Intermittent piercing pain in the base of the genitals with the sense that the focus of the pain is radiated upwards to involve the lower abdomen. Lowered libido; brain chunter brings on sudden impotence. Fear of impotence.

Urinary organs
Distension of the bladder causing considerable discomfort; feels that urging would become urgent. General feeling of heat when the bladder feels distended. Pains in the right kidney that come and go.

Back and neck
Sensation of a weight on the back of the neck and across the shoulders that presses downwards. Tension in the base of the spine. Tension felt in the left shoulder that extends into the right.

Extremities
Sciatica < from the top of the thigh down the whole leg to the heel < right side. Cramp in the muscles of the thigh which extends to the back of the knee. Pain that runs from the wrist, up the arm and into the shoulder on the left side: feeling as if the pain were in the marrow. A subjective sense that the left arm and the left thigh are one limb. Itching of the skin of the hands < night-time.

Considerations for the use of the remedy

Clear Quartz is a remedy to consider early on for any pathology of the eyes and vision. It is useful to help heal the harmful effects of laser treatment on the energy body of the eyes (see also **Ruby**). It has an affinity for the pituitary and thymus glands. When either or both of these are affected in a patient then it should be of service as a drainage remedy or in its own right as a constitutional remedy. It affects the cerebrospinal fluid, acting as a cleanser of this fluid vehicle of the hormone system. It is useful in the treatment of anyone who is suffering from memory loss and poor focus and concentration; this is particularly true of the elderly. There is a further affinity with the organs of the solar plexus: it balances the acid and alkali levels in favour of alkalinity; it cleanses the liver, gall bladder and blood and improves pancreatic functioning. As a drainage remedy it assists the lungs to release old emotions and it calms what amounts to fear held in the kidneys.

In terms of the energy channels of the body as expressed in traditional Chinese medicine, **Clear Quartz** is associated with the governing vessel and the conception vessel. This would confirm the remedy's association with the kidneys, the organs from which these vessels originate. It also holds true to its affinity for the structures associated with each of these vessels: back, spine, neck, head, eyes and brain (governing) and abdomen, chest, lungs, throat and face (conception). It is also one of the remedies most closely associated with restoring what cranial osteopaths describe as 'the midline', the integrity of the spinal column in relation to the energy that flows up and down, as well as the balance between the left and right sides of the body. (Other remedies in this category include **Oak**, **Silica**, **Calc-carb**, **Thuja**, **Sequoia** and **Ayahuasca**.)

NB It is sensible to recommend that a patient who is taking it for the first time should be careful not to lift anything awkward in bulk or heavy during the first week or so, as the remedy is often used by the system to readjust the musculoskeletal frame where there is any history of postural imbalance.

Clear Quartz can compare with and has affinities for other remedies:

- **Dolphin Sonar** which has a particular and special relation to the spine in that it can induce that state of absolute calm that characterizes the 'still point', the moment of stillness before movement. **Clear Quartz** is a remedy that precedes or follows **Dolphin Sonar** as it has an affinity for the energy that cyclically travels up and down the midline of the spine. This makes both remedies invaluable during treatment that involves cranial osteopathy.
- **Rainbow** is also complementary in that it has as strong an affinity for the pituitary and the cerebrospinal fluid (see page 438 of *Volume I* for a full explanation of the CV4 treatment). They follow and support each other well.
- **Carcinosin** is well supported by **Clear Quartz** not least as it may lessen any aggravations set up by the miasmatic remedy.

- **Sycamore Seed** is well known as a remedy of balance for the two sides of the body and for improving the function of the pituitary gland (see *Volume I*). It has less affinity for the organs of the solar plexus than **Clear Quartz** and has the ability to encourage the loosening of bony structures, particularly the sphenoid and the hips. **Clear Quartz** 6, 30 or 200 is useful in supporting a high potency of **Sycamore Seed**.
- **Sodium Bicarbonate** is one of the principle remedies for the rebalancing of acid and alkali in the body.

Clear Quartz can be used as a drainage remedy in low potency; it is best employed in combination with others chosen for their affinity for the particular organ under consideration. Here it will act well with kidney, lung, spleen, liver and bladder drainage remedies. For example:

- **CQ + Berberis Vulgaris + Lycopodium** 6x or 12x: kidney support.
- **CQ + Kali-mur + Lycopodium** 6x or 12x: lung support.
- **CQ + Ceanothus + Oak** 6x or 12x: spleen support.
- **CQ + White Chestnut Flower + Sepia** 6x or 12x: bladder support.

Esoteric therapeutics

The remedy has an affinity for all the chakras through its special relationship with the spinal column. It is a remedy that heals the physical and spiritual aspects of the spine, strengthening and improving the ease and quality of energy flow both upwards and downwards. This circulation gives **Clear Quartz** its particular association with the vagaries of time, time being an energy in itself; it is to the universe what blood is to the body. Time in the sphere of action of **Clear Quartz** brings first confusion and then clarity; the apparent distortion of time is mostly the result of the need for the patient to address issues that date back to previous generations' unresolved patterns of difficulties. One of the ways a patient becomes aware of the significance of the ancestral past is when they become aware of the esoteric meaning of their symptoms; it affords an idea of or the actual knowledge of the journey-purpose of healing. It is because of this ancestral aspect that the remedy is important in the treatment of conditions that affect the thymus gland (see *Volume I*). The use of **Thymus Gland + Ayahuasca + Clear Quartz** in either high potency or LM can be a means for the patient to get in touch with this aspect of their journey when indicated remedies fail to do all that is expected.

Kidney energy, in traditional Chinese medicine, is associated with ancestral energy. **Clear Quartz** is invaluable in supporting weak kidney qi, especially in those whose constitutions are weak either from miasmatic inheritance or from past emotional trauma. In terms of the elements, **Clear Quartz** should be considered in treating anyone who has a chronic excess of any one of them: earth, water, wood, fire or metal.

Chakras

Crown
The remedy eases the cancer miasm out of the crown chakra so that physical symptoms are less likely to manifest. There can be an enhanced consciousness of the spiritual purpose behind the patient's symptoms. Sleep is eased; dreams are calmed. For those who have difficulty in meditating, this remedy can facilitate quietening of the chuntering mind that tends to block access to the spiritual plane.

Brow
This is an important addition for the healing of the third eye. There is a greater sense of balance and flow between the intellect and intuition. Confusion and retreat give way to clarity and decisiveness. Doubts and cynicism dissolve as there is greater confidence in the power of common sense. Tension is eased in the head and vision (perception) is restored.

Throat
Self-expression may have been limited but it can now become very direct and uncompromisingly pertinent to the individual's purpose and growth. The ability to speak out without fear of disapproval from either one's family or associates becomes a major feature.

Heart
The ancestral connection can become apparent with the use of **Clear Quartz** and it derives from the way it works at this level. It is only by coming to terms with the harshness and hardness of experience that one can bring out the more yin side of the heart centre. There is a greater sense of security in this chakra so that it feels safe to be open and more full-hearted.

Solar plexus

Detoxifying the organs of the solar plexus supports and matches the clarifying of the mind and softening of the heart. Hence this remedy comes into its own as a support remedy when detoxification is necessary for parts of the body that would otherwise struggle to keep up with more general changes brought about by otherwise well-chosen constitutional remedies.

Sacral

This is chiefly a remedy for kidneys (particularly the right) and bladder at this level but there is a strong affinity for the male genital organs and the impact on them from the heart and mind.

Base

The remedy has a strong relationship with the spinal column in general and thus is central to the vitality of the body's core structure. It features in conditions of the bone: pains and problems related to ageing and miasmatic influences. It is also important to the functioning of the endocrine glands and to the eliminative processes. It is capable of encouraging the safe gathering and rising of the kundalini.

A Prover's dream

One of the provers had a dream that occurred on the night immediately following the proving that might be symptomatic of the remedy.

> 'I was in a room, unfamiliar to me, with another man of whom I was rather suspicious; he made me feel uncomfortable. He seemed over-familiar and gave me the impression that he was gay. As I became aware of his gaze, it was obvious that I had not done up the zip of my trousers. On looking down I saw that a piece of paper was sticking out. I removed it and realized it was a crisp new banknote. The note was beautifully designed but completely unfamiliar; a foreign currency. As I looked at it, the note became a wad. The immediate impression of good fortune quickly changed to frustration. Where on earth could I use such money? Who would accept it as legal tender? It was actually worthless. I might just as well throw it away. The sense of deflation and disappointment was acute.'

Case studies

1 'Female artist (59): a Libran born in the second decanate so very independent and can be stroppy. She's a long-term patient who uses homoeopathy as her main system of medical treatment though she supplements this with cranial osteopathy and acupuncture. She has a history of tilted pelvis, back pain and low energy. She tends to be angry and frustrated a lot of the time as she is often in opposition to close members of her family. She has done well on **Sulphur** and **Medorrhinum** in the past as she tends to live in her head and to have mood swings where she alternates between relaxed and laid back to furious, intolerant and irrational. She has been on an elimination diet to ease her acid indigestion and in order to lose weight which is now happening. Her digestion is working better (she is intolerant of wheat and dairy) but she still has poor energy and finds it hard to get to sleep. (She likes to stay up at night once she has the house to herself.) She is also complaining of what she herself has diagnosed as tennis elbow and carpal tunnel symptoms, all on the right side. There is an obvious internal rotation of her left shoulder which is mirrored in the hips. She has felt uncreative and unmotivated.

"'I want clarity in my brow centre. I've got lots of projects in mind but I just can't get into them." She was given **Clear Quartz** 30: one each week for eight weeks. "To start with I got a lot of energy out of them but it wasn't comfortable. I was too racy. I felt I was being made to do things. I wasn't in control. Then I had a serious relapse in my back and the osteopath told me my sacrum was tilted forward and that the whole of my right side was not in alignment just as it always used to be." She realized as she said this that she had been revisiting past symptoms.

"'My back is fine now. And I have much more clarity in my head. I know where I am going. I feel that remedy is almost too narrow. I want to be more expansive now. It felt like a rod for my back and I feel it needs to be spread around now."' **JM**

2 One of the participating homoeopaths at a seminar during which **Clear Quartz** and **Sodium Bicarbonate** were presented, sent an email describing her experience. She had arrived at the seminar feeling unwell

due to a dental problem that gave her considerable pain in the jaw. She explained that she felt 'out of her body' and she was clearly uncomfortable with making the effort to participate in the group. At the beginning of the lecture on **Clear Quartz** a bottle of the 30th potency was placed on the floor next to a clear quartz point in full view of the whole group.

'The first thing was that I was so out of my body because of the pain. This was confirmed when, during a preliminary exercise in learning how to read pulses, I was told, "You are not in your body". Having felt the beneficial effect of the remedy during the lecture (presumably due to the amplifying effects of the crystal) and having learnt that **Clear Quartz** helps one get back to one's midline, I thought I would take the remedy (there and then). Within moments I felt like I was back in. I had not felt like that for the seven days since the dental treatment. My pulse was taken again during the break in lectures which confirmed that I was now grounded and centred.

'The second thing [I remember] was that later on we were learning the remedy **Sodium Bicarbonate**. If I remember correctly the bottle [of the remedy] was open on the floor with the [piece of] clear quartz in front of the bottle. It was facing in my direction. My tooth pain became magnified and I had to ask for the quartz to be moved. The pain then calmed right down again.' CG

Two experiences with Clear Quartz

1 Between 17 and 20 May 2010 a course in evolutionary homoeopathy was held in London which was attended by the author of the following experience. At this seminar **Clear Quartz** was presented for the first time as a new remedy.

'On the first day, each participant was given a clear quartz crystal which had been programmed by Janice Micallef. My understanding was that the crystal had been asked to give each participant what they needed from the course. This crystal was in my pocket or on my chair throughout the course.

'Just before the start of the second day I shared with one of the other course participants the information that my own personal journey at present was focused on integrating my intellect and my intuition, something I had been struggling with for some time, as my rational mind always dominates.

'We then started the day with a qigong exercise in the garden. While performing the exercise I experienced an expansion of my conscious awareness. My whole being was merging with the grass and trees around me, as though the atoms of my body were melding with those of the earth. Afterwards, when sharing our experiences of the exercise in the group we discovered that another woman had had a very similar experience. My mind went to the crystals we had been given and Colin suggested we might be experiencing the remedy **Clear Quartz** which he would be teaching to us for the first time later that morning.

'The first lecture of the day was on cranial sacral therapy, specifically the cranial tides. As I sat listening to a beautiful description of the breath of life while also looking at a handout containing detailed anatomical diagrams of the human brain, I experienced a massive shift in consciousness. I could feel a fine trembling throughout my whole body especially at my throat chakra. Tears formed in my eyes and dropped down my cheeks. I felt as though a huge amount of information was being transmitted directly to me through my crown and higher chakras. Suddenly, I did not need to listen to the lecture. I "knew" everything that was being said. I recognized the esoteric teachings as Truth and I inexplicably "knew" the intricate anatomy of the brain. Moments later I experienced the presence of my maternal grandfather on one side of me and his brother on the other side. I also had a sense of their mother behind them. My grandfather was a civil engineer but also a spiritual healer, like his mother. His brother was a brain surgeon! I knew from family history that the two brothers were completely estranged following the marriage of my grandfather to my grandmother who is also a spiritual healer. This schism was never resolved and all contact was lost between the two brothers and those lines of the family are unknown to each other.

'I understood that I was being shown the ancestral origins of my own struggle between intuition and intellect. I also received the message: "If I did not heal this, my son would have to do so." This reference to my son made me weep and I had to leave the room. I was also a bit rattled by having such a spontaneous and profound experience during a lecture amidst a group of virtual strangers and needed to regroup!

'Later that morning, when Colin gave the lecture on the remedy **Clear Quartz** it resonated strongly with my experience described above especially when he described how the provers in the meditation circle had also experienced their own ancestral energy.

'Several months ago, after a series of vivid dreams and other inner work, I identified a need to achieve greater balance between my intellect and intuition. I sought to understand why I repeatedly allow my rational mind to override my intuition. I have turned away from hands-on healing in recent years in favour of more mind-based homoeopathy. All the inner work I was doing suggested I should be doing both, even blending them together but something deep within made me resist returning to more esoteric forms of healing. I have made progress with this but have been hampered by not understanding its root cause. I had put much of it down to the suffering my grandmother experienced as a direct result of being a spiritual healer both within and outside the family. Some of the resistance related to my own childhood experiences. I have identified and released a huge amount of the fear I held around this but some element of resistance remains. This profound experience with **Clear Quartz** has shown me that this inability to balance these two aspects is not entirely due to the events of my own lifetime but has an ancestral origin. This has a liberating feel to it and I don't feel quite so useless for not having been able to resolve it completely despite a huge amount of work. The sheer power of the experience will also serve to increase my trust in the non-rational mind. My path forward can only be illuminated by this as I continue to seek the transcendent quality that lies between intellect and intuition.

'PS I have *always* had the feeling that anyone involved in healing can see right through me and see all my secrets. Even as a child! I have yet to take the remedy!' **CAB (23 May 2010)**

2   One of the prospective participants of the same seminar who was unable to attend was sent a clear quartz point along with her refund for the course. Each student had received one of these points. The following is her experience.

'That crystal I got through the post is amazing. I woke with a vertex headache which ended up in my occiput yesterday morning. I had been to Woking for two days and coming home put my satnav on and it would not work – panic! I had no idea how to get home without it . . . So my partner had to guide me through the traffic on loudspeaker to get me to the M25 in the rush hour! So getting home was so stressful. When I eventually arrived home three hours later I had my dinner and a glass of red wine.

'As I said, I awoke with this awful headache and as I had a 9am patient on Friday morning I just took a paracetamol but it did nothing (no surprises there then!). I had not read the notes you had kindly sent through on this remedy but I just felt that I should put the crystal on my occiput – which I did for a couple of minutes and the headache went. Amazing in just a few minutes! Then I read the notes and it covers it. I also felt much more chilled out and more focused than in the morning when I was all over the place and that's not good when one is working on difficult cases!' JT

5

COTTON WOOL

The remedy was proved on 5 February 1999. Six women and three men were present. Each took a single dose of the 30th potency. Up until now the remedy has been available as 'Cotton' but this should be amended to differentiate it from **Gossypium**, the remedy made from the whole plant.

The Background

Cotton is a member of the *Malvaceae* and is known by its Linnaean name, *Gossypium herbaceum*. For the remedy made from the plant, it was the fresh inner root bark, chopped and pounded to a pulp that was used. The sample of cotton wool used for this remedy was taken from a field in southern Spain in November 1998 shortly before harvesting. The plant stems were blackened stalks with a tight ball of cotton wool. Only the white cotton was used.

Gossypium is an indigenous species of India though it also readily grows in southern Europe where the climate is warm enough for the crop to mature. (*Gossypium barbadense* is a similar plant but is native to America.) Mrs Grieve tells us that Gossypium 'is a biennial or triennial plant with branching stems 2 to 6 feet high, palmate hairy leaves, lobes lanceolate and acute, flowers with yellow petals and a purple spot in the centre, leaves of involucres serrate, capsule when ripe splits open and shows a loose white tuft surrounding the seeds and adhering firmly to outer coating; it requires warm weather to ripen the seeds . . .' She goes on to say that 'the crushed seeds give a fixed, semi-drying oil used to make soap, etc. The flowering time ends in September and a month or so earlier the tops are cut off in order to ripen and send the sap back to the capsules.'

To continue with Mrs Grieve: 'The herbaceous part of the plant contains much mucilage and has been used as a demulcent. Cotton seeds have been used in the Southern States of America for intermittent fever with great success. The root and stem-bark deteriorates with age so only newly harvested material should be used. The root-bark of commerce consists of thin, flexible bands of quilled pieces covered with a browny yellow periderm, odour not strong, taste slightly acid.'

The plant contains an odourless acid resin that is not soluble in water; the bark contains sugar, tannin, gum, fixed oil and chlorophyll. In the past the plant has been used as an abortifacient instead of ergot as the latter is far more toxic. It was favoured by the slaves of the southern States. The medicine causes contractions of the uterus in labour. However, it also was found useful in the treatment of heavy period bleeding that resulted from fibroids. Mrs Grieve also noted that a preparation of the seeds helped lactation in nursing women.

The modern farmed crop is a hybrid form of natural wild cotton. The latter has short, coarser fibres while the hybrid version produces longer and silkier fibres making the end product more valuable. There are many different varieties of cotton, some being adapted to low-lying marshlands and others to uplands. It seems to have originated in Pakistan and then been taken to the Mediterranean and then the Orient. Mexico had its own variety from which a fabulous textile handicraft developed that Cortes first encountered in 1519.

Cotton requires deep, rich soil in an area of plentiful rainfall. It suffers from frost, drought and wind. Though naturally it is mostly a perennial plant it is generally regarded by farmers as an annual crop. Flowering and fruiting is a continuous process from July/August until the first frosts of early winter.

Before the Industrial Revolution of the 19th century cotton was a labour-intensive cottage industry. Families of workers in poorer parts of the world would toil at the long process of cloth manufacture which required separating seeds from fibres, spinning, making thread, weaving and baling. The finished material was extremely expensive. In direct response to the early attempts to simplify, cheapen and speed up the cloth manufacture, machinery was invented that led to the Industrial Revolution – first the gin to separate the seeds from the boll, and then the industrial looms in the Lancashire mills. To maintain the supply of cotton, the slave trade in the southern States boomed. Between the 1790s and 1861 slavery became, in real terms, a bigger money-spinner than cotton growing. (It was only after the Civil War that it became apparent that it had always been possible to produce the requisite amounts of the crop without using slave labour.)

Historically, in the United States the farming of cotton was always a vastly wasteful enterprise. When it was first grown there by the colonists, land was 'freely' available (which meant that it had to be wrested from the native population) and as there was so much of it, rather than husband a chosen area of land, the farmers would continuously move further and further westward leaving behind large areas of used wasteland, denuded of trees and naturally occurring plant life. In the earliest years of cotton growing, slavery was unknown; it was a poor white man's crop. The mechanical gin encouraged the use of slaves and the decline of the white population's will to work creatively for itself. The development of black slavery matched the decline of the cottage industry in Britain and the development of industrial manufacturing towns with their serried rows of poor, congested housing. (The rise of such towns spelled the break-up of rural life and the fragmentation of families quite as much as with black people in the States.)

Keynote effects

Dispels inertia and clears the mind for intuitive thinking. It is a remedy to foster a sense of enlightenment. One is able to reject what is no longer necessary from the past; 'old tunes' that the mind has kept playing for years are let go. There is a return to basics; a search for a simplified life.

General symptoms

A state of dullness; all the body tissues feel dull and without spark. The remedy brings clarity, sharpness of thought and vision. Pituitary gland and pineal gland both affected. It encourages the release of the pituitary from sluggishness. Sleepiness and tiredness. Slow growth on any level: stunted children; difficulty in coming to spiritual awareness; blocked through emotional disturbance. It is said to be able to create new neural pathways in the brain. Useful in brain damage from difficult birth or traumatic injury: see **Thymus Gland** (*Volume I*). Also benign tumours that are slow growing; of the pituitary, of the thyroid. Precancerous states when it might be suspected that cell formation is becoming perverted; when cysts might turn cancerous. Heavy production of sinus mucus which threatens to block breathing or prevent sleep. All the facial sinuses can be involved as well as the ethmoid. Lack of oxygen to the tissues. General feelings of heaviness. Body clock is out of sync. Endocrine system functions poorly.

Shows a need to simplify life; to go back to basics. Useful after a stroke or in ME. Also in Parkinson's. Overweight or obese. Another remedy to help clear the radiation miasm.

Miasms

Psora, cancer and sycosis.

Mental and emotional symptoms

Dull and lifeless; torpor. A strong sense of waste. Dullness felt as a consequence of a weight of experience that has not truly been assimilated. Feels blank. Can't be bothered mentality; fed up. Paralysis of the emotions with a loss of connection between thoughts and feelings. Has lost the ability to use the intuition; feeling of being on autopilot without a guiding spirit. Has lost a grip on life's forward movement. Just going through the motions. Slow to make connections. Poor concentration; mind wanders off at a tangent to unimportant, mundane things. Mind is full of trivial ideas. Goes over old thoughts endlessly. Cannot adapt to change. Feels put out to grass. Commonly needed by retired people who can look back on their lives and see, despite material success, only a spiritual and emotional wasteland. Wakes in the middle of the night with chuntering brain. Becomes self-critical; intense self-examination; can't see any quality to life; turns to blaming self for events long past. Unable to make a balanced judgement about events in the past, feeling that it is oneself who was in error. (**Hornbeam** is complementary here.) Ailments from disappointment. Bereavement. Cannot visualize or project into the future. Abdicates responsibilities to others or to institutions. Loses sight of where true responsibility lies. Feelings of inadequacy and incompetence. Makes mistakes with words and calculations. Struggles to make sense of what they read or hear. Poor self-expression; difficulty in finding the right words to express what one feels. Finds it very difficult to communicate with others especially on an emotional level. A sense of being trapped; within oneself; within the situation one has created which creates a tearful mood. Wants to cry but cannot find the energy to do so. A sense of deep sadness; of wasted opportunity. A sense of failure. Feel that they struggle in vain to see the way forward but nothing that they do can clarify the issues that need to be resolved. The continuous effort causes pressure headaches. Know what they ought to be doing but cannot find the energy to get going nor the concentration necessary. Tendency to drift. Does not want to face the difficulties ahead. Can harbour morbid thoughts: wonder when they will die and whether age is catching up with them. Consequent desire for things to stay the same yet knowing that they cannot. Lack of self-confidence. Generally > after the full moon has passed. Inexplicable sense of fear. A fear of letting go. Inertia. Agitation and debility. Impatience. Jealousy as in 'oldest child' syndrome. There is also weakness and timidity following the experience of an episode of aggression, violence or rage. Reticent. Can be useful for those who have been through a 'system' (such as education) which has left them feeling unprepared to face the world despite the gifts and talents that they naturally possess.

Physical symptoms

Head

Feels full and congested. Sinuses all full of mucus. Thick and muzzy head. Pressure on the middle of the brow with a sensation of slow pulsation. Intense pressure in the third eye area. Headache in the brow area. Pounding head all over. Tingling on the vertex. Vertigo: a tendency to lean to the left. Clenching and tension in the occiput. Benign tumours of the pituitary gland.

The plant has: burning and then stinging from both temporal bones to the middle of the frontal bone; drawing pain over the eyes with stinging in the pupils. (W Boericke on **Gossypium**)

Eyes

Vision is dimmed, clouded or obscured. Cataract. Nystagmus. Colour blindness. Frowning from poor sight.

The plant has: drawing pains over the eyes with stinging pain in pupils. (W Boericke on **Gossypium**)

Ears

Thick wax which causes hardness of hearing. Glue ear. Deep pain in the right ear connected to the tongue. Tinnitus: ringing sound.

Nose

Thick catarrh which is difficult to dislodge. Mucus is sticky and heavy. Mouth breathing especially in children. Snuffly breathing.

Face

Frowning as from seriousness.

Throat

Thick mucus becomes stuck in the throat. Irritation and coughing. Catarrh can make swallowing difficult. (No taste to the mucus but has very little sense of taste at all.) Sore, tight throat with a sensation of clenching with a referred pain into the right ear. Thyroid problems: underactive but usually consequent on pituitary pathology. Thyroid and eye symptoms go together.

Respiration and chest

Pressure feeling over the thymus area. Want of oxygen makes breathing difficult. Shallow breathing with need to take sighing breaths from time to time. Lack of oxygen = sluggishness (physical and mental). Pressure over the heart area. Heart feels heavy. Asthmatic breathing especially with the accumulation of thick mucus in the larynx. Constriction of the upper chest.

Stomach

The plant has: nausea with a lot of salivation. Nausea of pregnancy with vomiting before breakfast. Rotating pain in the stomach. Anorexia especially < around menses. (W Boericke on **Gossypium**)

Abdomen

Distension not > for passing wind. Frequent stools. Urging to pass stools with little result. Heavy and dragging in the abdomen with the feeling that the digestive system is in need of detoxification. Piles; with little bleeding. Rx > rectal spasm.

Female

Ovarian remedy: sterility. FSH (follicle-stimulating hormone) and LH (luteinizing hormone) are insufficient to stimulate the process of establishing the corpus luteum thus rendering ineffective any pregnancy. Flocculent discharge, white. Gynaecological symptoms are often accompanied by discomfort in the digestive organs. Heaviness and dragging of the uterine region though not necessarily associated with the menstrual cycle.

The plant has: labia swollen and itching. Intermittent pain in ovaries. Retained

placenta. Morning sickness with sensitive uterine region. Suppressed menstrua-
tion. Menses too watery. Backache, weight and dragging in pelvis. Uterine
sub-involution and fibroids with gastric pain and debility. (W Boericke on
Gossypium)

Back
Stiffness and tightness at cervical region and across shoulders. Pressing pain
in the lower spine.

Sleep
Very sleepy even in the daytime. Sleepiness with heaviness in the limbs. Wakes
early (5am) and lies awake thinking confused thoughts.

Considerations for the use of the remedy

It is worth drawing an analogy with the natural history of the spider. In some
species of spider, the female carries her egg cocoon (that looks so much like
a piece of cotton wool) around on her back. If this is removed, the spider
becomes completely inert.

Cotton wool complements **Baryta-carb, Calc-carb, Sulphur, Silica, Phos,
Lyc** and **Carcinosin**. It also works well in relation to other new remedies:

- **Sequoia** which may follow when **Cotton wool** has begun the process of
  lifting brain fog as a period of developmental growth should begin,
  which Sequoia would enhance if the characteristic indications are
  there.
- **Thymus Gland** is sometimes indicated by similar symptoms of inertia
  and poor focus though it is usually to be thought of either in children
  struggling with development issues or those who never completed
  their natural learning during childhood (as if they had never finished
  childhood satisfactorily). For someone who has reached middle age or
  retirement age **Cotton wool** may be followed well by this remedy.
- **Rainbow** is a very useful remedy to complement and support **Cotton
  wool** as it encourages the cerebrospinal fluid to keep flowing and
  amplify the effects on the system of the hormone messages when this
  process has been difficult up to now. The lower potencies will not
  interrupt the work of a high potency of **Cotton wool.**
- **Sycamore Seed** in gynaecology cases can harmonize the pituitary and

the ovaries. In a case where there are menstrual difficulties, especially in the menopause, **Sycamore Seed** in a low potency will complement **Cotton wool** given in a deeper potency.
- Any of the radiation remedies are potentially related to **Cotton**, particularly **Plutonium**.

Cotton wool is a miasmatic remedy and is associated with psora and the cancer miasm though it also has an affinity for sycosis. It is used as a similimum in its own right or it can be used as a drainage remedy in medium-deep (12 or 30) potency repeated to work alongside and complement an indicated constitutional remedy. **Cotton** is not inimical to any other remedy with the possible exception of the viburnum remedies.[8] It can also be usefully employed as a constituent of combination remedies.

- **Cotton wool + Carcinosin + Arsenicum** helps to drain cancer from the aura (that is before it has reached physical manifestation). The indications for it would be anxiety about health, restlessness and lack of drive to sort things out in one who has recently retired or come to an impasse.
- **Cotton wool + Plutonium + Thymus Gland** is useful to clear the radiation miasm where it threatens to create a carcinogenic state. Indications include deathly tiredness, aching in the limbs, lack of mental acuity, greyness and passivity following a period of intense emotional upheaval.
- **Cotton wool + Arnica + Thymus Gland** 10M is a remedy to be thought of for brain damage after difficult births or traumatic accidents.

Esoteric therapeutics

All the layers of the aura are affected and are stultified and left as if paralysed. The remedy restores the balance between the base and the brow and encourages the vocal self-expression necessary through the throat centre. Pulse reading may reveal a somewhat thick nature to the pulses: sluggish and turbid. The elements that are most missing are air and fire.

---

8 See *Encyclopaedia of Remedy Relationships in Homoeopathy*, Rehman.

Chakras

Crown

Sleep is heavy and dreams are confusing. There is no place for cool reflection here as there is too much corruption of the higher mind with 'history' which will include disappointment and worry as well as inertia. The 'light receiver' of the highest centre is 'switched off'.

Brow

This centre becomes occluded and confused. The will and intuition lose contact which leads to too much material thinking. Loss of intuitive powers. A sense of being blocked from spiritual resources; spiritual darkness or wilderness. The remedy engenders peace and tranquillity; stillness of mind and body and an ability to sort the mental wheat from chaff.

Throat

Find it very difficult to speak uninhibitedly about their concerns which are deep and even tend to the morbid. The deepest thoughts may even manifest as congestion in the thyroid.

Heart

Sadness in this centre is mostly associated with grief for oneself: the grief of not having achieved much, if anything, and that it is now too late. It is also for those who feel that they no longer deserve appreciation of others. The perception that has led to this is usually unfounded and comes from a profound dissatisfaction with self. The remedy is one that can help to recover a person's sense of self-worth even into old age.

Solar plexus

There is not much fight left in the patient; they have faced challenges and dealt with conflicts but it has all left a rather poor taste in the mouth: dust and ashes. There is not enough brow-centred conviction to look for further challenges. Motivation is weak so the spleen is strongly affected and often needs support (**Ceanothus Ø**, for example, or **Golden Beryl** in low 'x' potency).

Sacral

Congestion and torpor create as much stasis in this chakra as they do in the brow and throat. Kidney energy may be weak if the mind is clouded.

Base

The kundalini energy fails to rise for any reason. There is a sense of impotency in the whole being that is nevertheless mostly felt in the brow centre. They are like the person who works on the top floor of an office block every day but does not know where the stairs are when the lift is broken. Work has been allowed to rule the base centre for too long and now there is little to replace it as a motivational force. Breakdown is less likely to be structural than hormonal and in the eliminative system.

Case studies

1 'Female 57, breast cancer. She had been given **Pulsatilla** 200c alternating with **Carcinosin** 200c using Dr Ramakrishnan's plussing method. These remedies were supporting her well and during the sessions with me we were working through lots of emotional traumas and untangling much of her history. She had grown up in a family of five children. She was the eldest and had taken huge responsibility in the upbringing of her siblings and the welfare of her parents. She had gone on to marry a kind but emotionally unavailable man who was also very needy and draining. She had five children of her own and had basically spent the whole of her life caring for others. All her life she has smoked cannabis to relax and help her sleep. She found it very difficult still not to be a slave to her family although very aware that she no longer wanted to be. She also found it very difficult to notice unkind remarks that family members made until days afterwards; they slowly sank in and she felt very hurt but unable to respond. Although she found it easy to express herself with me and get clarity about her healing process she said, "When I leave and I try to process what I realize here my head feels full of cotton wool. When I try to express my feelings at any time to my family it is the same. So instead I find myself just falling asleep or feeling very depressed."

'I prescribed **Cotton Wool** because she said her head felt full of cotton wool. (I always consider **Cotton Wool** as a remedy when a patient uses these words). Also this remedy seemed appropriate due to her history of suppression. **Cotton Wool** 30c was prescribed daily along with the original remedies and she really is thinking much more clearly, reacting much more quickly to remarks made and is generally far less depressed, drugged, stifled and foggy. Her whole demeanour is much lighter and clearer.' HJ

2 'Man, early 30s; came for regular treatment. Had been through long treatment for leukaemia for which he had had both orthodox and alternative medicine. He had been given the all-clear by the doctors though his immune system was being kept under surveillance. He was unable to get back into work and felt redundant. He struggled with disappointment about the way his life had gone. He arrived with a headache which he described as 'thick' and which made him feel confused and 'woolly in the head'. He was given **Cotton Wool** 200 early in the appointment. By the end of the session the headache was cleared.' JM

A Prover's experience

'I think I have been proving this remedy for several weeks. I have been completely paralysed with inactivity especially in this last week. I have got so much to do. We are moving on Wednesday and I have done nothing. I know what I should be doing but I haven't got round to doing it. I feel very spaced out and had difficulty even managing to do the shopping. Even when I had written everything down on a list, I was still coming out of shops with things missing. That improved after I saw the cranial osteopath last week but I have started to drift again.'

6

CURCUMA LONGA

Turmeric

The proving was carried out on 8 February 2008; 11 people were present: 7 women and 4 men. One of the women was Janice Micallef, the medium who acted as co-ordinator. ·

The remedy was made from a piece of turmeric root which was donated by Swami Atmachaithanya, a holy man from the region of Kerala in southern India. In giving the remedy to Sylvia Treacher to make up at the Helios pharmacy, he gave the following indications for its use: blood purification, the treatment of all skin diseases and as an aid in preventing the spread of cancer. When ordering the remedy ask for 'Turmeric (S Treacher)'.

The Background

Turmeric is one of the *Zingiberaceae*. In Sanskrit it is known as *haridra*. Its origins are obscure though it is likely that it comes from South and South-East Asia, especially from India. Today, India supplies 94 per cent of the world's turmeric. Brought West by Arab traders, it became popular in Europe and elsewhere as a replacement for the fabulously expensive saffron. It has been known for many centuries as herb, spice and medicine; writings dating back to the seventh century BC mention its value in the kitchen and the sick room. Apart from this it has other uses: it is a dye and creates the bright yellow that is so characteristic and, when mixed with alkaline fluids, a bright red. It is also used for cosmetic purposes as an anti-ageing substance.

Turmeric is unknown in the wild and is therefore a domesticated plant. The oblong leaves, shooting up from the fleshy rhizome, reach approximately one metre in height. The flowers are yellow-white and appear at the top of a spiky stalk. These flowers are sterile and render the plant unable to reproduce from seeds. The useful part is the rhizome which appears ringed where old leaf growth shows. It is boiled, dried and ground into powder. The flesh is sometimes used for culinary and medicinal purposes.

Turmeric has been and still is the focus for much scientific research. Many studies have been undertaken into its medicinal properties in the search for cures for conditions of the bowels, heart, liver, skin and for neurological disorders. Claims have been made for it as being beneficial in all these areas and for AIDS, Alzheimer's, Crohn's disease, cystic fibrosis and cancers among others. It is recognized to have all the following properties: antibacterial, antifungal, anti-inflammatory, antispasmodic, antibiotic, expectorant and analgesic. Curcumin, the chemical that gives the rhizome its distinctive colour, is also recognized as having anti-cancer potential.

Turmeric has been known as a natural medicine for well over 2,000 years but is particularly associated with Ayurvedic medicine. So popular has it become that it is now available in herbal and health food shops as a supplement in the form of capsules. It is used to strengthen and to warm the whole system. It is chiefly famous for its ability to calm a disordered digestive system; diarrhoea, dysentery, bloating, flatus and flatulence all come under its influence. The liver and gall bladder are also benefited: it is a medicine for jaundice and congested liver and for gall stones. It is a carminative and demulcent and a tonic for the stomach. It has been used for inflammation of the joints as one would find in arthritis; for diabetes and the reduction of obesity; to lower levels of 'bad' (LDL) cholesterol in the blood. Eye infections such as conjunctivitis have been treated with turmeric as have insect bites. It is a wound remedy: poultices with a paste made from the rhizome have salved and cured open sores, wounds and ulcers. It has even gained a reputation in history for healing leprosy. Practitioners have long used it for skin conditions such as dermatitis and eczema.

Turmeric is very much associated with Taurus for this is the sign that is most open to dietary abuse. Taurean patients may seem to require more swiftly increased potencies in drainage. It is also of great value in Scorpio, the most sensitive and potentially insecure of all signs, opposite to Taurus in the zodiac and requiring potencies at the other end of the scale. Patients may allow their fears and insecurities to get the better of their temperament and resort to using protective subterfuge to feel safe; what Scorpios fear most is the sense of loss not only in the emotional sense but also of material things. The remedy helps the patient to be more open and less ready to go on the attack. This is particularly so if the remedy is combined with **Ayahuasca** and **Syphilinum** and used at the 10M.

Keynote effects

Drainage and cleansing of toxicity that then creates the basis for clarity of intuitive vision, clarity of thought processes and greater tranquillity of mind. Restores balance to a system disturbed by poor nutrition caused by faulty dietary habits. It is seen to simplify complicated cases; it sheds light where there has been turmoil, stagnation and a gathering threat of deeper pathology. By primarily focusing its action on physical cleansing the remedy fosters a gradual clearing of heart energy so that this may open safely and lead to a greater awareness of a life path. There is a sense of being more at one with oneself and therefore greater optimism and strength in facing the next challenges. It has a strong effect on syphilitic and radiation miasms, helping to clear both from the system.

General symptoms

This is a cleansing and protective remedy for both vital organs and the chakras. Its action is chiefly centred on the liver and solar plexus. It will also affect the function of the spleen and pancreas by association with the liver. Enhances and strengthens the immune system. It is a drainage remedy for the liver and the blood. Whatever cleansing it does, initiates healing in other areas; its benefits radiate both upwards, towards the heart and throat and downwards from the solar plexus, towards the bowel and bladder. It enhances the secretion of bile. It restores damaged liver cells to integrity and aids in the assimilation of nutrition particularly in those who have used microwave cooking over a long period and elderly people who have resorted to convenience food. It works strongly on the liver and gall bladder meridians as well as the large intestine and stomach meridians. It is useful in relieving pains in the muscles and halting atrophy or rigidity in those with liver function problems. In those with hyperacidity of the system there is susceptibility to candida and parasites such as pinworms; situations in which this remedy will be of considerable use. It is an invaluable support remedy in patients who have digestive disorders with concomitant sluggish circulation. It may be indicated in those whose arteries are furred up or whose venous system is poor. It is indicated in those with menstrual problems such as dysmenorrhoea, amenorrhoea and damage from the Pill or HRT.

It is also said to help restore integrity to a brain fouled with hallucinogenic drugging or allopathic medicines. It has been suggested as a remedy for those damaged by cocaine; a system that has been artificially provoked to produce huge amounts of adrenalin and then left to recoup with sugar, coffee and other stimulants. It may also be indicated in those who have damaged brain cells; it may be of practical support in alcoholics. It works well on ulcers anywhere in the body but is of particular value in stomach ulcers. It is said to lower cholesterol levels especially when given in combination with other remedies with the same sphere of action. (See below for suggested combinations.) Is of value in cancer therapeutics: in the early stages of cancer or even before it manifests physically, it can be given in low potency over an extended period (t.d.s. for two months). It is also of use in more advanced cancer states when it helps to slow down the disease process, facilitating the action of the more constitutionally indicated remedies. It has been mentioned as a remedy capable of wound healing after the manner of **Calendula**.

Miasms

Psora, cancer and leprosy.

Mental and emotional symptoms

Depression; feel as if they carry the weight of the world on their shoulders. Feel they are old before their time. Feeling of being out of touch with the planet. A strong need for peace and quiet. After a long period of mental and emotional turmoil, especially in relation to struggling with worldly things, there is a weakness of resolve, a wish to retire and not to have to cope. There may be an absence of awareness of how other people are feeling or faring with their problems, not from want of empathy but from 'burn out'. There is a lack of clarity of thought and there is a loss of intuitive energy. Feels blocked on the mental level and this is matched on the physical plane by feeling sluggish, tired and lacking in motivation. The patient may even say they need a detox or that a week in a health spa might be a good idea. All this is of greater significance in one who feels that they have been struggling fruitlessly in an occupation that has had little meaning for them. There may well be a sense that they have not yet found what they want to do in life; there is no clarity about the essential soul purpose. This has made the daily battle seem particularly wasteful. There is an awareness that life has gone wrong but not of how or what to do about it. A sense that the future is empty. A tendency to rush into things with the consequence of blundering about. A history of aiming high but falling short. Irritability especially at one's own shortcomings; at not being able to understand what is going on; at not being able to communicate properly. Muddled thinking that contributes to shying away from all those things sent to try us. Fearfulness: of inadequacy; of speaking out about emotions. Strongly indicated by those who have been 'living in their heads'; life till now has been head- (and probably ego-) centred with more energy going into thinking than into maintaining the correct balance between the bodies. After so much energy has been invested in making critical judgements, the mental body has become, as it were, swollen, inflamed and weak. Too much reasoning and rationalizing has overtaxed the mind and the expense is borne by the physical body. The patient has become mired in habitual ways of negative thinking; everything tends to become intellectualized and causes introversion. Panicky feelings.

Physical symptoms

Head
Congestive headaches.

Face
Pain in the right cheekbone with swelling.

Throat
Blocked sensation < checked emotions.

Chest
Tension or oppression.

Stomach
Peptic ulcer. Acid indigestion; acid reflux. Incipient hiatus hernia.

Abdomen
Sharp, needle-like pain in the left side. Worms. Lack of balance of the bowel flora leading to candidiasis. Thrush.

Female
Dysmenorrhoea; amenorrhoea. NBWS the Pill or HRT.

Shoulders
Tightness of the muscles across the top of the shoulders that feels like cramp.

Limbs
Uncomfortable prickling and tingling in the buttocks and down the legs which is intermittent. Hot shins. Cold lower legs. Arthritic changes in the hands; joints become painful.

Muscles
Rigidity and pain: aching and atrophy from continued stiffness. Restriction of joints.

Sleep
Wakes with a headache between 5 and 6am.

Considerations for the use of the remedy

Turmeric may be compared with other constitutional and drainage remedies:

- **Orange** has similar mind and spirit states: both lack peace of mind and are desperate for it; both find that intuitive thinking is difficult if not virtually impossible; both have a history of using reason and logic too assiduously to sort a busy mind. What differentiates them is the use of **Turmeric** for states of toxicity and its burnt out condition which **Orange** does not have.
- **Cardamom** which is a remedy that is more concerned with the support and restoration of integrity of energy to the main vital organs

especially of the lower body. It is a chakra cleansing remedy and focuses on the interaction between the kidneys, spleen, liver and bladder as well as the adrenal glands, the gall bladder and pancreas. Like **Turmeric**, it is a remedy that is indicated by patients with faulty digestion due to dietary problems and is most useful where there is an acid/alkali imbalance. However, **Cardamom** also has a strong affinity with the heart from which its action radiates outwards (rather as the action of **Berberis** radiates out from the kidneys) while **Turmeric**'s action tends to radiate from the liver.

- **Hydrastis** is the most usual remedy to consider in those suffering from hyperacidity. It complements **Turmeric** and **Cardamom** on the drainage level and **Arsen-alb** and **Carbo-veg** on the constitutional level. It is also, like **Turmeric**, a remedy to consider in precancerous conditions. Its main action is on the liver and the connection with the mucous membranes.
- **Lycopodium** is a major polychrest that is often indicated early on in treatment of any individual who would benefit from **Turmeric** (or either of the above remedies). It is chiefly right-sided (though by no means exclusively) while **Turmeric** does not have a bias for either side.
- **Chelidonium** is far more specific in its indications as a liver drainage or constitutional remedy. It has a narrower field of application though when included in combination with other drainage remedies it does not need to be considered for its characteristic pain under the right shoulder blade.
- **Sodium Bicarbonate** is another very important remedy in one who is too acidic. It is usually a warm-blooded remedy (though by no means exclusively so) and is characterized by either a lack of thirst or a tendency to dehydration (with or without thirst).

The remedy is recommended to be given in the lowest potencies first and to rise in potency gradually. The 3x can be repeated over a long period followed by the 6x, 9x and 12x for organ drainage. The 30th to the CM provide a ladder of progression over an extended time. The LM scale provides an alternative to this strategy.

Turmeric is extremely susceptible to being used in triad combination remedies. These may be prescribed in the 6x or 12x potencies. The following are examples:

- **Turmeric + Cholesterinum + Hydrastis**
  A remedy to help the body to drain the cancer miasm from a toxic liver in someone with a strongly acidic constitution.
- **Turmeric + Yellow + Lumbricus**
  A remedy to drain the liver and restore the biochemical integrity of the connection with the intestines which have been subject to years of bad diet; the bowel may well be full of compacted faeces. This is a remedy to consider in one who needs enemas or bowel flushes.
- **Turmeric + Candida + Hydrastis**
  A remedy to consider in one who is susceptible or already has candida of the bowel. There is sluggishness, poor nutrition, tiredness, depression, constipation (or the opposite) and acidity.
- **Turmeric + Hydrastis + Arsen-alb (or Carbo-veg)**
  A useful remedy in cases of stomach ulcer and hyperacidity.
- **Turmeric + Cardamom + Golden Beryl**
  A remedy to act on the interaction between the organs of the solar plexus, the kidneys, spleen and points of elimination: anus and bladder. It is a balancing remedy for the spleen and liver and is particularly indicated in those whose motivation is very low.
- **Turmeric + Syphilinum + Ayahuasca** 10M
  This remedy is particularly useful in those who have Scorpio strongly represented in their chart as it calms the fears and the tendency to use attack as a means of security. It is calming of the fears of the moment which cause the patient to be so on guard; this calming allows the patient to measure things less critically and more in terms of their history and circumstances.

Esoteric therapeutics

Turmeric is a remedy that cleanses and protects the aura of each chakra. It is chiefly centred on the solar plexus though it is also one of the most important remedies for the strengthening and enlivening of the hara, the centre of energy in the core of the lower abdomen. It is linked with the lower dan tien that is the qi centre associated with the base chakra. Through the calming and recovery of this centre the patient is closer to being able to rise through the other chakras towards higher attainments of soul purpose. The remedy integrates the root of each chakra with the spinal column. It illuminates the purpose of karmic responsibilities and the role of ancestral energy. These are higher aspects of the base centre where the influence of Saturnian energy is most at play. By accepting the role of Saturn (the teacher through experience and through coping with all that is choiceless), the patient is offered greater freedom to broaden horizons and explore further potential. It enhances the connection between the base and the brow; seeing through the third eye becomes greatly facilitated with the result that the patient becomes more open-minded and more prepared to invest time and energy in new experiences.

Chakras

Crown

Depressive thoughts, with feelings of not being at one with anything, affect the connection with the brow and heart centres. Sleep is unsatisfying; dreams are fugitive and busy but with little achieved in them. The spirit feels laden with worldly matters. There is little inner peace to the point where the patient may simply want to shut down or, at least, shut off.

Brow

It is as if the electrical circuits of the brain have been fused; the mind is facing burnout. All this comes after a history of trying hard to achieve; ambition has come with a high price. It may be that the patient has struggled long and hard but without any real idea of what he or she might want to do; there is here the depressing state of having wasted time with the 'If only I had . . .' thoughts. No real clarity of third-eye vision; confusion and muddling through. Sometimes **Turmeric** is indicated by one who has never found what it is that they want to do because of the use of hallucinogens or, alternatively, by one who has thought that they knew what they wanted to do but has sought to enhance their performance with cocaine, a substance that has masked the true path of creative activity.

Throat

Easily choked up with emotions. Has little aptitude for expressing emotions though these underlie all issues of failure and depressiveness.

Heart

Disappointment after a long and fruitless tussle. A feeling of emptiness may pervade this centre that is a reflection of how bleak the future seems. There is also fear here: of being too involved with difficult emotions.

Solar plexus

The state of the liver may dominate the patient's physical health issues. The liver is too negatively active for any peace to be found in this chakra and it impinges on the stomach and spleen. Much of the challenge and conflict that are usually to be found in a liver remedy are mostly worked on in the mind in **Turmeric**.

Sacral

To date there is little evidence of disturbance to this chakra beyond the potential damage wrought by interfering with the natural cycle of hormones by HRT or the Pill.

Base

So much energy has been expended in the mind that the body has been left to fend for itself. The underlying structures of the physical body may not, in a good constitution, show many defects beyond what might occur in the digestive tract but in a weakened constitution there may be a lot of muscular soreness, joint trouble and excessive tiredness. The immune system may labour with frequent acute infections.

Case studies

1 '78-year-old female complaining of daily headaches. Patient quite confused following a mild stroke two years ago. **Turmeric** 6 given daily. One month later the headaches are less severe and there have been several days when she has been free of pain. The **Turmeric** 6 daily is repeated, as before. Three headaches occurred in the last month and the pain is much reduced. Patient is still on the medication.' LS

2 '55-year-old female complaining of IBS type symptoms such as "extreme indigestion and diarrhoea" and often complains of "bilious" symptoms. The patient leads a very stressful life: is a university lecturer, always attending conferences and seminars and is also going through a traumatic divorce. **Turmeric** 6 daily for one month. One month later: all the IBS symptoms have gone. She remains on the Turmeric 6 daily.' LS

3 'A man in his late 60s had begun treatment at the behest of his anxious wife. He wanted to be able to continue working for as long as possible which he feared he might not be able to do for much longer as he was running out of stamina. There was a long history of emotional trauma which he was rather dismissive and matter-of-fact about: his parents and siblings had all been emotionally dysfunctional people. He had been the only one who had made a satisfactory living but he had been married to a woman with bipolar problems who had committed suicide. He had had **Winchelsea Sea Salt** 1M which did little more than encourage him to be a bit more open about many further family difficulties that lay in his past though he showed little overt distress. He appeared rather more sarcastic than upset. He then had **Thuja** 200 followed by **Rose Quartz** 1M which he certainly felt created a greater response; he had found life difficult. After taking the **Thuja** he had woken up in the night and sobbed uncontrollably. When he returned he related how his father had recently died. He was bitter and angry with the doctors whom he blamed for negligence and he was equally resentful about his mother's role in the lack of parenting from his father. She had "poisoned my mind against him". He felt aggressive and depressed. He had felt like committing murder and declared that he had even visualized throttling his wife. He volunteered that he hated being left alone: "It's like being abandoned." He felt that the best part of his life was with the dogs which he took for frequent walks. He had had a lot of "whacky dreams". At one point he stated that he never wanted anyone to own him and at another he confessed to having been a womanizer. The interview showed up the sheer jumble of thoughts that was going on in his head. Running through the whole of this was a thread of dissatisfaction and regret that things had not worked out the way he might have wanted. He knew that he was good at his job but there was an underlying sense that he knew that he was not a front runner. He had **Carcinosin** 1M for the sheer diversity of patterns of negative energy that he held and shortly afterwards **Turmeric** 200: one each week for six weeks. It was after the **Turmeric** that he said that he felt much better: "I have felt much more sunshine – warm, happy, friendly. That carried on for some time." Though he went on to need **Med-am, Black Obsidian, Stramonium** and others, it was after the **Turmeric** that he was able to feel the positivity of the changes he was making. Before it he had been "going through the motions" more or less for his wife's sake.' CG

7

DOLPHIN SONAR[9]

The remedy was proved at the 36th potency by five women and two men plus the medium at the beginning of a week's lecturing on three-dimensional homoeopathy held at Duncton Mill, West Sussex in May 2007.

The Background

The remedy was prepared from 'captured' sonar clicks of a wild, Atlantic spotted dolphin (*Stenella frontalis*) 'in communication' with one of the provers. The prover, Maxine Harrison, had organized a trip to the Bahamas for several people who had wanted to experience swimming with wild dolphins. They reached a particular area in the Caribbean, near the part of the ocean where the Gulf Stream starts its westward sweep and where the sea floor rises up to a very shallow shelf, known as a place for migrating dolphins to congregate and breed. This part of the sea, only some three metres deep, is noted for its white 'sand' (actually not sand but the remains of millions of years of shell fragments), the strong current and its emptiness (comparatively few fish, birds or vegetation) that gives the place a sense of extraordinary and ineffable calm. Having spent most of the time searching for dolphins but without a sighting and noting that the weather was becoming increasingly threatening, the crew felt obliged to turn back to port. However, taking advantage of a break in the lowering storms around them, the party headed back to the most likely area for one last try. On arrival at the spot where the crew had witnessed dolphins on previous occasions, the company were finally rewarded by the appearance of a pod of several females and their male companion. Maxine dived into the water with a bottle

9 **Dolphin Sonar** was originally called **Dolphin Song**.

of ethanol and a clear quartz crystal. Her instructions had been to hold the crystal between a 'speaking' dolphin and the ethanol. She swam towards the pod that were feeding on the sea floor and one of the dolphins, the male, immediately turned, made eye contact and approached her from below at considerable speed and, within about three or four feet from the crystal she held out, started to make all the characteristic squeaks and clicks. At this point Maxine dropped the bottle from her hand. The dolphin continued to 'communicate' for some 20 seconds whereupon it turned and swam back to its companions. Though disappointed not to have been able to bring back the ethanol, she nevertheless put the crystal directly into a bottle of brandy. On her return to England she delivered the crystal and the brandy to the author who immediately put the crystal into a covered bowl of ethanol that was left in the bright sunlight for two days. One drop of this 'tincture' was then added to 99 drops of ethanol to create the first potency. From here it was taken up to the 36th potency by hand. The reason behind the choice of this potency rather than the usual 30th was intuitive but had more than a little to do with the sense that 30 is not, in three dimensions, a perfect number while 36 (12x3) is. Whether this makes any difference to the prescription of the remedy remains to be seen.

It may be of interest that on a further trip to the Bahamas in search of dolphins and when it seemed as if there would be difficulty in finding them, a few doses of the remedy were dropped into the water to 'call' them. Within just a few minutes they appeared and circled the boat.

It is also pertinent to mention the story of one of the people who took part in the first dolphin trip. This was an Austrian woman in her thirties who had been coping with terminal breast and bone cancer. She decided to go on the trip despite considerable weakness. She participated fully and was able to swim with the dolphins. On her return, not only did she appear to be considerably improved in health but she fell in love shortly after, conceived a child and gave birth to a healthy boy. She was able to live long enough to see his second birthday having originally been given just a few months to live.

Dolphins are sea mammals (Cetacea) belonging to the same suborder as toothed whales (Odontocetes). There are 26 species of dolphin including the Atlantic spotted dolphin and the best known, the bottlenose. Some species of dolphin can reach up to six metres or more in length but most are between two and three metres. They inhabit the waters of almost every sea and one species even lives in the fresher waters of large river systems. The Atlantic spotted dolphin lives in the area of the southern Gulf Stream which includes the Gulf of Mexico, up to the Florida coast, across the Atlantic to the African coast and south as far as the coast of southern Brazil.

Dolphins feed on fish and crustaceans such as shrimp, lobster, molluscs and krill. Some are migratory and others have restricted their lifestyle to the shallower waters of coastlines. Those which travel over larger distances, following shoals of their prey, can swim at relatively fast speeds: 24 kph with bursts of acceleration exceeding 32 kph. They achieve this by leaping and diving in and out of the surface water.

Dolphins are social animals and live in groups that are organized by strict hierarchy. Groups, known as pods, can vary substantially in number; anything from 2 or 3 to 30 or more. The major advantages of this are that they can hunt cooperatively and form a defensive team when threatened. Their greatest natural enemy is the shark but fishermen trawling for tuna, and pollution can be even more lethal. The South Atlantic dolphin that inhabits the Bahamas is less prone to these dangers.

Dolphins live, hunt and breed in the water just below the surface. Their eyesight is reckoned to be good though they have evolved a sophisticated echolocation system that allows for even greater efficiency. They produce high-speed, ultrasonic 'clicks' with their nasal passages which are focused and directed by the melon-shaped forehead. The returning 'bounced' sound is 'received' by the specially adapted lower jawbone and transmitted to the inner ear and thence to the brain. They also communicate with each other constantly in a continual stream of clicks and squeaks.

Dolphins live for an average of 20 years and sometimes more. They often bear the scars of shark attack or wounds inflicted by boat propellers. Such marks are used to identify individuals during marine research. Dolphins are subject to similar diseases as man. Respiratory disorders, heart disease, skin diseases, stomach ulcers, urogenital disorders and cancerous tumours have all been recorded. Science puts much of this down to pollution and bacterial invasion though with their enormously rich social life and highly developed brains it might not be far-fetched to consider that dolphins are subject to psychosomatic illness.

Dolphin intelligence is regarded as being almost comparable with our own. This is because there is a considerable amount of folding in the cerebral cortex suggesting that there is ample brain area to be devoted to thinking. Evidence of their prodigious ability to learn is displayed both by captive dolphins which learn to perform complicated 'tricks' for dubious entertainment, and by wild dolphins that have shown extraordinary courage and cooperative group thinking in saving the lives of swimmers in danger from sharks.

Dolphins have smooth, glandless skin with a thick layer of blubber beneath. They overcome any problems that might be caused by the inability to sweat by sloughing off their skin very frequently, some species doing so every few hours or so.

Dolphin calves are born live, tail first, with eyes wide open and aware of their surroundings through smell, sight, sound and touch. A mother aids her calf to the surface for its first breath. Milk is the calf's only sustenance for the first 12 to 18 months and the mother will actively care for her offspring for up to seven or eight years. Most dolphins produce one calf every two years. Calves are born either between February and May or September and November. Males become sexually active by about ten years but females are mature by five or six. Scientists have noted that there may be no regular, cyclical ovulation. Dolphins are not monogamous. Indeed, groups of males may herd females in order to ensure a greater chance of copulation. Scientists have also observed evidence of aggressive behaviour towards reluctant females that has even been described as 'gang rape' or kidnapping.[10] Marine biologists regard the apparently promiscuous social activity, which includes homosexuality, as equivalent to grooming among primates or gossip among people.

My own observation of dolphin behaviour would suggest that dolphins' reputation for curiosity and playfulness is not exaggerated. The dolphins we followed off Bimini not only hugely enjoyed running with the boat's wake but seemed to invite us to throw them seaweed which they flipped from dorsal fin to tail and back. They also appeared to play hide-and-seek: one moment they would be swimming alongside us and then they would disappear suddenly only to resurface after a few minutes of our searching for them. They also seemed to break off from their swimming among us by diving down to the bottom, keeping heads down close together as if in confabulation only to dart back up to leap out of the water in front of one or other of us. On several occasions they remained with us for two hours before getting bored and leaving. We had ample opportunity to notice how their moods changed; one day some of them would be 'laid back', even torpid and on another they would be skittish and unpredictable, though at no time did we have any cause for concern about their attitude to us. However, though the unwritten rule is that humans do not touch dolphins, it was sometimes difficult to avoid them touching us. Their habit of

10 www.scienceray.com/biology

eyeing people directly, side on, can be quite disconcerting. One has a strong sense of being shrewdly summed up by a sharp intelligence – only for the impression to be superseded by delight in some antic or gesture.

Keynote effects

The energy of this remedy represents the 'still point', that point in the fluid energy of the body where the flow between in-breath and out-breath changes; where the tide of the body turns. This still point occurs within the spinal column though it informs the whole being. It is the point of complete balance and harmony where stillness is absolute for the brief moment that it is held. The word that describes this state most closely is 'nothingness' and the remedy is most useful for fostering a condition of total surrender; surrender to the inevitable and the relinquishing of the fears that accompany our journey into the unknown whatever the situation.

General symptoms

The greatest number of symptoms was manifest in the head and the central nervous system. A feeling of having been drugged was evident. There was even, in one prover, a sensation of having died. Pain or discomfort was experienced along with sensations of expansion and inflation; parts of the body or the whole felt as if blown up like a balloon. Tingling and prickling and even stabbing pains were also felt in various parts of the body. Heat in the head was concomitant with freezing feet. There was also a sensation as if a vibration was sent through the body. Use of the remedy has demonstrated its value in treating the terminally ill: it brings peace and stillness to those who are on morphine to quell pain but which slows down and hampers the dying process. Anecdotal evidence shows that patients who have lingered on when they might have been expected to pass over but are lying, so to speak, in limbo are able to go with peace as this is one of the very few remedies that is able to 'cut through' chemical medication. Seasickness with nausea and vertigo, heaviness of limbs and enervation were also noted.

In the first case study below, the remedy was used to treat a boy suffering from Asperger's and ADHD. It is more than possible that this case, though far from 'cured' by **Dolphin Sonar**, illustrates another and different aspect of the remedy. South Atlantic dolphins are friendly, entertaining, mischievous, playful, communicative and inquisitive. They travel in family groups and appear to be quite discriminating about who they show interest in. They are also creatures of habit. When contact with people and a boat is made, it appears that one or two of them act as scouts before the whole pod becomes involved. One of the features of their behaviour with people is that they do a lot of circling, wheeling, diving and disappearing only to reappear suddenly out of the blue. Much of the time their behaviour is active and restless but there are also moments when they can become languid and as if content to float alongside while there is no apparent trigger for the switch in mood. Experience, as illustrated by the case study, will tell us if any of this has a bearing on the nature of the remedy.

Miasms

Psora, cancer, tuberculosis and leprosy.

Mental and emotional symptoms

A strong desire for peace and stillness; also light, especially sunlight. Feels alien and as if on a different plane. Does not want to be here; disappointment that one is here at all. Finds life disagreeable; too confusing to cope with it. Feels out of focus and adrift though without a sense that this is a negative thing. Momentarily feels a sense of fragile energy that would best be fostered by peace and quiet; as if this energy has a spiritual connection with a desire to be quiet and still. Has nothing to say; feels blank and disconnected though not distressed by this; on the contrary, wants to persist in this state. Thoughts are fleeting and fugitive. Feeling as if one had died but had not got to the light and the spirit world yet. A sense of being in transition. A sense as if it is only the head and what usually goes on in it that prevents complete serenity; has had enough thinking and wants to switch it off. A feeling as if the throat is blocked and unable to utter any sentiments or thoughts. 'I was aware that time had stopped,' yet there was also a keen sense of anticipation, excitement almost. Sadness but without knowing why or from where. Homesickness but without any desire to go home. A feeling of being neither here nor there.

Physical symptoms

Head and neck

Tight band across the forehead. Throbbing and pulsating in the forehead. Feels as if the brain is expanding inside the cranium, as if the brain were blowing up like a balloon. Felt as if 'my head is going to be blown apart, centred in my brow'. Pain in the occiput: stiffness of the neck with a hard ache in the nape and occiput as if there were a weight there and a need to move. A feeling that one wants to 'click' a bone in the neck to free up movement. Discomfort in the cervical spine as if it is heavy. A sensation as if someone had struck the back of the head with a heavy blow. Pain across the top of the head. Feels as if something wants to explode out of the top of the head. Pressure on the back of the neck which is irritating and needs to be shaken off. 'If only I could get rid of this thing on the back of my neck.' Head feels full though this symptom was not reported to be unpleasant having something like anticipation associated with it. Hydrocephalus. Consider in torticollis where other remedies fail.

Throat

Sensation of blockage that prevents expression. Sensation of the larynx being inflated. 'It feels as if someone is trying to stop me speaking. Not strangling me. As if (there's a) huge restriction in my throat.' Tingling in the throat around the voice box. A sense of there being something to say that can nevertheless not be expressed in words. Tickling in the throat leading to cough that aggravates the pain in the back of the head and neck.

Heart

A sensation as of a tight band around the heart.

Abdomen

Aching in the spleen.

Back

Stiffness, pain and vibrations felt in the spinal column. A remedy for healing the spine where others fail despite indications. Scoliosis, lordosis and kyphosis.

Hips and pelvis

Pain in the buttocks.

Extremities

Sharp pains in the wrists; pricking pain in the bones. Wrists and legs feel as if they want to float. Very cold legs and feet with hot hands. Sweating hands. Lower legs feel tingling. Tingling all over coming from the legs.

Considerations for the use of the remedy

The words of the medium best describe the sense that all the provers had from taking this remedy: 'There is no intellectual understanding of this remedy. All is still and quiet and yet much happens. There is great benevolence of spirit: forgiveness, humility and there is calm and union with all beings on all levels. (The remedy) refines the spirit which is wounded, the mind that is tortured, the heart which is broken, the planet that is tired and forsaken.' The blankness that everyone experienced is perhaps best described as the sensation of blackness that comes with a general anaesthetic.

A comparison with **Opium** is worth making. Both remedies have blankness, forgetfulness, a sense of being far away and feelings of heat. However, **Dolphin Sonar**'s blankness is one of emptiness while **Opium**'s is one of forgetfulness. There is a desire to forget in **Opium** which is not present in the other; **Dolphin Sonar** has a desire to remember how to achieve equilibrium, peace and stillness in order to arrive at a setting-off point. **Opium** wants to blot out what has been shocking and devastating; **Dolphin Sonar** wants to lift the oppression of whatever is preventing the spirit's progression. **Dolphin Sonar**, like the remedy **Opium** itself, is an antidote to morphine and opium poisoning. It is also able to get through chemotherapy to provoke movement in a patient's vital force even in terminal situations. If **Dolphin Sonar** has proved useful in such extreme states then it is highly likely that it will also be of value at the opposite end of life: the birth experience. It also appears to have an increasingly important influence on children suffering from symptoms that occur anywhere on the autistic spectrum. Here it has been likened to the maverick energy of dolphins with their habit of sudden playfulness or spurts of unpredictable energy; their hypersensitive states of awareness; their provocative and sometimes overtly sexual precocity.

Esoteric therapeutics

The nothingness of this remedy encourages stillness of mind and a silencing of the mental chatter that disturbs the harmony of the brow centre and keeps us all going at a rate too fast for essential healing. It is a remedy for the refinement of consciousness; for the bringing to bear on our awareness of ether, the infinity of space within which all things have fluid movement and encounter moments of surrender; it is a place of no emotion but of deep feeling.

Chakras

Crown
The remedy brings forward the connection of spirit to the brow and heart centres in those who are seeking spiritual transformation that is temporarily blocked by chemotherapy, shock or ceaseless mind clutter.

Brow
The brow is confused, cluttered and in need of calm. It fosters the acceptance by the intellectual mind of complete surrender to the imperative force of Nature in her demand that we keep moving toward a more refined and spiritual goal. It is indicated often in those who have spent a life of emotional turmoil that has led to stagnation on all levels of the being with the consequence of terminal pathology that is painful and that invites suppression. The prospect of such an end mirrors the strong refusal of the patient to seek emotional resolution before physical pathology has caught up with them.

Throat
A sense of strain and constraint occupy this centre; it appears in those who have much to express but now have no means of doing so that is meaningful.

Heart
A burdened heart with much left unresolved but which is nevertheless accepting of what must come.

Base
The remedy is one for the release from the Saturnian constraints of this centre. Even for those who are not in a terminal state of decline, it is a remedy that encourages the calm acceptance of what must be when there has been fear and trepidation.

Peculiarly, this remedy has so much concentrated in the crown, brow, heart and base chakras, and yet we received nothing for the solar plexus or the sacral chakras.

Case studies

1 Sue Baker, a homoeopath who is accustomed to working closely with a cranial osteopath, sent in the following report in reply to a request for anecdotal evidence.

'Lesley and I treated a little boy of nine years who was diagnosed at four years with Asperger's and ADHD. His mother suspected vaccination damage. She said he changed overnight after the MMR vaccination. He was a very sensitive boy with feminine tendencies and liked girls much better because they were more gentle than the boys. He had two younger brothers and he could be quite aggressive to them. I saw him first but felt that a joint treatment would have a deeper impact. He was always all over the room with Lesley trying to catch up with him and me trying to put remedies on him! He had an obsession with mermaids and the cartoon character, SpongeBob SquarePants, which all live under the sea. So one day we were in desperation and tried **Dolphin Sonar** and he just lay still for 20 minutes quietly. Unheard of! Mother was shocked. He was after that much more open, peaceful; had better communication and was not so restless in class. He was most pleased to have had **Dolphin Sonar** and asked for it on subsequent visits (as well as anything pink which was another obsession). Mother was desperate to keep him in mainstream school and after this he was definitely in with more of a chance.'

In a subsequent email Sue added that 'he did make lots of squeaking noises too'.

2 'Girl, Emma, aged nine, foster-child adopted by a family with four children, two of whom, the boys, were on the autistic spectrum. Parents were very clued-up about children with autistic spectrum difficulties having spent time learning skills and strategies for coping and parenting. All the children were home-educated. Emma had a history of a traumatic birth and fostering prior to her present placement. She remained convinced that something bad would happen to her: for example, she slept on the edge of her bed, ready to escape in the event of fire. She suffered from appallingly low self-esteem coupled with rage that could be violent and focused on "you can't make me!" She had had **Lac Humanum, Thuja, Medorrhinum** and **Mag-mur** which settled her

beyond recognition but left her caught between daring to trust and default of rejecting everyone especially her adoptive parents. Apart from the difficult behaviour patterns she suffered from irritable bowel syndrome with acute pains and diarrhoea. She was given **Dolphin Sonar** 200, 1M and 10M: each one given night and morning on consecutive days.

'The mother emailed with the following update: "We've had an interesting time with Emma since the **Dolphin** remedy . . . seemed like it had really shifted something. She became so much more grounded, calmer, more connected, more flexible . . . even her reading and calculating seemed to suddenly take off somewhat. There was a surety about her that we hadn't witnessed before. It felt like she was finally accepting the here and now and wanting to be part of it. However, since yesterday she's been kind of losing ground again. She's not been sleeping very well and her IBS has kicked in a bit again. Then something strange happened last night, we think: I got up this morning to find a box of chocolates I'd brought home, opened and half the chocs eaten! I 'confronted' Emma this morning (about what might have happened) but she seemed to have no idea what I was trying to get at . . . I can normally work out when she's covering up stuff. Anyhow, she has spent the whole day unanchored; she looked and behaved like she was completely lost, disconnected, like she didn't really have any certainty in anything, kind of living in the past and going on about loads of past stuff which she hasn't done for months. [She's] not angry, just disgruntled and insecure, muddled and confused."

'I wondered if this were a case of a return of old symptoms or if the remedy had been interrupted by the chocolate incident. Considered using **Dolphin Sonar** 50M but opted to wait and see whether any further developments would occur.' CB

3   This email was sent to me by a colleague who had been present during a lecture in which **Dolphin Sonar** had been referred to in passing:

'I am writing to let you know about an experience I have had with the remedy **Dolphin Song**. I attended a lecture you did on cancer . . . and **Dolphin Song** (**Sonar**) was mentioned as a remedy able to cut through morphine.

'I remembered this recently when my mother-in-law was diagnosed with terminal cancer. She was in hospital for several weeks and then moved to a hospice after refusing further palliative surgery. Various remedies and flower essences helped her with her dying process, particularly letting go of material things and people, but her physical suffering was great and she was on very high doses of morphine-based drugs. She seemed ready to die and complained daily that it was taking so long.

'I am also a hands-on healer and I spent many hours with her over the weeks leading to her death. The more the morphine increased, the harder it became for the healing energy to penetrate this heaviness that I perceived to be like a "fog". When I realized I too was being affected by this heaviness despite the remedies that were helping me in other ways, I remembered the remedy **Dolphin Song** from your lecture and which I had ordered when she was diagnosed.

'I took some (10M) to the hospice. As she was sleeping when I arrived I sat by her bed and decided to take the remedy myself and felt an immediate shift in my own energy. When she awoke my heart sank a little when I realized she was so weak that her gag reflex had failed and she could no longer drink. I put the remedy into the water I was using to wet her lips and mouth with a little sponge and gave it to her that way. I also put the dissolved remedy onto the pulse points on her wrists. She fell asleep shortly after that and I left her for the day. When I got home I suddenly realized that I was playing with my five-year-old daughter in the most childish, silly, joyful way imaginable – something I had not done much of at all in the preceding weeks.

'My husband visited his mother shortly after I had left and found her sleeping peacefully. Not long after he got home (just five hours after the **Dolphin Song**) we received a call from the hospice to say her breathing had suddenly changed. By the time we got there 20 minutes later, she had already died, much to the surprise of the nurses, slipping peacefully away without waking up since I had left her.

'As with so much in homoeopathy, this is of course anecdotal but I believe that the **Dolphin Song** helped her escaped the "morphine fog" and hastened her transition, confirming the indications for the remedy. I also had a strong sense that her transition was successful and that no soul retrieval work would be necessary.' **CAB**

4 'N. (age 40) was born in France to an alcoholic father and a suicidally depressed mother who told her she was unwanted. Her mother threatened to blow up the house with them all in it. She was sexually abused at the age of three by a family member; her mother later refused to believe her. She was school phobic and suffered from fits induced by anxiety. These were so severe that on one occasion the whole right side of her body became black (like an enormous bruise) with no feeling and no response at all. She spent five days in hospital and was put on anti-depressants for three years. She was in a car crash at 18 when her skull was cracked and her nose was broken. She was "not with it" for three months. (She couldn't remember whether or not she lost consciousness.)

'She left home for England as soon as she could and married a man who bullied her. She was homesick for several years. She had four miscarriages followed by a son, followed by male triplets born after IVF treatment. With no support from anyone she barely coped; the triplets were quite out of control and she screamed at them all the time. She was constantly hysterical: loud and very angry. This was made worse by one disaster happening after another. She was stroppy, belligerent and indignant – even her laugh was like the cackle of a witch. Her elder son started truanting at 11 and as the years went on he caused more and more trouble.

'Her husband finally left her for her best friend after a long-term affair. Her elder son discovered them having sex with all their "toys" and started drinking, stealing, being violent at home and getting into trouble with the police. Despite the fact that N. found a boyfriend who adores her and started dancing with a passion, her tension, stress and shrieking grew worse because for the previous four years there had been weekly disasters with her son, worries about money, having to find a job teaching that added more stress. Homoeopathy has, for years, just made improvements in her physical symptoms and kept her relatively sane.

'She had **Dolphin Sonar** 6x twice daily for a month (although I doubt she took it very often) and she seemed calmer, quieter: 7/10, instead of the 10/10 before. A further month on **Dolphin** and she marked it 5/10 and said she felt as she had before the car crash: more mellow, grounded and as if a weight had been lifted from her shoulders. Although she was obviously very anxious as a child and teenager, she often said that she had felt "different" ever since the accident; there was a change in her personality. Not only had it been immediately noticeable to herself on her return home but the rest of her family and friends had remarked on it.

'Following the Dolphin Sonar she also had the return of old symptoms.

- Her tongue began pulsating or vibrating; this used to be the precursor to the fits.
- Her BP was dramatically low (it had been very low as a child) and she felt very light-headed. She had only one episode of this.
- She was also absolutely exhausted which continued for about six weeks.

'The case continues but it was **Dolphin Sonar** that took her back to the self she was before the accident.' **WW**

8

ELETARRIA CARDAMOMUM

Cardamom

Cardamom was proved by the meditation group on 4 April 2008. The medium and ten provers were present: seven women and four men. The remedy was made only from organic, dried, whole cardamom pods. No other part of the plant was included in the remedy. The original tincture was made from pods steeped in ethanol in a bottle that was left in sunlight for a month. One drop of this 'mother' tincture then provided the initial step to potentization. What is unique about the remedy is that at the 9th, 19th and 29th potencies one drop of the mother tincture was added to the potentized remedy before taking it further up the scale. Though a normal run of the first 30 potencies was also made, it was this 'reinforced' remedy that was used in the proving. In ordering the remedy from the pharmacy it is necessary to specify which is required. (See 'Esoteric therapeutics' below for further information on this aspect.) It should be noted that the mother tincture and, to a lesser extent, the 1c potency both were obviously scented with the characteristic sweetish aroma of the spice. This was also true of the 9th, 19th and 29th potencies that were 'reinforced' in the way described.

The Background

Eletarria cardamomum belongs to the Zingiberaceae (ginger) family. It needs to be distinguished from the brown and black varieties that are larger and closely related and which have also been used in similar ways in cooking and healing. The plant grows from a large and fleshy rhizome. It has long, lanceolate leaves with blades of 45 to 60 centimetres in length; the whole plant of up to 20 shoots can appear from 2 to 6 metres high. The leaves are dark green on top and paler green and glaucous (hairy) beneath. The flowering stems spread horizontally near the ground and produce racemes of small white flowers with a yellowish or pale green tinge with one white petal that is violet lipped. The fruit is a pod of three chambers with two rows of dark brown aromatic seeds. The pods are gathered and stored in this state until they are to be used as the taste and aroma are diminished once the seeds are powdered.

The chemical constituents of the seeds include volatile oil, fixed oil, potassium, starch, nitrogenous mucilage, fibre and resin. The volatile oil is made up of terpenes, terpineol and cineole, and is readily soluble in alcohol. The high value of the spice and the comparatively small amount of volatile oil it produces has left cardamom with a history of usually having been adulterated before it reached the open market. It was often mixed with cinnamon, cloves and caraway as well as being substituted by other species of plant.

Cardamom originates from the Western Ghats of southern India. It grows abundantly in forests several thousand feet above sea level. It is now widely grown commercially in India, Sri Lanka and South-East Asia. It has always been viewed as a valuable commodity and is one of the most expensive spices in the world, perhaps second only to saffron. It has also always been viewed as having medicinal properties; Ayurvedic medicine ensures its place in the medicine cabinet to the present day. Traditionally it has been used as a stimulant and a carminative. It is useful in flatulence, colic and other forms of indigestion; halitosis and infections of the teeth and gums; congestion of the lungs, bronchitis, asthma and pulmonary tuberculosis; urinary infections; inflammation of the eyelids (blepharitis). It is also a preventative for throat infections. It carried a reputation of being an antidote to snake and scorpion venom. Cardamom mixed with honey has been valued as a means of improving eyesight. Furthermore, cardamom is regarded as a detoxifying agent in those who take too much caffeine. Cardamom is sometimes added to coffee in Turkey and Arabia not least as it is said that it eliminates the harmful effects of caffeine.

Methods of prescribing cardamom are various. Mostly it is given as a tincture or as an infusion. It might also be mixed with other ingredients such as neem and camphor (a preparation for congested nasal sinuses). It has been used as a gargle to prevent sore throats and as an ingredient of cough sweets. It is a flavouring agent in pharmaceuticals and the pods have been added to tea to ease stress and depression.

Keynote effects

The main keynote word for **Cardamom** is 'balance'. It creates balance in the hormone, nervous and water systems when these have become unsettled by stress, emotion, trauma or accident. This is particularly so when there has been a period of overheating and inflammation of the system or a part of it from such events; when there has been too much fire at the expense of water. It balances the interaction of the vital organs: liver and kidneys, gall bladder and intestines, stomach and pancreas, spleen and heart. It is most likely to be of service in one who has arrived feeling spent and is left with little energy, little motivation and a sense of disconnection from everyday life. It is a remedy that offers protection through integration of the functions of these vital organs.

General symptoms

The organs of the solar plexus are particularly affected: poor digestion and poor elimination lead to toxicity, particularly toxicity as a result of loss of vital energy and lowered morale. The digestive system is likely to have suffered from dietary abuse; the whole system may well have suffered from addictive abuse of smoking and alcohol. Tends to be warm especially after food. Assists in rebalancing the pH levels in the body. Acid indigestion (see **Sodium bicarbonate**). The large intestine may well be lined with a build-up of plaque. Mental activity is dulled or compromised by the level of toxicity. Kidney and gall stones. Sepsis: abscesses and boils; is of service when other indications are present. Neuralgia particularly of the teeth, face and head. The teeth affected may well be connected by way of the meridians with the organs of digestion. Hormonal imbalances especially in those who have been given other remedies for this (such as **Sepia**) that have failed (see **Rainbow**). For conditions of the lungs: congestion, acute infections; may prove to be of value in tubercular conditions. Throat infections especially when **Mercury** has been indicated and failed (see 'Considerations' below). The remedy has aphrodisiac effects (see 'Mental and emotional symptoms' below) especially in those whose organs of the sacral centre are compromised or weakened by an existing pathology such as diabetes.

Any pains are likely to be sharp and neuralgic. Pains shift and shoot about the body; they are brief and fleeting. **Cardamom** is a remedy with a marked one-sidedness to the symptom picture; there is no bias to either left or right but one side is out of balance with the other and the patient is usually not aware of the anomaly. It has been suggested for the relief of radiation toxicity. This is also a remedy for the history of trauma to the bones; the memory of traumatic accidents to the physical body is held in the tissues of the bones and flesh even if the patient is unmindful of the actual events. Poor healing and discoloration of the skin from old wounds or lesions.

Miasms

Psora, cancer, syphilis, radiation and tuberculosis.

Mental and emotional symptoms

A feeling of disconnection as a result of combined enervation, stress and lack of care of oneself. Where there has been turmoil, **Cardamom** can bring peace of mind and the ability to view things calmly and dispassionately especially in one who puts on a brave face or who presents a tough exterior that belies the tension beneath. Underlying trauma that carries emotions such as grief and anger will form part of the indicating picture. Poor memory; the patient complains of this a lot but indicated remedies will have done little to improve the problem. Senility: early stages of failing mental powers. **Cardamom** is a chronic remedy of **Staphysagria**; see **White Chestnut Flower** which shares this distinction but mostly to do with the abuse of the sacral centre. The remedy allows such traumas to be expressed in time without any damaging outbursts of anger; there is the release of tension quietly and without bitterness. Irritability such as with all toxicity cases: frustration, disappointment and loss of confidence, typical of gall bladder and liver pathology. The impatience and irritability are most likely to be seen when the protective barrier of stoicism is undermined or breached in some way, usually by tiredness. There is a lack of courage and a loss of vision about what is needed or wanted. Poor motivation after grinding away for a long time without recognition or while being harassed by the expectations of others. There is a strong desire for recognition from both peers and colleagues but also an inner recognition of what and who one is; a need to feel reminded why one is on the path that has been chosen. Tends to work automatically, without any enthusiasm; feels scattered and out of sorts.

Loss of confidence which may be general or specific to sex; lack of libido and impotence. Hyperactivity: patient tends to rush around frenetically without much effectiveness; hyperactive behaviour with inefficient but reactive digestive system. Hyperactive children who rush about and eat either fast food or food likely to speed up the adrenals. Such children may appear to be fretful or fearful. Longing for peace and quiet which it never seems possible to achieve. Makes choices that lead on to further activity and turmoil before realizing that there has, once again, been no thought of self-preservation. Very serious mood; seldom thinks of doing anything that is for sheer enjoyment; has to be persuaded to relax and do something different.

Physical symptoms

Head
Headaches especially when < with menstrual cycle. Sharp pain in the right frontal lobe.

Eyes
Conjunctivitis. Blepharitis. Soreness of the eyes. Vision seems to be deteriorating. Wounds to the eye.

Face
Trigeminal neuralgia.

Mouth
Sharp, neuralgic pains in the jaw and teeth. Toothache especially in teeth connected to the organs of digestion through the meridians (chiefly the molars). Pain in the upper jaw shoots up into the cheek. Sepsis in the mouth: abscesses especially with sharp, neuralgic pains.

Throat
Sore throat and swollen glands; painful or difficult to swallow. To be considered when **Merc-sol** fails or to complement it in difficult cases.

Heart, chest and lungs
Shooting pain in the heart (left side) followed by a shooting pain in left temple. Asthmatic breathing. Congestion in the lungs which may shift sides.

Digestive system

Gall bladder: discomfort in the region of the left side of the liver. Diverticulosis. Irritable bowel syndrome. Acid indigestion. Diabetes: Type 2. Tension held in the thoracic diaphragm.

Male

Low libido; remedy may act as an aphrodisiac especially in those who have diabetic problems.

Back

Shooting pain in the right kidney area.

Limbs

Sharp pain in the right axilla, shooting down the underside of the right arm into the elbow. Numbness in the right hand from the fingers to the wrist; sensation as if the hand were wearing a glove. Nerves of the hand tingle.

Skin

Eczema: lower extremities; behind the knees. Wants to scratch till it bleeds.

Considerations for the use of the remedy

Cardamom is a warm-blooded remedy but this should not prevent its use in those who are chilly especially in elderly patients or children. If the patient is a chilly person then there is likely to be a slight but necessary aggravation of the symptom under consideration once the remedy has been administered; if the patient is warm-blooded there may be no aggravation apparent.

It is most useful in one who has had too much of the fire element in the system which has left them 'burnt out' or having suffered from too much heat especially in the heart centre or the upper digestive tract. It can be used to calm an overwrought nervous system after anger or fear; to ease the nervous system after a period of intensity; to settle a digestive tract after a bout of inflammation; to 'cool' a nervous system after any sort of feverishness.

When the homoeopathic indications are there, **Cardamom** can be used:

- as a constitutional remedy in high potency
- as a support remedy in those whose energy is undermined by a physical condition such as an irritable bowel or a compromised heart

- in low 'x' potency as a drainage remedy when an organ or a system is compromised as in liver toxicity or diabetes
- as a rebalancing remedy in one who symptomatically indicates lack of equilibrium in the endocrine system
- as a support remedy in a patient who has been given **Merc-sol**; it enhances the action of this other remedy and does nothing to undermine its action.

It is useful to compare **Cardamom** with other remedies:

- **Baryta-carb** has the same degree of dullness, memory loss and lack of morale but it is usually more shy and retreating than **Cardamom** which seeks recognition even if there is no obvious outward sign of that. **Baryta-carb** is also usually chilly and not so marked for toxicity. Both, however, have a desire to reclaim lost ability and have a similar frustration over loss of brain power. **Baryta-carb** is a much slower energy than **Cardamom**.
- **Blue** is also for those with an underlying pattern of exhaustion and depletion. It is chiefly concerned with the organs of the sacral and throat centres while **Cardamom** is more associated with the vital organs and their interaction. There is more likelihood that the patient needing **Blue** is chilly and any period of intensity endured would have been some time in the past. The energy of **Blue** is slower than **Cardamom**.
- **Sulphur** can appear to be very similar in its general state of exhaustion and torpor but is differentiated by its usual symptoms of modality. **Cardamom** has few fixed modalities of time and reaction; it is too changeable for such patterns to become established. **Cardamom** is almost as good a grounding remedy as **Sulphur** though it should not be forgotten that one is vegetable and the other mineral; it is the latter that would establish a longer-lasting and more permanent state of constitutional and psoric groundedness. If **Sulphur** is the remedy of choice to be given after an acute disease to restore full vitality, **Cardamom** is the remedy of choice after an accident, operation or romantic relationship once the indicated remedies have been given for the trauma.
- **White Chestnut Flower** is also known as a chronic of **Staphysagria**. Both **Cardamom** and WCF are indicated by abuse of the sexual organs

either through a traumatic relationship or surgery. Differentiation has to be made by looking at the rest of the picture. **WCF** is more likely to be needed when the patient suffers terribly from damaged innocence while **Cardamom** is more likely to be indicated when there is world-weariness and a buried sense of anger. They are complementary and follow each other well.

Esoteric therapeutics

The keynote of this remedy is balance. It fosters balance throughout all the chakras and on all levels of the auric field. The balance here is not about the equality of left and right, top and bottom (**Sycamore Seed**) but about the balance between vital organs and endocrine glands that must be in harmony to maintain biochemical integrity and full functioning of the autonomic nervous system. It is a remedy for the release from grief that is held deep in the auric field of the vital organs, and that has upset the natural balance between them; for grief held there chronically from the patient's past or even from ancestral habit, and often unacknowledged or unregistered by patient or practitioner. It is a protective remedy for these same organs on an esoteric level; it is particularly noted for its protective influence on the digestive tract. For all those who have problems stemming from difficulties with the stomach meridian (that is those who have trouble with nurturing themselves or who are repelled by what they perceive the world has to offer them) **Cardamom** may afford relief.

Chakras

Crown

This is a remedy that is most valuable for children when prescribed on this centre. It helps to clear the malignant energies of modern technology and those influences that would disrupt the true nature of their karmic journey: ultrasound scans, microwave radiation and the like, as well as vaccination and medical drug intervention, all of which can disturb the subtle connections in this chakra between the physical incarnation and the soul purpose. Helps to foster a quieter, more restful sleep pattern.

Brow

Balance can be restored in this chakra between the left and right sides of the brain after a period of intensity either of fever or feverish activity; eases a restless or feverish mind. It is also helpful in those who have lost sight of their intuitive gifts after a long period of intellectual study or of being subjected to the strong influence of a rationalist education; for those whose minds are skewed to favour a too materialistic view of life. It is a remedy that helps the practice of meditation by calming the mind. It is also for those patients who are not 'mindful' of the disturbance to vital organs (especially the heart and those of the digestive tract); the remedy is a 'reminder' of the need to take care of oneself and not to allow self-neglect to be part of a maintaining cause.

Throat
Encourages the patient to be a listener rather than a talker. Difficulties expressing hope.

Heart
Encourages the patient to be a receiver and not just a giver. The remedy warms and protects the heart centre and softens any hardness that has developed as a result of trauma. Thus it is a heart protection remedy. What is initiated in the heart is then passed on to other vital organs; the heart-warming effects radiate out to the organs of digestion, the kidneys and the lungs. It is also a remedy for re-establishing the vital connection between the head and the heart so that whatever is undertaken is informed with wisdom.

Solar plexus
Soothes the stomach that is used to having to put up with the ingestion of inappropriate food and drink. This is one of the remedies to create a better acid/alkali balance (see **Sodium Bicarbonate**). It is likely to be useful in one who has had a disordered digestion for years and as a result has built up a lot of plaque on the bowel walls that contributes to toxicity in the liver and disturbance of spleen energy. Congestion in this chakra can lead to brain fog and depressive tendencies with irritability. Continued use of the remedy can help the patient to dissolve gall stones that in turn releases more energy for taking creative decisions.

Sacral
Helps to prevent the gathering of gravel in the kidneys and bladder. Balances the water system in one whose heart chakra is out of balance. Calms the system that has become used to being driven by emotional demands.

Base

Relaxes the tension of an overwrought nervous system. Tones down the activity of the adrenal glands in those who are in overdrive. Eliminative processes are set on a path of recovery. Protective of the etheric body in general and in particular of the vital organs.

Case studies

1 'This brief description of reaction was from a patient who had been prescribed **Cardamom** 30, once per week for four weeks after she had explained the difficulties she was experiencing in her marriage. Theirs was a passionate relationship characterized by confrontation and some jealousy. The patient wanted there to be more heart energy between them but felt that her husband was unaware of how to achieve this.

   '"After 1st dose: huge crying session after argument with my husband. Felt a big release. Woke next day with left ear pain (return of old symptoms). Difficult to swallow on left; diarrhoea and cystitis! (Cystitis: return of old symptom.) The next day felt physically better but no motivation. Looking back at this I think the reaction was exaggerated by being premenstrual.

   '"After 2nd dose: very restless sleep, lots of dreams of difficult things. Woke feeling very bruised! Could feel the remedy working on the back of my throat chakra, I haven't ever felt anything working at this depth of this chakra before (sorry! struggling to describe the position of it). Also felt the energy moving freely down to the heart chakra too."' CG

2 'An Anglo-French woman of 48, a Virgo and a counsellor with 12 years' experience, came for constitutional treatment. She is married with two daughters and has long been exasperated by her husband who is unable to do anything right. "I know; he can't win! If he does what I want I despise him and if he doesn't, I'm angry with him." She is very easily overwhelmed by all that she has to do and admits that she lacks the courage to make all the changes she needs to in order to feel better about herself. She feels inferior and lacks confidence. She has slight tendencies

to paranoia. She would love to take part in community activities but she is afraid of the judgement of others. She has a lot of tension in her lower spine and across her shoulders. She spends much of her time rushing around after other people. She has had many remedies from other homoeopaths already; she has had **Nat-mur, Staphysagria** and **Causticum** as well as **Tub-bov** and **Carcinosin**. She was given **Cardamom** 200, a single collective dose. She became extremely angry. "I went into melt down!" For 12 hours she continued to be in an inexplicable rage after which she became very tired. As she came out of the mood she realized that she wanted to give up seeing her clients and devote her energies to the family and to the house "and blow everyone else!" She felt the return of old symptoms and took various remedies for them which had ameliorated them in the past. She also decided that the family needed to go back to France where she had been brought up and where the remaining members of her family still lived. "I need to trust the choice I made years ago about the man I live with."' **JM**

9

EPILOBIUM ANGUSTIFOLIUM

Rosebay Willowherb

The remedy was given a double meditative proving at the Guild of Homoeopaths' Summer School at Duncton Mill in May 2007. There were two groups of provers, A and B. As well as the 12 participating students in each group, the two circles consisted of Janice Micallef, the medium who led the circles, Jill Wright, who introduced the remedy to homoeopathy, and Diane Pitman and Nick Griffith who acted as medium supports. The remedy was taken in the 30th potency on the night before the meditations and at the start of the circles.

The Background

Rosebay willowherb has a second scientific name: *Chamaenerion* (or *Chamerion*) *angustifolium*. It also has several common names including: fireweed, blooming sally and great willowherb. The name *Epilobium* is derived from the Greek *epi* (upon) and *lobos* (a pod). It is called 'willow' herb as the leaves are reminiscent of the Salix family, the willow tree. (Blooming sally is the Irish name where 'sally' is a corruption of 'Salix'.) The plant belongs to the family Onagraceae which makes it a relative of evening primrose. It was introduced into Britain from America in the 18th and 19th centuries as a garden plant. It is a perennial that spreads by seed or by a creeping rhizome which is white and fleshy. It has become naturalized due to the ease of propagation.

The plant is very tough being hardy to approximately minus 20°C. It likes moisture-retaining soil which is well drained. It can thrive in partial shade but is happiest in a sunny patch. Open woodland is where it thrives most. The plant often reaches two metres in height. It is usually found in large clumps especially where there has been a woodland fire or clearing by foresters; it seems to specialize in colonizing ground that has been burnt. So prolific is it that it is now regarded as a weed and viewed by many as a pest plant that needs to be eradicated wholesale in areas of cultivation. This is despite its elegance; it is a tall plant with a spire of pink open florets growing above a smooth stem that features pointed, lanceolate, hairless leaves that are arranged alternately. These leaves turn red and yellow in the autumn before the whole top-growth dies back. The raceme of flowers develops through June to August. Each flower consists of four notched petals from the centre of which droop a group of stamens. The long slender fruit capsule matures to split lengthways into four, revealing seeds that are covered with white feathering that assists in wind propagation.

The flowers are hermaphrodite and are much favoured by bees. The pollen is said to produce excellent honey. The edible parts of the plant include the leaves, flowers, root and stem. Apart from using the leaves as a tea, young shoots and leaves can be used either raw or cooked in salads. Only young leaves should be used; there is a warning from some writers that an infusion of leaves causes stupefaction. The young shoots are claimed to be a substitute for asparagus. The stems are said to be laxative. The root contains tannin, starch, sugar and mucilage. An infusion of the leaves has been used in the treatment of leucorrhoea, menorrhagia and uterine haemorrhage. It is also of topical use in treating ophthalmia, mouth and throat ulcers. A poultice of leaves has been used to heal long-standing skin ulcers and a poultice of the peeled root has been recorded as healing for boils, burns, sores and swellings. Because of its antispasmodic properties it is regarded as a remedy for pertussis, asthmatic cough and hiccough. As an ointment it has been applied in skin conditions of infants. It also has a reputation for the easing of summer diarrhoea as well as some conditions of the prostate gland.

Keynote effects

Rosebay Willowherb is a remedy that is indicated in those who have reached 'a dark place' in their karmic journey. It positively influences the cancer miasm though, like most plant remedies, it is multi-miasmatic. It heals those who suffer 'disconnection' on any level. It encourages those who have closed down and shut off (and who have a tendency to hide in any aspect) to reconnect with their self-healing energy and it galvanizes their motivation to make positive change. It is a remedy to make people feel safer about being in their physical vehicle. It also encourages self-reflection.

General symptoms

This is a very carcinogenic remedy and has a significant impact on the cancer miasm. It should be considered in anyone who has lost connection with their life's path and creative purpose; who suffers disconnection between the body, mind, emotions and spirit; who is in thorough denial about their state; who does not see that serious pathology may be the only option left to the body to focus on the necessity for change; whose chakras are all out of alignment; who lives a life in which there is no protection for the etheric body from malign external influences; who is in a state of continual suppression of the spirit, emotions and physical bodies.

Rosebay Willowherb is useful in the treatment of those who have cancer; it is indicated in those with cancers that are likely to metastasize quickly; it can help to ameliorate the pains that result from metastasis. It can be used as a cancer drainage remedy when given in low potency. It is said to help the body to shift cancerous cells out of the lymph system and into the eliminative channels. It is indicated in those who do not manifest physical symptoms of cancer but who appear to be heavily carcinogenic while hiding any physical manifestation of the disease. (Such people are often in complete denial about their physical and emotional health.) It is a more generalized lymph drainage remedy as well. This is especially true of anyone who has had cancer of, say, the breast and has had a mastectomy. It is to be considered in those who are diagnosed with cancer of the ovaries particularly, or of the other generative organs. This is another remedy that is able to cover the susceptibility to cancer triggered by years of taking the Pill or HRT, the morning-after pill or fertility treatment. (Should be compared with **Tiger's Eye, Senecio + Tyria** and **Folliculinium.**) It should not be forgotten in male patients: prostate and testicular cancer (cf. **Pomegranate**). In men the remedy is indicated when symptoms are right-sided; in women symptoms are likely to be left-sided.

If the practitioner senses something insidious about the pathological energy of the patient then the remedy may prove to be of great service despite the almost exclusively intuitive reasoning for the choice. It might be said of this patient that his or her 'light has gone out'. In this context it is worth considering in those who found it an appalling struggle to be born; there is a history of birth trauma and difficult incarnation, perhaps so difficult that full incarnation was not possible. It is for those whose life force struggles to flow along the meridians. Stasis is a keynote of this remedy; it may occur in any part of the system but is most likely in the lymph, circulation and digestive processes apart from the emotions. It can be of service in those who suffer from food intolerance; it can 'educate' the system to recognize what is harmful and what is not. (This becomes useful in those who refuse to believe that such things as gluten and dairy food may be harming them.)

The remedy also works well to restore integrity to the central nervous system even when it is affected with gross pathology. It is useful in disturbances of brain function. When the patient feels that they cannot function properly in their brain; where there is disconnection. Spasticity and paralysis may both crop up in a patient needing the remedy. It is of use in multiple sclerosis especially in those who seem not to want to get better; it may be indicated in Parkinson's. A lack of balance is likely to be a main feature of the whole case: the imbalance may be in any sphere but will have a lot to do with darkness, heaviness, denial and inertia. Motivation is very poor especially to get better; loss of motivation suggests that the spleen energy is weak. The remedy is also useful in supporting the heart and circulation. It works on valvular heart disease; this pathology requires low potencies given repeatedly over a long period. Where there is arterial or venous stasis, use in lower potencies. (It has a good working relationship with **Lachesis** and can be used to support this remedy.)

The remedy may be regarded as principally left-sided but this can be deceptive especially among men with deep pathology. Pains appear on the left side in the breast, the spleen, the scapula, the neck. There is a tendency to be overheated and this may come on with a sense of claustrophobia. Heat can be localized and manifest as burning pains (especially in the left breast).

Miasms

Cancer, psora, syphilis and tuberculosis.

Mental and emotional symptoms

Rosebay Willowherb is particularly useful in those who face dealing with health issues in an emotionally disconnected state. The patient is in denial and, in particular, is in denial of the emotional body; if they thought that they were suffering from a threatening illness they might well seek advice upon which they would hand over responsibility for their health problems to others. They might well choose suppression over the hard work of real recovery. Feels sad, stuck, confused and in a dark place. 'I have this sense of separation between my higher self and my lower self. I feel fed up. There is this great sense of stasis and stuckness; great feeling of disappointment and cannot be bothered; I feel very detached from the emotions as if I am observing them and not really feeling them.' The sense of separation, unlike **Thuja**'s and **Medorrhinum**'s, is less with reality and more within the self; it exists between the psyche and the persona. There is a sense of wanting to cry but of not knowing whether to or not. Sadness but without any sense of its cause. A rising sense of frustration and impatience but not much enthusiasm for making any change. There is a desire to go home, to get out (of the situation or of the place) or to go away. The remedy has the energy to reintegrate the emotions with the psyche so that natural and real feelings are restored even if these are painful and cause weeping and anger. The patient recovers the ability to use their emotional 'vocabulary' or gets in touch with their emotions making it possible to express and thus eliminate unresolved issues. This is most likely to be needed in one who has a heavy karmic journey (many life lessons to learn) but who has always fought shy of facing problems or has attempted to do so but with little success (usually because there has been a lack of guidance in the family background). The history of failure to come to terms with difficult circumstances has led to an increasing sense of a heavy burden. This might be so dire as to make the person feel as if life is not worth living at all. They feel 'it would be easier to go than to continue on any level' and this is why 'often these souls go into dark places where they wallow in their sadness'.

There is a sense of mental numbness; emptiness where one is divorced from the emotions. Being emotionally 'in the dark' can seem like a form of madness. The patient may even say that they have felt sensations of growing bigger as in *Alice in Wonderland*. Anxiety and desperation might accompany the sense of dislocation or separation. A strong desire to fall asleep which is really a wish to avoid issues. Vagueness. Unwilling to participate. There is a feeling that things are not quite right despite appearances that suggest otherwise. A sense of unease which is easily dismissed. Anxiety can reach a pitch where there is a need for company. There is a dread and anticipation that someone might leave and not come back.

There is a physical sense of being jittery, nervous, anxious, fidgety, 'buzzy' and/or irritable with a state of being calm, detached and unable to feel the emotions associated with the state.

Difficulty in using words; in remembering words.

Physical symptoms

Head

Sensation of spinning in the head especially around the temple region. Sensation as if head is separated from the body. Sensation as if the head is growing bigger. Heaviness in the head with a sensation as if there is a pulling backwards from the occipital area. Pain in the head worse over the crown as if something were stuck in there. Pain in the head moves to the right eye and the heart. Intense pressure in the head worse from the crown to the throat. Outward pushing pressure sensations accompanied by jitteriness and restlessness. Headache on the left side of the head. Pains in the back of the head with tightness and tension. Headache may alternate from one side to the other or migrate from one place to another. Pains in the head may migrate to other parts of the body especially to the left side in general or to the heart. Feeling 'floaty' and light-headed.

Eyes

Tingling sensation around the right eye. Watering eyes without emotional expression. Burning sensation. Itchy eyes < inner canthi. Right eye keeps watering.

Ears

Clicking sensation in the left ear.

Nose

Prickling around the nose. Sneezing and runny nose (experienced by hay fever sufferer).

Face
Dry heat. Pain in the left side of face.

Mouth
Sensation of tingling in the lips. Disgusting taste in the mouth with other symptoms of throat and chest.

Throat
Sensation of a lump in the throat: globus hystericus. Choking and coughing caused by unexpressed emotions. Constriction felt in the throat especially when followed by palpitations, breathlessness and choking feeling (yet without a sense of fear). Tickling sensation on the right side. Sensation of excitement caught in the throat. Dryness in the throat especially with symptoms in the heart and left side. Phlegm with muzziness of the head < left upper forehead. Tonsillitis with pain < in the pharynx. Sticking sensation in the right side. Constriction on the right side of throat so that swallowing is difficult and then with a sensation of a crumb at the back of the throat. Tongue feels like sandpaper with strong thirst. Throat eased by drinking scalding hot water.

Respiration and chest
Pain in the left breast: burning. Heat felt in the chest. Mucus in the lungs which can be coughed up. Sharp pain in the middle of the chest which is better for rubbing and pressure. Tenderness in the sternum area < coughing. Heavy cold with copious mucus and coughing and a general sense of bodily heaviness especially after a night disturbed by sweating.

Heart
Sensation as of something circling around the heart with palpitations. Palpitations as if excited. Excitement felt in the heart (and the throat). Strong sense of anxiety felt in the heart area. Palpitations with breathlessness. Right ventricle of the heart becomes the site of potential pathology.

Digestion and stomach
Sensation of warmth in the stomach area and in the spleen with circling sensation and excitement felt in the heart and throat. Pain in the spleen after pain in the left breast. Waking from heartburn. Heat felt in the solar plexus. Nausea with strong thirst for cold water. Nausea with desire to eat to relieve

the symptom. Nausea especially after chemotherapy. Nausea with a desire to bend forward. Spasms in the stomach. Rumbling in the stomach without any hunger. Spleen feels clenched. Stabbing pain in the spleen as if a knife were being pushed in. Gurgling in the stomach which then extends into the abdomen < left side. Tremendous aching in spleen and stomach. Pressure build-up in the descending colon. Pain in the left side of abdomen shoots up into the left scapula. Strong thirst for water. Flatus and flatulence with stasis in the liver, spleen and pancreas. Microbial parasitic infestation of the intestines which has been an underlying factor in the patient's chronic ill health and which they have been in denial about for a long time.

Female
Symptoms may generally manifest at the menopause. Chronic pain in the right ovary. Polycystic ovaries and fertility problems. NBWS abuse from the Pill, HRT, fertility treatment and the morning-after pill especially where the patient is in denial of the potential damage. Menstrual flow is stronger at night. Slight ache in the right groin with period. Pulsation in the left ovary (which may be accompanied by pains extending down the legs; < left leg. Endometriosis. Pubic bone feels burning. Gynaecological symptoms are likely to be more on the left side.

Male
Prostate cancer. Symptoms in this sphere are more likely to be on the right side.

Urinary organs
Spasms felt in the bladder which wake the patient or while sitting. Urging to pass water < 10–12 at night; more frequent urging before sleep.

Skin
Open wounds that require stitches. Possible necrosis of wounds.

Neck and back
Left scapula and shoulder feel sore. Soreness under the left scapula. Pain at the lumbar-sacral junction < right side. Intense, deep, burning pain in the lower back < all over the coccyx and from the waist down. A strong sensation in the neck 'like a square thing' that constricts movement and which extends round to the front. Pain in the left side of the neck extending into the left shoulder. Itching on the left side of the neck. Pain in the back generally > for stretching

backward. Stiffness and tightness in the neck making movement difficult and painful. Sensation goes up into the occiput. Pulsations felt in neck with the stiffness; feels as if the neck is gripped in a vice; symptoms extend into the jaw which in turn becomes stiff. Cramping pain under the left scapula.

Hips
Pain in the hip worse on the left which is much worse for lying on it. Deep ache in the muscles and the bone.

Extremities
Left arm aching with strong burning pains in the left breast and aching in the left side generally. Fluid retention with sore knees. Legs become numb and it is difficult moving them; legs will not obey the mental instruction to move < from hips to feet. Weak musculature. Legs feel very heavy. Shaking in the limbs. Hands begin to contract < right side. Hands can burn with heat; may be accompanied by copious sweating. Sensation as if someone is clenching the left arm tightly, causing pain: a very deep ache. Tingling in the fingers; also tingling in the feet and arms while the face feels dry and hot. Sweating of the hands: greasy. Burning pains in the feet as if scalded.

Sleep
Strong desire to sleep. Dreams of desire for a married man. Dreams of being unfaithful but with little emotion on waking.

Considerations for the use of the remedy

- **Conium** shares the weakness, heaviness, stuckness and tendency to cancer or paralysis. The jitteriness and restlessness of **Rosebay Willowherb** is less likely in **Conium** which has trembling in the limbs. The defining differentiation lies in **Rosebay Willowherb's** sense of separation between the spiritual centre and the rest of the whole body. **Conium** is far more locked into routine and anxiety about the little things in life. **RBWH** is in denial about the important things in life. **Conium** is sad from a known cause of grief, from overwork or the loss of physical contact with a loved one. **RBWH** is sad without knowing particularly why; it has lost contact with the causes of the growing tide of potential pathology.

- **Carcinosin** falls midway between **RBWH** and **Conium**, sharing as it does many common symptoms. It works well alongside, before or after both of the others and, indeed, should be considered in this way. **Carcinosin** will be indicated in any case of **RBWH** where there is a lot of suppression of any of the three bodies: physical, emotional and spiritual. It provides grounding for one who has so lost touch with their base and their ancestral energy. In cases of frank cancer, **RBWH** can be given frequently as it bears repetition well. It encourages the slowing down of metastasis or it can relieve the pains of terminal cancer.
- **Lachesis** has a passing resemblance to **RBWH** in the left-sidedness, 'pressure from within, out' symptoms and the heart symptoms. **Lachesis** is clearly differentiated by its mental and emotional picture but this should not preclude consideration of its use as it may be of service as a drainage remedy. The need for it may well stem from a buried emotional history that the patient is unable fully to manifest yet.
- **Latrodectus Mactans** shares many of the heart signs and symptoms. It remains the remedy of choice in acute heart attack but for those who are suffering from chronic angina with the heart symptoms manifest in the proving, **RBWH** may be the constitutional state out of which the urgent need for the use of **Latrodectus** grows. Giving **RBWH** in an LM or in a maintaining dose of lower potency with the instruction to use **Latrodectus** in a high potency when the pains and symptoms of the heart become more frankly acute, may turn out to be good practice.
- **Thuja** and **Medorrhinum (Americana)** both have feeling of separation but in these two remedies it is more to do with being or not being in reality. **RBWH** lives in reality but denies what is going on within it. The feeling of separation comes either in the sense of the head not being attached to the body or in the sense that the spirit and emotions are separate from the rest of the system. **Thuja** may not be in denial; it just finds life very uncomfortable because of the lack of security and trust in reality. **RBWH** just cannot 'connect'. It is said that **RBWH** is a remedy of sycotic origin and it not only can be but should be given, where appropriate, alongside **Medorrhinum**. **RBWH** will help to clear the sycotic influence in a case that is generally carcinogenic.
- **Yellow** and **Clay** are also indicated in cases where there is stasis with a

compromised lymphatic system. In **Yellow** there is also the tendency to go towards the cancer state and it is useful in cancer drainage especially when it is put into combination with other cancer drainage remedies. However, **Yellow**, though there is often a feeling of ungroundedness and disconnection, has muddle and confusion, a lack of confidence and fearfulness; it is not a remedy state of being in denial. It is very complementary with **RBWH** and can be used in combination with it in low potency: **Yellow** + **RBWH** + **Chalcancite** or **Yellow** + **RBWH** + **Nat-sulph**, for example. **Clay**, on the other hand, is easily differentiated as this remedy is terribly earthbound, resentful and indolent. In **Clay** there is no sense of separation between spirit, emotions and the body; there is scant acknowledgement that the spirit is of much consequence anyway.

- **Folliculinum** may also be compared as it is so well known for NBWS hormone drugs. Both remedies can be exhausted and are 'drained' states emotionally and may be 'doormat', **Carcinosin** types but **Folliculinum** has a stronger picture of ovulation and period symptoms as well as modalities such as ++ sweets and sweet food; ++ carbohydrates; < heat; > fresh air. There are also far more likely to be mood swings in **Folliculinum**.

RBWH follows **Carcinosin**, **Folliculinum** and **Thuja** very well. It also complements **Black Obsidian**.

Esoteric therapeutics

Rosebay Willowherb is a crown centre remedy in that it is so strongly associated with the cancer miasm; it is through the crown centre that the energy of cancer infiltrates the physical body from the etheric. It is only when the base centre is so compromised that cancer energy is able to manifest in the physical body; **RBWH** has a strong influence on encouraging the patient to work on their base chakra as a starting point of general healing. There is a disconnection between the crown, brow, throat and heart centres which means that the patient is unable to create a healing momentum from within. Integration of the chakras is, perhaps, the first thing that needs to be addressed. One of the main problems for the patient who requires this remedy is that not only might there be a denial of the emotional body but there is a denial of or refusal to accept karmic lessons; this is a patient who may not want to get better. Just as the patient has closed down the higher centres for protection, so this remedy affords protection to the etheric body.

It may well be hard for the patient to understand or realize the reason for which they have incarnated; so far from knowing their life's purpose might they be, that they do not realize that incarnation has had purpose for them. There is spiritual inertia as well as mental and emotional stuckness. In the extremity of this remedy state, it may be said of this person that 'they don't want to be here'.

The patient's energy that courses along the meridians between the chakras may well not function properly. (They may have tried acupuncture but have found it aggravated severely or did not work at all.) A prescription of **RBWH** should help the patient to feel a lot less vulnerable in their physical 'vehicle'. A thorough investigation of root causes should reveal that the patient has had a history of emotional trauma stretching back into childhood and even beyond into ancestral history. It is often as if the patient has incarnated with an intrinsic sense of failure. It may seem that this patient has travelled this road many times before and has never really 'got it right'.

RBWH is associated with the astrological significance of Pluto, a very dark energy indeed and one that influences unexpected, traumatic events that upset the routine patterns of life. The remedy can afford protection at times when Pluto is in a patient's chart.

It is also a remedy that will expose deceit or corruption. It can be used to reveal truth when there is an absence of frankness.

Chakras

Crown
The connection between the crown and all the other centres is absent (never having been forged) or broken. The remedy will help dissolve the denial of the spirit's role in the life journey. The desire for sleep to avoid dealing with the world is gradually replaced by normal sleep patterns.

Brow
There is little perception that inner vision is obscured; there is little idea that suppression of the personality has led to a lack of keen judgement. The patients are unaware of lying to themselves about emotional and spiritual

matters. They are unaware of the lack of communication between the head and heart thus making expression extremely difficult or untrustworthy.

Throat

The pathology of the throat suggests the need to express emotions a lot better. Thyroid malfunction even where there is a dearth of symptoms.

Thymus gland

RBWH is complementary to the thymus and can be put into combination with it plus one other indicated remedy. It is particularly useful when ancestral trauma has contributed to a fracturing of the bodies so that the physical, emotional and spiritual do not seem to be integrated. Possible combinations include **RBWH + TG + Plutonium** (when there is inherited shock and trauma that the patient is in denial about); **RBWH + TG + Carcinosin** (when the patient is in complete denial about the emotional negativity that they carry).

Heart

Much grief is held in the heart centre sometimes without the patient's awareness. They find it hard or impossible to communicate their feelings as the connection between heart and throat and brow is absent. However, the patient will carry the burdens of grief even if unable to express them so that a sense of heaviness or emotional darkness will be obvious.

Solar plexus

Spleen energy is gravely lacking; there is a sense of lost aspiration. There is a no motivation beyond day-to-day functioning which is a struggle. This puts a burden on the liver which has a reluctance to cope with more than the essentials. Hence there is a build-up of toxicity in the liver and the lymphatic system. The pancreas also struggles and there is little of the joy and 'sweetness of life' that should be associated with this organ.

Sacral

This centre may well have been the subject of much chemical abuse since the Pill, HRT and other drugs. The expression of this chakra – the excitement of exploration and the expansion of awareness – is shut down.

Base

The lack of grounding is the most evident aspect of any case indicating this remedy though it is always accompanied by the sense of denial of the emotional body. The patient is simply unable to make the connection between their constitutional state of ill health and their shut-down emotions. This affects everything to do with this centre: the sense of security, the ability to maintain adrenal flow, memory, the ability to organize and to make creative use of routine. The lymphatic system threatens to block up and cause toxicity. As with so many other remedies with a lack of integrity in this chakra, there is a deep sense of fear, particularly of change – there is the fear that change may spark off conditions that threaten an already unstable state and introduce events that seem emotionally impossible to cope with. It may be necessary to prescribe priming remedies for the base such as **Oak** in order to create a preliminary semblance of stability.

Case studies

1 'A 71-year-old hypochondriac woman who always had to have something to complain about, continued homoeopathic treatment because it was the only therapy she was prepared to stick with. It was as if she liked to be ill; she had a range of symptoms which kept switching about. She would always lament, "Why me?" She usually did well on **Pulsatilla**, **Arsen-alb**, **Thuja** or **Silica**. She was given **Med-am 200** followed by **Thuja** 10M after which she said that she did feel a lot better. However, she then seemed to shut down again. She led a charmed life; she had a delightful husband and a supportive family about whom she complained the whole time. At this point she was given **Rosebay Willowherb** 30 o.d. for four weeks. The effect was remarkable: "I feel better than I've ever felt before!" Her daughter rang up especially to ask what she had been given as her mother had made such a radical shift. The remedy seemed to have removed a karmic block in her brow and crown chakras and she was able to move out from under the depressiveness that had been hampering her life for so long. She was given **Sac Lac** for the next prescription as the remedy was clearly working still. However, the next time she did need **Pulsatilla** and then **Thuja** both

remedies worked far more thoroughly. Furthermore, she began to tell more of the truth about her past.' JM

2 'A Sagittarian man of 35 with a long history of promiscuity came for a treatment. He never appeared to be entirely in his body. He was a chronic procrastinator and in permanent emotional denial. He always had to be right; he was selfish and disorganized. He lived in his head; he was a thinker and made no link between thought and action. He was a typical **Sulphur**. He started to manifest symptoms in the prostate and had recently been catheterized in hospital for a sudden tenesmus of the bladder. In the past he had been given **Sulphur**, **Morgan**, **Manganum**, **Fluor-ac**, **Med-am** and **Syphilinum** all of which had made improvements only for him to slip back. He was given **Rosebay Willowherb** 200 – 1M – 10M over 24 hours. When he returned his aura was completely different. He had found a job which he enjoyed and was committed to. He began a relationship with a girlfriend and felt more content than he had before. His prostate was now showing no symptoms and its energy and that of his heart chakra were spinning in the correct direction.' JM

10

GREEN

The meditative proving of **Green** was made on three separate occasions by two different but related groups. The first was 5 April 1996 with 4 men and 5 women and the medium. The second happened on 19 April 1996 where 2 men and 7 women plus the medium were present. The remedy was made by Katherine Boulderstone, one of the homoeopaths associated with the Helios Pharmacy in Tunbridge Wells. It is well worth quoting Katherine's article for *Prometheus* (Vol.10, June 1999) in which she describes the initiative for creating the colour remedies.

'Seven and a half years ago I embarked upon a personal journey of exploration of the colours. I happened to answer the phone at Helios one day to Melissa Assilem asking if we could make **Blue** for her. The same week Ambika Wauters walked in with some colour tinctures she had made using colour filters and sunlight and I ran them all up to 200c by hand over a period of some months . . . Only some of us were involved with these colours and as far as I know nobody took up the challenge of doing a full Hahnemannian proving of them although some of us were tuning in and noting down our experiences.

'The colours sat on the shelves at Helios barely being used for four years except by a few practitioners, notably Ambika and Melissa. Then three and a half years ago an old friend from college, Gill Dransfield, appeared out of the blue saying that she had a group of provers all ready and she wanted to do the colours. I felt that the colours needed to be remade from scratch and asked for guidance. I was told to make them from sunlight refracted through a prism which I duly did for each of the seven rainbow colours. Each time I was stunned at the brightness and purity of each colour. Each time I did my own meditative proving of it and noted in my diary what was going on in the world or in my world at the time. Sometimes it was quite personal, for example starting a period on the day I made **Red** or going into labour a few days after **Violet**. Sometimes the whole nation seemed to be involved in some kind of mass catharsis (Dunblane just before I made **Green**, the funeral of Princess Diana while I was making **Indigo**).'

Katherine opens her article on **Green** by quoting the words of the medium of the two circles: 'Each colour has its own crystal energy, its own elemental energy and its own sound and harmony.'[11]

She continues, '**Green** is the colour associated with the heart centre, the colour created on earth by the light of the sun through plant life. It is a calming and revivifying vibration, associated with both earth and water.' It is important here to note that the colour in question is emerald green rather than the dozens of variations available today. The precious stone, emerald, is the mineral analogue of **Green**.

The Background

The word 'green' is derived from the Old Norse (*groenn*) and from the old Germanic languages (*gruoni*), the original meaning of which is 'to grow'. Green, the colour, is most associated with spring and new growth; freshness and burgeoning vitality. In this context, the colour is associated with growing towards the light; in terms of the forest, this is the competitive struggle for sufficient space in the canopy of leaves to receive sunlight as the initiator of a

11 There are precedents for relating colour to harmony in the history of music. Scriabin (1872–1915) invented a cycle of colours and their associated harmonies based on the cycle of fifths: C – red, G – orange, D – yellow, A – green, E and B – bluish white (pale sky blue), D flat – violet, A flat – purple/violet, E flat and B flat – steel colour with a metallic lustre, F – dark red. In his *Prometheus, The Poem of Fire*, this colour scheme seems to have determined the base line of the music thus providing the work with an integral part of its basic structure. Professor Alexander Wallace Rimington (1854–1918) invented an 'organ' on which lighting effects could be 'played'. He arrived at his invention through being intrigued by the concept that colour and music shared similar vibrational qualities.

fresh life cycle. However, green has come to have other and different meanings, each of which sheds light on the colour that sometimes suggests its use for healing purposes:

- 'to be green': unskilled, untutored, unsophisticated, innocent, new to something and even ignorant; essentially immature or not yet full grown
- 'green-eyed': to be motivated by jealousy
- 'to be given the green light': to be given the go-ahead.
- 'the green man': the mythical figure of legend who represents the forces of Nature, forces that can be of either benefit or harm to us
- 'the Green Party': the political party that stands, in part, for a return to the natural order of things
- 'greenhorn': a simpleton or ignoramous; untutored
- 'greensleeves': a young woman who has stained her clothing on grass while out with a youth. Also 'a woman of an inconstant disposition in love affairs' (1580).

Green also has the meaning of unripe and immature; fresh and untouched; virginal. The Greek word for 'green' is associated with pallor. The 'green sickness' was the term for pubescent girls who became pale, wan and anaemic and who went an unhealthy green colour: chlorosis. This condition is partly the result of poor oxygenation of the blood and poor lymphatic drainage. (Deoxygenated blood is bluish and lymph is yellowish.)

For practitioners of colour therapy green is a vibration of harmony, balance and calmness. As the colour that is associated with the heart chakra, it lies in the middle of the spectrum thus holding a balance between the two extremes of the colours of the base and of the crown. It particularly balances the emotions and aids in the recovery from emotional trauma that has left everything out of equilibrium. It has long been used to assist in the healing of broken bones and the regrowth of damaged tissues.

Keynote effects

The main theme to this remedy is balance after a disturbance to any part of the physical, mental, emotional or spiritual bodies. It acts much as a keel does on an ocean-going boat. This may be needed either at the start of a journey (as in the young) or to restart a journey that has become fraught with impediments. The main disturbance is most likely to be manifest in symptoms that occur above the diaphragm even if the exciting cause happens to be a trauma to a part below it. Like its counterpart, **Emerald**, it is an 'ego healer'. Removes the tendency to inertia.

General symptoms

Green affects the whole system. It encourages the regrowth of tissue after damage. Nerve tissue regeneration after trauma or surgery. Useful in preventing keloid tissue. Encourages mucous membranes to secrete normally especially where they have become dried out or blocked through the use of drugs. Helpful in the growth of bone and muscle especially in the young who have irregular growth spurts with consequent lapses of vital energy, or in those who have broken bones (especially greenstick fractures). (Works well with **Calc-phos** and **Thymus Gland**.) In pathologies with green discharges it can purify the lymphatic system and encourage the elimination of toxicity. (Follows **Yellow** well here when that remedy has started off the elimination process.) Is very useful in cases of hyper-sensitivity of the nervous system (see **Apple Tree**) with any degree of depression. **Green** affects the pineal gland and can help to stimulate the production of serotonin. This is linked with the digestive system and the uptake of nutrients by the liver. Where **Green** is indicated there is often poor nutrition and a lack of vitamins in the body. A serious lack of the B vitamins can be a strong indication for **Green**. This lack of nutrients, vitamins and some trace elements can be indicated by poor functioning of the nervous system. Anaemia, tremors, cramps, tics, patches of inexplicable skin sensitivity and poor nerve conduction all come into this category. Sycotic: it covers proliferation (that is keloid tissue, benign growths, excessive catarrh, etc). Also tubercular especially in asthma cases where there is an emotional component to the condition. Is a major shock remedy most particularly when the shock has brought the patient to a point of standstill: inertia after a shock. Can be given to expectant mothers who are about to undergo amniocentesis; it is suggested that it protects the growing child from trauma though **Aconite**, **Ledum** and **Hypericum** may also be thought of in this context. Often needed in conditions where copper is a problem or lacking. < Pollution; < cigarette smoke. **Green** is thought to be of value in cancer therapeutics as a remedy that fosters balance and harmony as the patient goes through the gruelling process of treatment, or as a remedy to help the patient lift the miasmatic energy out of the physical body.

Miasms

Psora, sycosis and tuberculosis.

Mental and emotional symptoms

Excitable and full of anticipation. Hopeful about circumstances. Expectation of change. Yet, also the opposite: slothful, with inertia and lacking in resolution. Allow things to build up round them and then feel weighed down by it all. Inertia (especially of alcoholics) and a 'can't be bothered' attitude. Tendency to vegetate; to ruminate. Difficulty in meditating; cannot settle to it. Confusion. Jealousy, greed and envy when feeling overwhelmed by responsibility and circumstances; gives in to these feelings in reaction to feeling so burdened. Finds conflict of interests in a lot of things. Feels constrained and restricted by the clutter of circumstances; wants to break free of it. Would like to follow a less routine existence but cannot summon the energy to throw away the daily agenda. Has a strong sense of what they really need to do but too irresolute to follow anything through that might initiate change. Lack confidence in their ability to carry through plans. Identifies with a more natural lifestyle but is unable to do anything about change; thus there is a sense of unresolved duality. This can raise the sycotic miasm. (**Green** works very well in support of **Thuja** and **Medorrhinum**.) A sense of living in chaos. Chaotic and shambolic lives; never on time, forgets things, says things out of place and inappropriately. Often searching for things lost or mislaid. Has to write things down to remember them or gets others to remind them of what they need to be doing. Irritability. In children there can be disobedience and unwillingness to cooperate; feelings as of a spoilt brat: throws things away in a tantrum. Alternatively, there can be a facile compliance that suggests that the child is giving up too much potential to parental domination. Often useful to citydwellers who lack so much awareness of 'green-ness'.

Physical symptoms

Head
Headache from blow to the head.

Eyes
Eyes are burning and sore.

Nose

Green catarrh; thick and purulent; hard to blow out or copious.

Throat

Irritability in the throat with choking that is < from breathing in too deeply. Coughing with choking.

Chest

Discomfort and sense of restriction in the chest < right side. Tightness in the diaphragm which restricts a full intake of breath. Asthma and asthmatic breathing. Sensation of the inside of the chest shrinking. A feeling that there is not enough oxygen. Green mucus that is coughed up in spasms. A feeling of hollowness in the chest.

Heart

A sensation of tightness around the heart as if there were indigestion. Physical pain around the heart.

Kidneys

Twinges in both kidneys.

Extremities

Aching in the joints < elbows; stiffness in the fingers with aching in the hands. Joints feel weak; easily sprained. Tremendous itching of the sole of the right foot.

Considerations for the use of the remedy

Perhaps the first and most common application for **Green** is in traumatic injuries. It is worth considering it after trauma to any part of the body. However, its role is specific and not always immediately apparent. It is most useful when the trauma has affected the patient in any aspect of growth and/or development. If the patient's physical growth or mental/emotional development has been affected then **Green** will almost certainly be of benefit in the long term. It complements **Arnica** and **Aconite** as well as **Rhus-tox** and **Ruta**; it also complements **Oak** and **Thymus Gland** in this aspect. It often does its best work after an initial dose of these well-known remedies has already been prescribed on their indications but has not entirely cleared up the symptoms. Sometimes **Green** is required to clear a case that has not been well since a traumatic injury of many years standing. The body has the ability to make use of this remedy historically, so to speak. What may emerge in some cases is that **Green**, having been given for such a trauma, reveals that the patient has 'needed', as it were, to go through the problem in order to highlight that his or her life is full of muddle and confusion or some other aspect of the **Green** psyche.

During the proving it emerged that one use of **Green** is to support any of the overtly sycotic remedies such as **Medorrhinum, Thuja, Nat-sulph, Nit-ac, Pulsatilla, Aurum-mur**, etc. It should prevent aggravations from the chosen remedy becoming more than a mild reaction and deepen the beneficial effects so that understanding of the process of change is enhanced.

Thuja, Med-am, Syc-co, Phos, Lach, Puls, Calc-carb and **Nat-sulph** are all complementary remedies. So are most of the tree remedies; especially **Oak** and **Fagus-purp**. Can be given in the 6th potency as a support to any of these remedies. It can be useful in combination with **Thymus Gland, Thuja, Med-am, Lycopodium, Calc-sulph, Calc-phos, Sequoia, Holly** and **Bay Leaf**. A useful combination is **Green** + **Calc-phos** + **Thymus Gland** 30 for children who are growing slowly or in fits and starts. Also **Green** + **Thuja** + **Med-am** 30 for strongly sycotic states where the combination can support the indicated main constitutional remedy.

Esoteric therapeutics

Green is the result of mixing blue and yellow which are the colours of the first two chakras. It is the colour that most readily represents the discovery and quickening of one's karmic purpose; the green growth out of the yellow earth and blue waters. (Hence it can be very useful when given to young people on the threshold of maturity.) Green is the colour of the lower heart chakra. This centre, when clear of negativity, is the root of hope, positive anticipation, innocent excitement, unconditional acceptance of life challenges, emotional receptivity and determination to live life to the full. It is also the centre of selfish love; the upper heart centre is concerned with the aspect of unconditional love. The 'earthing' of energies from the higher chakras is achieved as they pass through and are filtered by this lower heart centre. When the lower heart chakra is negatively charged then it is the root of envy, jealousy, gossip, suspicion, some fears, sloth and destructive ill humour. This is also the centre which can take on the negative energy of others as green is an absorbent colour. (The thymus gland is the other centre that absorbs negative energies and it works in tandem with the lower heart centre. The former becomes a fathomless 'black hole' and the latter becomes heavy, dark and festering.) The remedy is needed to encourage us to grow towards sources of positive light. It is spiritually soothing and calming. It is a remedy that links the emotions with the nervous system thus making emotional reactions easier to bear. Hence **Emerald** and other green crystal remedies are exceptionally good at calming an agitated system. When the remedy is indicated then patients do well if they heed the advice to get out into Nature more or become involved in activities such as gardening. There is the surrender to the forces of Nature which often needs to happen in those who feel the need to be in control all the time. One indication is a reluctance to get on with the journey of spiritual growth: inertia and irresolution on a spiritual level. There is a spiritual sitting on the fence; they know which way to go but they won't take it. The remedy also opens lines of communication between all the centres facilitating the flow of energy between them. It follows **Yellow** and **Blue** well when the lower chakras have been particularly stuck and cleared by these remedies first. It can also precede them when energies flowing from the higher centres cannot reach the base. In this circumstance **Green** follows well after **Purple** and **Orange**.

Chakras

Crown

This centre is chiefly apparent through its absence; the patient has neglected this energy centre or is unaware of its significance. **Green** is most usefully employed here in one who is or seems likely to be affected by the cancer miasm: when skilfully prescribed, **Green** can be instrumental in turning the path of one who would otherwise embark on such a negative journey.

Brow

Imbalance in this centre can reflect disturbance that already exists in the heart centre though it may also be necessary to settle a disturbed mind that is struggling with the inertia sometimes felt after trauma. **Green** can act on this centre much as a gentle walk in a quiet woodland in spring might.

Throat

Rather than encouraging the verbal expression of emotion as some throat chakra remedies do, **Green** tends to quieten or still the voice and to give it more personal authority; it helps the patient to be clear in what needs to be communicated so that others are in no doubt of what is meant or needed. Damage to this centre from pollutants (including inoculations) and radiation should be repaired.

Heart

The remedy 'allows us to feel compassionate towards others who have hurt us. It heals the abuse of trust and love. It brings forgiveness.' (Quote from the proving.) For the heart centre that has become lodged in doubt and pain from troublesome circumstances associated with others who were or were felt to have been an influence or support. See **Olive** and **Peridot** to compare this aspect; **Green** follows or supports these remedies well. Green is also the colour of hope; where this has been lost through serious and threatening illness, the remedy may well serve as a support to this centre while other indicated and complementary remedies do their work.

Solar plexus

Green is complementary to the colour of this chakra: red. The negative energy that can be held in the lower heart centre very easily invades the solar plexus causing toxic liver energy to rise, resulting in acidity, tension, irritability and physical discomfort from a disturbed digestive system. These symptoms will be of the lower heart centre in origin. Dirty, reddish green can easily represent the vibration of an uncomfortable gall bladder.

Sacral

If shock to this centre has led to stagnation of energy in any way then **Green** can be of service here. Physical symptoms that may be manifest on this level will cause the water element to become stagnant; mucus and pus may form as a sign that there is too much stale earth energy mixing with the flow of old emotions.

Base

Green is very much an earthing remedy though any obvious imbalance will be manifest in the heart centre principally. The patient possibly feels a sense of disconnection from what is significant and important in life; from what is held most dear or what has been of most value and beneficial influence. This may be a person, an institution or a place.

Case studies

1 'Woman, a spinster of 76, small, neat and precise with sharp, intelligent eyes who had been a long-term patient, came during the winter of 2002 complaining of having pulled a muscle in her back that had gone into spasm causing her considerable discomfort. She felt massage helped and had taken **Rhus-tox** which ameliorated the problem temporarily. This had been compounded by a fall she had sustained. "I felt my right knee go and I went down just like that!" She hit and bruised her head. Her right side was also considerably bruised. She felt rather shocked so took several doses of **Arnica** 200. She also felt that the physical effects of these two problems had caused her some distressing sensations in her chest. She was aware of pressure and tension in her mid-chest: there was a sensation of a painful lump in the precordial region and she was having fluttering sensations with shuddering through her core. The pain in the centre of the chest tended to radiate towards the left axilla. In addition, she was having unpleasant dreams that were disturbing her sleep. She was given **Latrodectus Mactans** 6 to be taken each night, **Rose Quartz** 1M (a single collective dose) and the combination of **Crataegus** Ø + **Cactus** 3x + **China** 3x: three drops twice a day.

'The chest and heart symptoms and the bad dreams were quickly eased away. However, the muscular pains continued. Further **Rhus-tox** doses achieved nothing. She rang to say that the bruising had not gone; that she still felt that she was "in the fall"; that she still felt a lack of confidence; that since the fall she had been light-headed. She was sent **Green** 200, a single dose followed by **Rhus-tox** 200 b.d. for five days. The net result of this was that she felt "wonderful!" She had been feeling so much better that she tended to overdo things and then get tired.' CG

2 'A woman of 47, a Leo, trained as a music teacher but a restless, wandering spirit, complained that she had begun to feel abnormally devoid of feelings. She had been through various traumas involving

relatives and relationships and had recently lost a friend who had committed suicide. She also mentioned how much of a mess her own life was: her daughter was seeing an unsuitable man and smoking too much dope; she was unsure whether her own new relationship was working out or coming to an end; she was in a quandary about her ex-husband's family. should she get in touch with them to find out how her children's father was or should she leave things alone? She still felt numb that she was no longer married to the father of her two girls. "What a mess! How did that all happen? Why didn't I do anything about it?" She was given **Green** 1M: single collective dose.

'She wrote an email to describe the result of taking the remedy. "After I took the remedy I was unable to sleep. I was still awake at 4am. Then I fell asleep at about 5 and had a dream. I was with my husband at a food demonstration. We were surrounded by smiling, friendly people. He was talking to those on each side of us and I was watching everything going on. Suddenly the demonstrators told us we should try all this amazing food; it was so rich and delicious. I didn't know where to begin! We all stuffed ourselves. I ate so much that I didn't notice anything else but suddenly I felt alone; everyone had gone and I felt abandoned and so ashamed. When I woke up I couldn't stop crying. As I came to I realized that it wasn't the world that was in a mess, it was me! I knew I had to get some control back in my life. I have to lose some weight and eat properly; I realize that I have lost my husband – not that I blame myself for that – but that I still have to care for the children who do need me. I've let everything drift. I can't do that any more." JM

3   'A man rang to say that he felt deeply shocked since witnessing a robbery. He felt "frozen" in the moments of the event. He felt unable to do or say anything at the time even when the police wanted his account of what had happened. He said that he realized that he had always felt easily overwhelmed by events and that he felt like a coward. He was now feeling really guilty. His self-confidence was even shakier than usual. "It's affected everything. I can't seem to see my way out of it. Everything is confused. I'm confused. It's as if I don't know how to do anything properly." He also said that he used to feel like this at school where he wanted to be unnoticed in case anyone asked him anything. He was given **Green** 200: one each night for three nights. He

reported that he felt much calmer after the remedy; it gave him a sense of security. Not long after that he began recalling other events in his life in which he had felt as he had after the robbery. He then had **Green** 10M which, he said, gave him a lot of peace of mind and restored his confidence.' CG

4 'A woman in her early 60s who was a long-term patient came in a state of agitation. Though it was not outwardly apparent – she is a person who rarely shows deep emotion on the surface – she was distressed by having forgotten to collect two children she had promised to be respon-sible for from school at the end of the day. She had been driving towards the supermarket when she had suddenly realized that she should have been at the school half an hour before and that it would take her at least twenty minutes to reach there. The children were foster-children whose foster-parents had had an appointment at the local hospital and had asked her to look after them. This had occurred three weeks before and she could not shake herself out of her feeling of guilt, shame and confusion. She continued feeling rather shaky despite the fact that the children had been looked after by the staff and were at no risk and were not distressed. On taking a pulse reading her kidney qi was low and she agreed that she had felt as if she were on the edge of a bladder infection – something to which she was prone. **Green** 200: one every two hours, was given. When she returned for her next appointment she said that she had forgotten all about the incident very quickly and she had not had any bladder or kidney symptoms since the last visit. Her pulses showed no problem with the kidney qi.' CG

11

GREEN JADE

Green Jade was proved by the circle on 2 June 1995. The group on that occasion consisted of 6 women, 4 men and the medium. The remedy was made from the gem essence and was taken in the 30th potency. In ordering the remedy it is necessary to make clear the differentiation between the gem essence and the triturated stone.

The Background

Jade is otherwise known as either nephrite or jadeite. These two are not the same; nephrite is the silicate of calcium, magnesium and iron and contains fluorine and hydroxyl while jadeite is the silicate of sodium and aluminium. Nephrite's chemical formula is $Ca_2 (Mg, Fe)_5 Si_8 O_{22}(OH)_2$; Jadeite's formula is $NaA_1 Si_2 O_6$. Despite their chemical differences, both are termed 'jade' and have been deemed more or less the same by those who seek it except in their relative value. Jadeite is rarer and therefore of greater monetary value. Nephrite, which is the stone that was used to make the remedy, is found abundantly in Siberia, Turkestan and New Zealand and in smaller quantities in many other parts of the world. It appears on Mohs' scale at 5 – 6. It is a strong stone that is eminently suitable for carving. It is formed in masses metamorphically during the formation of actinolite slates.

The original term '*lapis nephriticus*' (kidney stone) was superseded by the word 'jade' which is derived from the Spanish '*hijada*'. The modern Spanish '*ijada*' means 'flank' or 'side' (of the body). This etymology reflects the age-old belief that jade is a stone that heals the body of all kidney diseases; it was also known as 'colic stone'.[12] Sir Walter Raleigh, writing in 1595, mentions the 'kinde

12 *The Shorter Oxford English Dictionary.* Clarendon Press, Oxford

of stones which the Spaniards call *piedras hijadas* and we use for spleene stones'. Jade's history goes far further back than Raleigh. It was much prized in ancient China; 'it poetically expresses to them all the virtues of many precious stones blended together'.[13] In pre-Christian times jade represented the nine accomplishments of early Chinese spiritual philosophy: charity, goodness, virtue, knowledge, skill, morality, divination, rectitude and harmony. The Chinese word for jade, '*yu*', can be loosely translated as 'courage' and the stone was thought to epitomize five virtues: bravery, charity, modesty, equity and discrimination. 'Jade is the concentrated element of love which protects the infant and the adult and preserved the bodies of the dead from decay'.[14]

From Li She Chan's Chinese encyclopaedia of 1596 we learn that a 'divine liquor of jade' can be brewed: equal parts of jade, rice and dew water were put into a copper pot and boiled and filtered. The result was 'said to strengthen the muscles and make them supple, to harden the bones, to calm the mind, to enrich the flesh and to purify the blood. Whoever took it for a long space of time ceased to suffer from either heat or cold and no longer felt hunger or thirst'.[15]

Jade was valued for its intrinsic healing and magical properties in ancient Egypt. It was held to be effective in cases of hysteria. Later Pliny wrote of the '*Adadu-nephros*' or 'kidney of Adonis' which linked jade with Venus and the parts of the body influenced by the planet. Indians saw jade as being the 'divine stone' and used it to cure kidney gravel and epilepsy as well as a charm to protect against animal bites and poisonous reptiles. 'It was also said to remove thirst and hunger, to cure heartburn and asthma and to affect favourably the voice, organs of the throat, the liver and the blood'.[16]

Jade stones were worn against the skin in the region of the kidneys to effect cure. The Maoris of New Zealand valued the stone as sacred; they used it as a charm, for tools and weapons and as medicine.

As a crystal healing stone, jade is a 'stone of fidelity' and a 'dream stone'. According to several sources jade 'improves one's remembering of dreams and assists in 'dream solving'. It is used to release suppressed emotions via the dream process; for this activity, a piece of jade is placed under the pillow prior to sleep'.[17]

13 *The Magic and Science of Jewels and Stones, Vol. II* Isadore Kozminsky
14 Ibid.
15 Ibid.
16 Kozminsky
17 *Love is in the Earth*, Melody

The historical background to the verb 'to jade' may also be of interest. According to the *Oxford English Dictionary*, the meaning in the early 17th century was '1 *trans*. To make a jade of (a horse); to exhaust or wear out by driving or working too hard; to fatigue, weary. 2 *intrans*. To become tired or worn out; to grow dull and languid; to flag.' Old, worn-out horses were often referred to contemptuously as 'jades' as were loose women in Tudor days.

Keynote effects

This is a remedy to soften a heart centre hardened through negative experience and walled off from further crisis. It is most often indicated on the emotional level during times of turmoil, not within but externally, in the circumstances of the patient's life. It brings one closer to peace of mind through the softening of attitude and emotion. It has been referred to as a 'homoeopathic tranquillizer' in its ability to engender serenity. It may also 'unlock' the voice so that it becomes easier to communicate how one is truly feeling.

General symptoms

The main focus of pathology is on the throat, lungs and heart. It also has an affinity for the spleen, kidneys, parathyroid and thymus gland. There is general heaviness with sensations of swelling in local areas that is either to do with the endocrine glands or from water retention. The thyroid and the thymus glands may become enlarged; the spleen may also show signs of hypertrophy with discomfort. Sensations of constriction may affect the throat or other parts such as the lungs or parts of the extremities that are affected by sluggish lymph drainage. Asthmatic breathing; congestion of the lungs < left side. With the sense of weight and sluggishness there is a feeling that something is being held in within the body; as if there should be an outlet for the draining away of excess fluid. Despite these general symptoms there is, nevertheless, acute and potentially painful sensitivity to noise; this may be transferred to sensitivity to smell and taste as well. There is a bias towards left-sidedness throughout the system even though this should not, on its own, be a determining factor. **Jade** has a profound effect on the endocrine system through its affinity for the thyroid, principally, and the pituitary, thymus, parathyroid and spleen. It stimulates these glands into 'communicating' better with each other; they function 'in concert' and encourage the system to maintain a better circadian rhythm. Palpitations with discomfort are felt in the heart. Paralysis agitans and Parkinsonism may occur after years of being in a state indicating **Jade**; the remedy can support such long-established remedies for these conditions as **Nat-mur, Causticum, Zinc** and **Conium**. Internal agitation and restlessness with exterior calm. May be of use in the treatment of patients suffering from the long-term effects of smoking especially if this includes 'tobacco heart'; **Jade** is complementary to **Lobelia Inflata**.

Miasms

Psora, tuberculosis and sycosis.

Mental and emotional symptoms

The patient complains of feeling the cares of the world on their shoulders. Seriousness; poker-faced (see **Blue**). Has the sense that there is too much going on around one; that they can't bear to hear about any more trouble; that there is no peace; that the expectations of others weighs too heavily. 'It is like standing in the middle of Piccadilly Circus and trying to talk to someone; so much noise. I just don't feel like bothering (with the struggle).' Yet has the sense that they are part of the general problem and that they are 'holding up the traffic' in some way. Has the feeling that their lack of contribution to the emotional turmoil is preventing the situation from being resolved; is being waited for by others to express feelings that have long been buried or walled off. Feels weighed down by a feeling of expectancy though the habit of years of keeping things to oneself is the real problem. Stubbornly truculent; refuses to vocalize deeply held feelings. Unaware of how strongly defended against the world they are. Hard-hearted and cynical. Indifference yet there is a tumult of activity in the mind; brain chunter. Has a sensation that in lacking any emotion to express, they have a wooden heart. Has a reluctance to hear what others have to say; 'there's none so deaf as those who don't want to hear'. Grief: there is a delayed reaction to deep grief or it has been put off indefinitely. Like **Arnica**, the **Jade** patient may say, 'No, leave me alone, I'm fine.' The heart may have been deeply wounded but the results are still in abeyance. There is a refusal to let emotions closely associated with a traumatized heart interfere with daily life. Helpful in the treatment of obstructive teenagers who are unwilling to grow up, hold grudges and are in a negative cycle of recrimination with parents (see

Ruby, *Volume I).* Asthmatic breathing aggravated by lack of emotional expression. Various comments about **Jade** patients are useful to bear in mind. 'He doesn't suffer fools gladly.' 'He should be treated with kid gloves.' 'She suffers in silence.' They feel as if they don't speak the same language. The adjective 'jaded' is often apposite with this remedy. Some **Jade** patients might well feel that they are 'outsiders'; they do not fit in and tend to be isolated.

Physical symptoms

Head
Heaviness in the left side of the head. Head feels full. Light-headed with sleepiness.

Ears
Acute hearing with sensitivity to noise.

Nose
Acute sense of smell with sensitivity to unpleasant odours.

Throat
Cough from constriction in the throat. Sharp, pinching sensation under the right jaw and in the area of the parathyroid gland. Swelling of the left side of the thyroid. Constriction in the throat especially associated with the thyroid. General sensation of heat in the body when the throat feels constricted. Tension in the throat yet lack of any emotion.

Chest
Deep cough from congestion in the lungs. Lungs feel heavy < left side. Asthmatic breathing with cough from emotional suppression. Difficult breathing and cough from years of cigarette smoking.

Heart
Palpitations with discomfort felt in the heart. General heat with palpitations. Heart problems consequent on smoking. Feels heavy in the heart (see **Cardamom**). Hardening of the arteries. Racing heart when there are emotional demands. Heart feels wooden. Heart block.

Kidneys
Water retention; hands and feet retain water. Urging to pass water at night. May pass more water than is drunk. Dehydration from lack of thirst.

Extremities
Swelling of the fingers from water retention. Sweat on hands; clamminess. Restlessness of the limbs; jerking and twitching may be observed.

Sleep
Wakes from disturbing dreams. Children have regular nightmares. Dreams that seem to have no relevance to the dreamer; that seem to defy interpretation.

Considerations for the use of the remedy

The two remedies that stand most comparison with **Jade** are **Nat-mur** and **Sepia**. However, **Lachesis**, **Arsen-alb** and **Conium** are also worth considering in the context of **Jade**'s symptoms.

- **Nat-mur** has a similar mental and emotional picture though it is more inclined to bear grudges and does not necessarily have the same internal sense of agitation. It is more inclined to be brittle and waspish than **Jade** which does not share the typical thirst for water and craving for salt. **Jade** is more obviously hard-hearted and wary of being drawn on any emotional subject. The defences of **Jade** are more obvious and almost as if overtly external; to defend the whole person while **Nat-mur** has more of a 'preservation order' on the heart itself. Neither type of patient finds receiving easy though **Nat-mur** is better at giving.
- **Sepia** may well be confused for **Jade** at the menopause as both are exhausted, heavy and fed up. However, **Jade** is more obviously affected by the family at large and the world in general while **Sepia** is more likely to be affected by either her husband or children who are demanding. The heaviness of **Sepia** is generally of uterine origin with much more slackness and weight felt in the pelvic region while **Jade** has its weighty discomfort in the heart, lungs and throat areas.
- **Lachesis** is an obvious one to compare in terms of the throat symptoms. They both have left-sidedness as well as constriction of the throat; both have symptoms of oppression elsewhere. Both cover mental confusion though **Lachesis** has more obvious non-consecutive

thinking and is more rambling in thought processes. **Jade** does not cover the purple quality of skin symptoms and it is not so loquacious; a **Jade** patient would find a **Lachesis** patient far too much to cope with.

• **Arsenicum** has the internal agitation and restlessness but it is a 'doer' who either gets on with what needs to be done or presses for things to be done by others. **Jade** tends to lack motivation and prefers to be stubbornly uncommunicative.

• **Conium** is another remedy that can clam up and not express the grief it carries with the result of becoming emotionally paralysed. However, it is far more likely to be sweeter natured and it doesn't suffer from the feeling of turmoil brewing all around.

Jade is complementary to **Nat-mur** and **Sepia**. It precedes **Nat-mur** well and helps to limit any aggravation that a dose of **Nat-mur** might cause. It is useful to use **Jade** as a support remedy for a high dose of **Sepia** especially during the menopause, a time of more change than hormonal rebalancing could account for. Indeed, it would not be surprising to see a prescription first of the **Sepia** and **Jade** followed at the next appointment by **Nat-mur**.

Some of the history of a patient indicating **Jade** might well include past, acute episodes that would cause the practitioner to think of **Staphysagria** and **Colocynth**, both remedies with a very strong link to **Nat-mur**. The other remedy in this group that might also be evoked is **Causticum**.

Esoteric therapeutics

The three chakras that are primarily influenced by **Green Jade** are the heart, throat and brow. It eases the heart that cannot receive or give much; it gives voice where there is little or no means of expression; it balances the siege mentality of those who feel full of turmoil due to the perceived clamour of the close world outside. It is contraindicated in anyone who is not influenced by some form of external hectic energy that mirrors the internal mental state. This can be missed in consultation as the patient may be stubbornly resistant to relating the origin of his or her problems.

Chakras

Crown
Sleep is disturbed by difficult dreams which are often unremembered or muddled and busy. There is little ability to pause for reflection; patients may not want to be reflective in their desire to opt out of their predicament.

Brow
The intuition is geared to the defensive and the intellect is occupied with coping with routine. There is an imbalance in the esoteric function between the left and right sides of the brain: the left wants to make life as quiet and easy as possible and the right cannot think of being creative and imaginative while there is so much turmoil. Shies away from taking in any more information; the brain refuses to take on any more. Perception is limited to immediate things though they are quick to register emotional issues that might arise to cause upset. They use avoidance tactics. Clumsiness in the use of words or in movements may result.

Throat
The voice is seldom if ever used to express the depths of what the heart actually holds. Expression is limited and may be non-committal or even mildly aggressive. The parathyroid gland that represents the highest degree of creativity is blocked which can lead to a sense of frustration though the patient is likely to be tired enough not to complain of this.

Heart and thymus gland
Blocked heart centre, weighed down by unexpressed emotions that lie too deep to be released without the sense that it would be too traumatic to accomplish. It has the sense not only of not 'belonging' but of 'not wanting to belong'. Jade is no exception to the list of remedies that feel outsiders in that there is the feeling that it is more difficult to break down the ramparts of emotional protection than risk the uncertainty of positive change.

Solar plexus
Motivation is lacking as the spleen is weak. Musculature may reflect this in easy strains, physical weakness and loss of perfect control.

Sacral

Weak kidney energy leads the patient to want to conserve strength as much as possible.

Base

Fear of emotional overload and consequent breakdown leads to a need for control or an exit strategy. The use of **Jade** aligns all the chakras and strengthens the midline (the energy circulating up and down the spine). It is related to the middle pillar of the Kabbalah (itself coming out of the base centre) so helps to hold the balance at the heart centre (Tiphoreth) between the weakness of too much openness and too much harsh and oppressive judgement.

Case studies

1 'Female, 51, menopausal and diagnosed recently with an underactive thyroid. She was prescribed 150mg of Thyroxine daily but still struggling with lack of energy, weight gain, low body temperature, hair loss and absence of outer third of the eyebrows. There was no family history of thyroid disease, no strong exposure to radiation, no obvious trauma, so I felt that the thyroid problem was due to unexpressed emotions which the menopausal process was trying to cleanse. However, she was not in any way open to this idea. My constitutional prescription was **Calc-carb** but there was little change. I prescribed **Jade** 30c on her third visit because she was wearing it as a necklace. It worked like magic. She opened emotionally, discussing her very unhappy marriage and her difficulties with her two daughters which were really quite serious. Within three months she had asked her husband to consider a trial separation to which he agreed and this resulted in her moving out permanently. All symptoms disappeared. The issues with the daughters also resolved as all the females overcame the "suppression". They all remain very friendly as a family – still sharing outings, holidays, etc. It appeared that the whole family healed.' **HJ**

2 'A five-year-old boy was brought for treatment because he wouldn't speak. He just would not speak at all; he was afraid to. His hearing was

fine; he had had the hospital tests. His comprehension was not a problem either. There was a family history of dyslexia and dyspraxia. He had deep, dark circles under his eyes. He was taken to a speech therapist but the experience set him back and things got worse. He appeared absent and unhappy. He had low energy and his throat chakra was not well. Any attempt to help was resisted. **Baryta-carb, Thuja, Silica** and **Ayahuasca** all improved things for a while but could not hold. **Opium, Syphilinum** and **Thyroidinum** had the same effect. Then he was given **Jade** 30: one three times a week. When he returned he was far more present and his heart chakra was beginning to open. He was less timid. The **Jade** was repeated and he began to speak.' JM

12

HIMALAYAN CRYSTAL SALT

The remedy was proved on 10 March 2006 by 10 members of the circle and the medium; there were 5 men and 5 women. The 30th potency was used. One dose of the remedy was taken for 7 days before the meeting where a further single dose was taken before the meditation began.[18] After the circle the participants were instructed to take the remedy daily for a further month.

The Background

Pure crystal salt or halite occurs in isometric crystals which are formed over millions of years under enormous geological pressure. It appears on Mohs' scale of hardness at 2 – 2.5. The crystals are found in a variety of colours: white, pink, blue, red, orange, yellow or grey or can also be colourless. The colour variation is due to naturally occurring impurities. (Himalayan crystal salt is pink.) These perfectly formed cubic crystals are created from vast beds of sedimentary evaporated minerals formed when lakes and inland seas dried up. Such salt beds are often hundreds of metres deep. Salt domes form where they are trapped in rock strata that exert stress as they shift and buckle upwards to form land masses and, in the case of the Himalayas, mountainous regions. Halite can be found in such diverse parts of the world as the United States of America, Canada, Germany, Spain, Romania, Iran and Pakistan.

18 This proving was undertaken after the 'world proving' had taken place: groups of provers around the world were coordinated to take the remedy at the same moment and report on their subsequent dream experience. None of the 10 in the present proving took part in the 'world proving'.

Himalayan crystal salt is a form of halite. Organic, unpurified crystal salt such as this is not just sodium chloride but a naturally formed source of a salt structure that is invested with some 84 of the necessary trace minerals required by the body's biochemistry. The balance of these minerals is very similar to that found in human blood. Unlike ordinary table salt, Himalayan crystal salt is not harmful to the body.

Table salt is 'purified' sodium chloride (NaCl) with most of the trace minerals removed from it. It can be damaging to health when consumed in excessive quantities because the body cannot recognize the biochemical value of it; it becomes a 'poison' that can cause damage to the blood, the water balance, the skin, the brain, the heart and circulation. The body is only able to deal with a small amount of un-ionized salt per day: as little as 5 grams. Any more than this will cause the body to take water from its own cells in order to surround the salt to ionize it into sodium and chloride so that it is easily excreted. This causes dehydration that then leads on to excessive acidity. Once this has gathered pace, oedema is established which in turn raises the risk of cellulitis. Uninhibited use of ordinary rock salt will eventually cause the body to create uric acid in its attempts to handle the crisis; unfortunately it binds to sodium chloride and forms new crystals that are then deposited in the joints causing gout and rheumatic arthritis. Halite, already in an ionized state, does not cause such harmful biochemical reactions. Indeed, it is readily assimilated by the body's cells and can help to maintain healthy cell structure. Thus Himalayan crystal salt is deemed a food rather than just a condiment and has a huge following eagerly promoted by health practitioners. Not only is it recommended as part of a healthy, balanced diet but it is also believed to have cosmetic properties; adding it to bath water is said to be beneficial for the skin and to improve the body's ability to eliminate waste.

Himalayan crystal salt, in its material state, has been credited with assisting the body in the following ways:

- regulating the body's water balance
- optimizing the hydroelectric energy of cells
- promoting a proper pH balance especially in brain cells
- correcting blood sugar levels
- helping to reduce blood pressure
- Maintaining the integrity and improving the condition of the arterial and venous system as well as of the sinuses and mucous membranes

- reducing the risk of muscle cramping
- maintaining bone strength
- optimizing the respiratory function
- optimizing the absorption of nutrition in the intestinal tract
- regulating sleep
- maintaining libido
- limiting the early signs of ageing

Keynote effects

The remedy casts light into the darkness held at exceptional depth in the heart by any residual emotional trauma or shock. It is said to have the ability to initiate healing where even **Nat-mur** and **Winchelsea Salt** have been unable to reach. It assuages the pains of the deepest sense of disappointment.

General symptoms

There is a marked tendency to dryness of the skin and mucous membranes as well as difficulty in maintaining the water balance necessary for perfect bio-chemical homoeostasis. Constipation and oedema may result from this tendency. The tissues of the heart can be affected by a general state of slug-gishness; atherosclerosis becomes a possibility as do such heart conditions as valvular incompetence and hypertrophy of the heart muscle. High blood pressure is a further likely manifestation. Respiration is shallow; poor exchange of gases. Muscles are prone to fatigue, cramp and pain. Skin is prone to eczema and dermatitis as well as herpetic eruptions; herpes simplex of both the face and the genitals. The remedy may be of use in treating intractable fungal infections of the feet and nails where more commonly indicated remedies fail to complete the cure (such as **Baryta-carb, Graphites, Thuja, Silica** and **Syphilinum**). Skin shows signs of wrinkling and early ageing. Oedema of the lower legs, thighs or under the eyes. Sluggish liver function with raised acidity levels. Dehydration with strain on the kidneys. Chilly though can become uncomfortably hot with clothing and heating; heat which quickly dissipates when the heating is turned off or layers of clothing are shed. Coldness > from a hot bath.

Miasms

Psora, tuberculosis and leprosy.

Mental and emotional symptoms

Deep sense of grief of long standing. Disappointment on the most profound level often associated with dashed expectations in personal relationships. Unresolved trauma or shock strong enough to have diverted the patient away from their life's true course. The mind tends to hold sway over the emotions: marked tendency to think rather than to feel. Confused feelings with a mind in turmoil. Suffers episodes of stormy thoughts which leave one feeling exhausted and either anxious or bewildered. Strong desire for peace and harmony; feels too emotionally 'attached'. Lack of feeling especially in those who have suffered 'broken lives'. A strong sense that everything so far understood about one's life has been thrown into question. Poor sense of personal boundaries; easily drained of energy by other people (energy vampires). Restlessness of mind and emotion (also physical). Contradictory states of mind; the character has become coloured by various conflicting aspects that have arisen through turmoil of emotional circumstances. Feel that they lack inspiration; no imaginative spark any more. Strong feeling of having lost one's way.

Physical symptoms

Very few physical symptoms were actually experienced during the proving though several were reported as a result of taking the remedy before and afterwards. However, the main interest and value in proving **HCS** is for the mental, emotional and esoteric information. Just as **Winchelsea Sea Salt** covers virtually all the symptoms of **Nat-mur**, so it is reasonable to assume that many of the symptoms exhibited by these other two salts may also appear in the materia medica of **HCS** but see below in 'Considerations for the use of the remedy'.

Head

Light-headedness and dizziness with a sense of detachment from the body. Brain feels numb.

Eyes
Dimming of vision. Sees poorly in the dark; night vision is affected causing difficulties with driving at night.

Nose
Congestion of the mucous membranes of the nose. Thick catarrh that is not particularly infected; albuminous.

Mouth
Herpes on the lips. Dryness and soreness of the lips.

Throat
Difficulties with swallowing. Choking. Cough from dryness of the throat. Throat symptoms < for emotional turmoil.

Chest
Sensation of pressure which makes one feel as if they have got something 'to get off their chest' though they are unaware of what that is. Shallow breathing. Awareness of the heart and the aching that is there from time to time. Feels 'unsafe' in the heart area.

Back
Pain in the back associated with and at the level of the heart, between the shoulder blades.

Skin
Dryness. Chapping. Eczema. Eases symptoms caused by radiation.

Considerations for the use of the remedy

HCS is a multi-miasmatic remedy though it has a strong affinity with the cancer miasm particularly. It supports the use of **Carcinosin** or may follow it when it has not done all that was expected in cases of deep emotional trauma. HCS may be considered in any pathology affecting the heart that arises from long-held emotional trauma in much the same way as **Nat-mur** and **Winchelsea Sea Salt** are considered. Daily doses of **HCS** in low potency are recommended in cases of compromised valvular function. In this form it is also useful following a heart attack to strengthen damaged heart tissue; its use will not adversely affect any necessary chemotherapy. In higher potency it is recommended for babies who have been through traumatic births and aftercare; when the start to life has been dramatically compromised. **HCS** complements and follows well after other birth trauma remedies such as **Blue** and **Ayahuasca**. For a general comparison of grief remedies see Appendix II.

Triple salt or three salts

A remedy has been made of the combination of **Himalayan Crystal Salt**, **Winchelsea Salt** and **Natrum Muriaticum**. This remedy implicitly carries the attributes of the three individual remedies and can be used as an alternative to any of them. It has been used with success in acute circumstances of potentially appalling grief (it follows **Ignatia** and **Chalice Well** very well) as well as in chronic cases. The choice of this combination remedy over the individual salts is necessarily dependent on intuition.

Esoteric therapeutics

The three chakras most affected by **HCS** are the heart, brow and base. The depth of emotional turmoil hidden in the heart also affects these other two centres so that the patient is unable to make significant progress in life due to lack of true grounding and an inability to discriminate between the truly lasting and the superficial. The practitioner gets the sense of a lack of movement in meaningful growth; there is an impediment to any life progress. There is a strong desire for peace and equilibrium in one who thinks more than feels. There is a lack of true joyfulness that can be felt throughout the whole being.

Chakras

Crown
Cancer diathesis.

Brow
Heals confusion and obfuscation in the brow resulting from deep trauma that has left the patient unable to focus any of their creative energy or to develop instinctually through wisdom gathered from experience. NBWS witnessing a terrible trauma/accident. Awakens the conscious mind to the spiritual path and

draws it into the heart from the base and the brow. Wakens ancestral energies (fosters the further resolution of past familial traumas). The practitioner will need to use intuition more actively in order to prescribe this remedy as it is often very hidden.

Throat

Patient is susceptible to the radiation miasm. (Salt is non-radioactive.) The voice is an unpractised medium for the expression for the heart centre so this chakra becomes a focus for persistent symptoms.

Heart

"It is said that this remedy is pure peace and harmony.' It 'opens the deepest gateway to the heart'. NBWS deep bereavement; forgotten grief; < grief from past generations (who never were able in their lifetimes to resolve any of it). The grief may be dark in character. Emotional aggravations from other remedies which the patient cannot handle or shake off (particularly **Japanese White Oleander** which can persist in aggravating skin symptoms). As if the patient is more comfortable with the aggravation than with the potential for release and resolution; more security in what they feel as habitual than in letting go and moving on. Remedy encourages optimism, joy and a return of a sense of humour. Heart pathology develops: valvular disease; arrhythmia and pulse irregularities. The remedy can be prescribed alongside remedies that are indicated for heart pathology such as **Latrodectus, Kalmia, Naja,** etc.

Sacral

Retention of water in the body with dryness of the eyes and mucosa; poor distribution of body fluids.

Base

NBWS birth trauma; can be given soon after birth (monthly for six months has been suggested, a prescription that maintains the baby's contact with the 'source' from which he or she came and helps them to carry the 'light' with which he or she is invested). Is said to encourage thorough grounding and foster the revelation of intrinsic aspects of the individual that would otherwise remain covered or become suppressed. Genetic skin disorders. The patient may say: 'I've never been well since I took such and such a remedy.'

Case studies

1 'Female: 47. Long history of failed, abusive relationships. Beautiful, sensual woman but constantly putting herself into 'victim' mode. Had done very well on **Natrum-mur** but I felt it hadn't quite gone deep enough because the relationships were still dysfunctional albeit less abusive. Gave her **Himalayan Crystal Salt** 1M in a split collective dose on 11/1/08. Saw her again on 22/2/08. The guy who she said was the 'love of her life' who had 'broken her heart', bumped into her in the street outside her house and said he was so sorry he'd ever hurt her (very unusual for him do that).

'She'd joined an Internet dating agency and had had 400 replies! Met a man through it, who was the first man she'd ever gone out with who had a good job, was well off, not an alcoholic or heavily into drugs or married! He was loving and very supportive. My patient gave up her job after the **HCS** (she'd been wanting to do this for ages) and bought a three-month round trip to India and Thailand. People at work cried when she left (that had *never* happened before to her). Some were even sobbing. "I feel so strong and confident. I can feel my power and others can feel it too. I feel so magnificent yet so humble. I can do anything I want. It's there for me – universal energy. I'm buzzing with it. I dreamt about a UFO last night; it was so beautiful!"

'She later sent me a wonderful card to say thank you for helping her to become the person she always knew was deep inside herself. I asked her permission to publish this and she said, "if anyone can feel how I feel from taking this remedy I would be honoured to have been part of helping that to happen." **PB**

2 'Female: 54. I gave **Himalayan Crystal Salt** 1M to a patient who had done well on **Carcinosin** and **Nat-mur**. She was very resentful towards her family and her ex-husband. After the **HCS** she rang to say that she had come to terms with how they were, had realized that they were never going to live up to her expectations (which she realized were unrealistic) and so there was no point in continuing as she had been. She said she felt very peaceful and realized that her sister, who had sat ignoring her at Christmas, reading a book, was actually a great role model for her (as she constantly used to get really stressed out by rushing about

trying to fuss over everyone and trying to keep everyone happy, and yet failing!). Her genital herpes attack (regular symptom) abated after HCS as well as cystitis.' PB

3 'A woman of 69 who had had a heart attack consequent on valvular disease came for treatment for never feeling at peace. She was forever helping other people but never found any tranquillity. It was as if she carried shock in her heart centre. Her husband had died when he was still young and she had been left to bring up the two children on her own. She had also suffered other traumas. She was short of breath most of the time. She had **Nat-mur** which helped somewhat and then **Opium**, **Lachesis** and **Statice** all of which made an impact but not in any impressive way. She was then given **Nat-mur** again as it had helped before but this time she went into a panic and her symptoms became exaggerated. At this point she was given **Himalayan Crystal Salt** 10M and all her heart and lung symptoms disappeared. The HCS was repeated over the next two months and she has reported feeling well and much more at peace within herself.' JM

4 'A man of 19 came with an unusual condition. He had always wanted to be a girl though he was not gay. His mother was very controlling. He had already arranged for the medical route; he was due to start taking the necessary drugs and the operation was already scheduled. He was given **Himalayan Crystal Salt** 10M based on the fact that he was never happy; there were few other indications as he was otherwise well. The result was that he cancelled the drug protocol and the operation. He said that he now wanted to remain a boy.' JM

5 'A woman of 23 with leukaemia came for treatment. She had had chemotherapy but with a negative prognosis and she felt that she wanted to use homoeopathy to help her die peacefully. Her spleen was very enlarged but **Tub-bov** and **Ceanothus** Ø brought this down. She was then given **Himalayan Crystal Salt** 10M one each week. She went into a state of complete acceptance of her death and felt at peace with both the world and herself.' JM

6 The following three cases illustrate the use of **Triple Salt**:

   i) 'R.M. 55-year-old female: kids gone to university, and husband having a midlife crisis. The marriage has jogged along amicably for years, but both of them find it impossible to communicate on a deep level. Patient feeling resentful and focussing on her job. Rx: **Triple salt** 10M.

   'The day after the remedy, husband started communicating with her; he has been seeing a much younger woman. As time went on, the two of them started talking about things they should have discussed years ago. They communicated more in that month than in the previous 10 years. Rx: **Triple salt** 10M, repeat dose.

   'Husband's midlife crisis continued, and the marriage eventually disintegrated. Patient much stronger now, and is getting on with her life.'

   ii) 'S.L. 60-year-old female, caring for her disabled husband. Prior to his illness, husband was the dominant partner; patient liked "peace and quiet". The caring is making patient very frustrated, she can't do what she wants and is "on-call" 24/7. Rx: **Triple Salt** 10M.

   'Patient coping better with life but occasionally "flips". Still feels trapped. Lots of family crises that she is having to sort out. Rx: Wait.

   'Patient now able to express herself calmly and is beginning to find ways of having time for herself.'LS

   iii) 'A.H. 42-year-old female. Her elderly dog died and her husband asked for a divorce in the same week. (They have been separated for a couple of years.) Feels very insecure without her dog as she lives alone in an isolated area. Very tearful and withdrawn. **Ignatia** helped initially. Rx: **Triple Salt** 10M.

   'Took a week's holiday and returned feeling much more positive. Trying to sort things out by correspondence with husband. Has been looking on the Internet for a pup, the same breed as the one she lost. One month later, she is exercising; is very motivated; has bought the pup and the divorce is going through.' LS

7 'A woman in her 60s came after an operation to fuse the bones in her foot, a procedure that had become necessary after decades of lameness from having suffered polio as a child. The operation had gone well and she was healing physically. Nevertheless, she was suffering from the grief

she had always felt about her disability and how it had so deeply influenced her life. She had become very tearful and was "finding it hard to be brave". She was given **Triple Salt** 10M: a single collective dose. Not only did she feel much happier in herself but the foot began to heal even more quickly.' CG

13

HYACINTHOIDES NON-SCRIPTA

Bluebell

The remedy was proved on 22 May 2009. The 30th potency was used: one tablet was placed on the tongue and the tincture was dabbed onto the wrists and brow of each participant. Though the remedy is exactly the same as the bluebell remedy already familiar to us, **Agraphis Nutans**, a new version was prepared at the Helios pharmacy by Sue Baker and Lesley Suter who had collected the specimens used from a wood in Patching, West Sussex. Both Sue and Lesley were part of the proving group. Several members had taken the remedy throughout the week preceding the proving.

Lesley Suter wrote the following about her experience. 'When Sue and I harvested the plant, it was in torrential rain yet we felt perfectly happy out in the woods. When we went to Helios to make the remedy up, again it was very heavy rainfall. While making the remedy neither of us was able to count to 20 (drops) so we both ended up counting out loud together to make sure we got it right. No concentration at all; just deliriously happy! A lovely floaty feeling; as if out of the body and looking down on what was going on. We were much longer there (at the pharmacy) than anticipated due to our mental faculties failing us, and our return journey was started at something like 12.50; I had to be in clinic for a 2pm start. We had planned on having lunch out before journeying back but there was no time. Did we care? Somehow, despite the heavy traffic and torrential rain, we were back in Littlehampton by 1.50 and had bought sandwiches to eat on the way. (The outbound journey had taken us something like 2¹/₂ hours!) We were really happy and chilled out for days.'

The Background

The common bluebell, named by Linnaeus, *Hyacinthus nonscriptus*, has an extraordinary number of names from different parts of the world. In England it has been known as calverkeys, auld man's bell, jacinth (which is Elizabethan), wood bells, adder's flower, blue goggles, crow bells and crowpicker, cuckoo's boots, dog leek, granfer-grigglesticks, locks and keys, squill, wood hyacinth and many others. Such names reflect local legend or ancient myth. In the language of flowers the plant symbolizes constancy, regret and solitude. No doubt these meanings reflect the sorry mythological tale of Hyacinthus, the beautiful youth loved by both Apollo, the sun god, and Zephyrus, god of the west wind. Hyacinthus preferred the affections of Apollo which caused Zephyrus to seek revenge in a fit of jealousy. During a game of quoits between the youth and Apollo, the wind god blew a quoit off course so that it struck Hyacinthus dead. In grief, Apollo raised a purple-blue flower from the boy's blood; on the flower was traced the exclamation '*Ai, Ai!*' thus immortalizing the god's cry of woe. Perhaps evolution has played us a trick for no such lettering appears on the plant; for this reason the secondary name of *Non-scriptus* ('no mark' or 'no writing') was also given. The other Greek-based name, *Agraphis nutans*, is derived from the similar meaning of 'not to mark'.

This nomenclature may be important to those who are considering using this remedy. Though there is absolutely no difference between **Agraphis Nutans** and **Hyacinthoides Non-scripta**, being one and the same plant, the remedies come from different sources and different times. The former is the familiar remedy known from Clarke's *Dictionary* and most famed for its influence over adenoids while the latter was freshly gathered in this century and, since its proving, has been credited with a far wider range of influence and application.[19] It may well be that there is no difference whatever between the

19 In one case of a girl who suffered from adenoids and who had done well on
  Agraphis Nutans 6c on a daily basis but who was showing signs of a diminished response, the patient was given **Hyacinthoides Non-scripta** 30c which caused no improvement and a short-lived aggravation. However, the case was heavily miasmatic, a fact that may have had a heavy influence on the negative outcome of using the newer version of the remedy.

two in their effects even though the proving of the former is woefully inadequate, being restricted as it is to a few details about the mucous membranes of the throat and ears. It is not strictly speaking, therefore, a 'new' remedy; nevertheless, the meditative proving has brought out aspects of its curative potential that bring it into that category.

Bluebell belongs to the Liliaceæ. 'The Wild Hyacinth', says Mrs Grieve in her *Modern Herbal*, 'is in flower from early in April till the end of May and, being a perennial and spreading rapidly, is found year after year in the same spot, forming a mass of rich colour in the woods where it grows ... From the midst of very long, narrow leaves, rising from the small bulb and overtopping them, rises the flower-stem bearing pendulous, bell-shaped blossoms arranged in a long curving line. Each flower has two small bracts at the base of the short flower-stalk. The perianth is bluish-purple and composed of six leaflets.' She goes on to inform us that the bulbs contain inulin, a chemical substance $(C_6H_{10}O_5)$ that is white and starchy and that is present in Elecampane (otherwise known as Inula), a famous folk and herbal medicine for tubercular cough. Bluebell, when dried and powdered, has been used as a styptic, a substance that halts haemorrhaging or fluid elimination by causing contraction of tissue fibres. Mrs Grieve quotes Sir John Hill (1716 – 1775) who said that there was hardly a more powerful remedy for leucorrhoea though the maximum dose of three grains should not be exceeded. Sir John is also the source of the information that 'a decoction of the bulb operates by urine'. While no medicinal use has ever been found for the flowers, the juice, according to the poet Tennyson, is adequate for snake bite. The bulbs are poisonous in their fresh state though this does not seem to deter the wild boar that now roam free in the woodlands of southern England from digging them up for a snack. The bulbs are full of mucilage, a viscid juice that is also abundant in the rest of the plant. This was used as an alternative to starch in the laundering of stiff ruffs in Elizabethan days. It was also used by bookbinders as a gum; it is stronger than paper, once dried. From around the same time it is recorded that choirmasters prescribed a distillation of the bulb to their choristers in order to prevent their voices from breaking; such a procedure might well have resulted in a distinctly adenoidal sound from the choir stalls.

The bluebell, which is associated with England's patron saint, St George, is protected by the Wildlife and Countryside Act (1981) which forbids the sale of wild plants and seeds. A different form of threat appears to exist in the advent to Britain of the Spanish bluebell, an ornamental variety that readily propagates with the wild plant. The habitat best suited to bluebells is slightly acid soil in shady or dappled woodland though it is tolerant of open ground and basic alkaline soil as well. It is reasonably hardy and is not affected by frost. The flowers are hermaphrodite and are chiefly pollinated by flies and beetles. Occasionally white bells will appear among their coloured siblings. The sweet scent of bluebells is enhanced by the warmth of the sun; a fact that perhaps gave rise to the Greek myth.

Symptoms of poisoning by Hyacinthoides include diarrhoea, abdominal pain and a depression of the heart rate causing a slow pulse. The mucilaginous sap causes dermatitis-like symptoms on the skin. Dr Clarke, in his dictionary, tells us that **Agraphis Nutans** has a curative influence over adenoids, catarrh, deafness and diarrhoea. The sticky nature of the sap lends credence to the first three (the deafness being due to catarrhal interference) and the fact that bluebell is known to be a styptic (causing contraction of tissue) suggests that abdominal pains might ensue from ingestion. Clarke's paragraph on the remedy is worth quoting in full:

> **Agraphis** is one of the remedies introduced by Dr Cooper. It partakes of the characters of the lilies and corresponds to catarrhal conditions. Obstruction of the nostrils, especially from adenoids, and throat deafness I have frequently seen relieved by the remedy. The action of it is felt towards the root of the nose. The plant grows in sheltered places and Dr Cooper gives > from shelter as a leading indication. It also corresponds to chill from cold winds and is very like Silica in this. I regard it as one of the leading remedies in cases of adenoids. Dr Cooper gives: 'Adenoids with enlarged tonsils; frequently accompanying dentition.' He has cured with it mucous diarrhoea following suppressed cold.

Clarke further cites **Allium Cepa**, **Allium Sativa** and **Scilla** as having a relationship with **Agraphis**. **Calc-iod**, **Calc-phos**, **Hydrastis**, **Squilla** and **Sulph-iod** all bear comparison in his opinion.

Taking his cue from Boericke and others, in his *Synoptic Matera Medica II*, Frans Vermeulen adds other leading symptoms:

- mutinism of childhood unconnected with deafness
- speech wanting in childhood
- mucous diarrhoea following suppressed coryza
- diarrhoea after cold drinks.

Further, he asks us to compare the remedy with **Calc-carb, Lycopodium, Dulcamara, Calc-phos** and **Verat-alb**. Clarke, Boericke, Phatak and others have not recorded any symptoms other than physical generals. The following description seeks to flesh out the whole picture of this remarkable remedy by adding a mental and emotional dimension. For the sake of completeness, the information on the physical aspect that we already know is included below in 'Physical symptoms' in italics.

Another and more conventional proving was carried out by Stuart Deekes in April 2002. He had been led to study this remedy by one of his proving group becoming overwhelmed by sadness and tearfulness while walking through bluebell woods. The proving was carried out on 7 people; one took placebo, three took one dose of the 30th potency and three took one dose of the 200th. In his write-up of the remedy Stuart found that the major themes were:

- sadness and grief
- fear with a sense of foreboding
- nausea alike to nausea of pregnancy

The general condition manifested as:

- wanting to withdraw, to hide
- < consolation or attention
- suffering from the polarities of fear or trust, upset and agitated or a sense of calmness
- headaches, especially in the temples, dry mouth but not thirsty, bitter taste in the mouth, especially at the back of the tongue, palpitations, mucous discharge, nausea.

Other effects from the remedy that were recorded included self-doubt, self-deprecation, drifting mind and lack of concentration.

Keynote effects

This is a remedy that in a period of acute crisis affords the patient who is full of fearfulness and lacks self-confidence, a sense of being able to cope and a fillip of hopefulness. It encourages the patient to stay in the present moment in times when they might otherwise be easily distracted. It is also one to ease the spirit body back into complete relationship with the physical body when there has been any traumatic incident that has disturbed the balance sufficiently to cause a dislocation between the two. On a physical level, the remedy is one of several that are indicated in a system that is acidulated and much affected by damp, cold and wind. It also affects the liver so that the general tendency to produce mucus and catarrh is lessened.

General symptoms

There is susceptibility to damp, cold and windy weather, any or all of which can cause colds and catarrhal conditions. Mucous membranes become overactive and produce thick, sticky phlegm and catarrh that is difficult to remove from tubes and orifices. The tubes and funnels of the body, most particularly those of the ears, nose and throat but also the Fallopian tubes, are affected by the excessive accumulation of thick mucus. Heavy production of thick mucus and catarrh following childhood vaccination; 'glue ear'. The central nervous system is affected either locally or generally; sensations of tingling that may or may not be associated with emotional states. Can bring about repair to damaged nerves; even the myelin sheath is positively influenced. The brain is subject to strange sensations and there is an imbalance in the hormonal activity of the pineal, pituitary, thyroid (either hypo- or hyperthy-roidism) and thymus glands. The right half of the brain may be more affected by symptoms than the left. Vegetative states, cretinism and lack of development all come under its sphere of action. The patient may appear to be vacant and not at all as if in the present. The valves of the heart and those of the veins may become incompetent. There is acid indigestion with congestion of the liver and consequent problems of poor acuity of brain function. Gall bladder problems. Vaccination may be a signal cause of the accumulation of mucus and this may be most evident in tubercular patients or in those who have had reactions to the BCG inoculation. Joint and osteoarthritic changes may develop in those who have lived through emotional crises without much outward expression; the remedy assists in turning the process of rigidifying tissue back towards dealing with the originating emotional problems. The senses of hearing and smell are both profoundly affected and the patient suffers emotionally from the limitations thus imposed. Sensations of enlargement or tingling may affect different parts; pains may be pricking or accompanied by sensations of fullness of the part concerned. Heat may be experienced in parts or in flushes or through the body. Perspiration may occur with heat particularly when feeling nervous or at a disadvantage. Vertigo with dizziness and nausea. Peculiar sensations of elongation or shrinking; shortened limbs with a long body. Feelings of being deformed.

Miasms

Sycosis, psora and tuberculosis.

Mental and emotional symptoms

Fearfulness, especially in one whose family members have suffered similarly in the past. Phobias of different kinds: < closed spaces; < open spaces. Claustrophobia; must be in the open air. Panic < in acute situations. Scattered thinking and dulled mental acuity; dementia. Appears cretinous. Despondent and lacking in motivation. 'I can't be bothered' feeling. Depressive. Weeping > depression. Feels buffeted between two or more opposing forces; < in circumstances where there are demands on attention and energy from different quarters in a difficult situation. The patient feels pulled towards one extreme or another which makes decision-making an emotional trauma. A remedy for those caught in an acute dilemma in which others are playing contrary parts. Feels that mind and body do not quite belong together; the body is on autopilot and the mind wants to wander off to a more comfortable zone. Feels reticent in responding which makes the patient seem either aloof or distracted. Wants to avoid participating in anything; would prefer people to keep their distance. Feels mentally blank; unable to muster the intellectual energy to do anything to break the cycle of negativity; feels the brain is shutting down. Easily distracted; loses concentration and focus which can lead to a sense of growing panic. Does not feel firmly established in the present. Mental imbalance in one who suffers from musculoskeletal problems; the patient has put the energy of unprocessed trauma into their physical structure. Head feels as if full of cotton wool. When asked for an explanation or description of anything, tends to ramble and lose the thread. Can be loquacious; rambling speech. Tearful with tiredness. It is also a remedy for those who are tempted into taking recreational drugs such as cannabis, cocaine and party drugs and who also have a loose attitude to sexual relationships and become susceptible to sexually transmitted diseases. It will also be indicated in those with a history of the same. The remedy is able to bring back into balance an endocrine system that is disturbed by an exaggerated libido.

Physical symptoms

Head

Brain feels dull and filled with cotton wool. Brain feels as if expanding; head feels swollen. Bursting sensation in the brain as if it would get bigger than the cranium. Head does not feel big enough to contain the brain. Headache in the occipital region; pain in the neck rising to the occipital protuberance. Pituitary malfunctioning; low thyroid-stimulating hormone. Tension from the head down into the solar plexus causing a contracting sensation with a sense of numbness and heaviness. Dizziness with tension headache in the back of the head.

Ears

Cannot hear well even though there is nothing wrong with the ears. Hearing may be < in the right ear. Catarrhal deafness. 'Glue ear'. Noises in the ear: popping and cracking but there is no improvement in hearing.

Nose

Thick catarrh that is hard to shift. Child has difficulty in blowing the nose.

Obstruction of the nostrils especially from adenoids with throat deafness. The action of (the remedy) is felt towards the root of the nose.

Mouth

Burning sensation under the tongue. Pain in the teeth (upper left jaw) which extends into the head. Adenoids.

Throat

Thyroid insufficiency. Thyrotoxicosis.

Adenoids with enlarged tonsils. Throat deafness. Mutinism of childhood unconnected with deafness.

Heart and chest

Heart feels as if it is contracting; as if knotted. Cannot take a deep enough breath when feeling tense and oppressed.

Stomach

Acid indigestion; heartburn.

Abdomen

Discomfort in the liver region. Congestion in the liver with sluggish digestion. Gall bladder pains.

Rectum

Mucus diarrhoea following a suppressed cold.

Female

Fallopian tubes are congested with either pus or mucus which can be a cause of discomfort or pain or infertility.

Male

May be of service in young men who are slow in maturing when there is a history of catarrhal congestion in the body. Also for those who have congestion of the testicles and epididymis following a history of gonorrhoeal disease.

Urinary organs

Weakness of the kidneys < right side especially in one who has a congested liver. Weak bladder; has to get up several times in a night.

Back

Pain under right scapula. Pains in the upper spine < cervical area. Tension in the spine.

Extremities

Osteoarthritis and rheumatic pains < cervical spine.

Considerations for the use of the remedy

This is a remedy that is indicated in anyone who has a history of suppression by or influence from one or more of the following:

- drugs that have encouraged the production of mucus
- vaccination that has caused the same thing (often it is the diphtheria, whooping cough and pertussin inoculation that is to blame)
- a phase of enjoying hallucinogenic or 'designer' drugs
- excessive dependence on acid-forming foods such as cheese, carbohydrates and fast foods.

Though the remedy appears to be mainly sycotic, the syphilitic state lurks beneath; the self-destructive element can manifest in adults with the characteristic history. Furthermore, it is not unusual, especially in children with mucous problems, to see the need to prescribe **Tuberculinum** in order to encourage continued response to the remedy though **Medorrhinum** may well be indicated for the same reason; differentiation depending on the usual miasmatic factors. **Medorrhinum** is also likely to be required by patients in middle years when rheumatic and mood-changing symptoms arise.

Hyacinthoides can be usefully compared with other remedies:

- **Baryta-carb** has a similar tendency to go into mental retreat and not wish to communicate and it is also found of service in those with congenital problems such as cretinism. Both remedies also have swollen glands and catarrhal mucus which causes congestion. However, **Baryta-carb** is more backward, chillier and more susceptible to slowness while **Hyacinthoides** is more muddled and confused and prone to inner feelings of panic; it is not as childish and it has more will power rather than obstinacy.

- **Thuja**, just as sycotic but there is much less evidence of trauma and internal panic than can be manifest in some **Hyacinthoides** patients. **Thuja** is more chronically worried with a feeling of being unsafe in some way not necessarily specified; **Hyacinthoides** is more concerned to keep its head down, not be involved, be left alone and not challenged.

- **Thyroidinum**: the question of thyroid trouble may arise in a case indicating **Hyacinthoides** which means that it is helpful to compare it with **Thyroidinum** and other thyroid influencing remedies. **Thyroidinum** is a sycotic/tubercular/psoric remedy which is useful in those who have poor concentration, depressiveness, irritability and metabolic disorders. So far the two remedies are similar. However, **Thyroidinum** covers symptoms of the skin (eczema particularly in children and psoriasis especially in the overweight) which so far do not appear in **Bluebell**; nor do grumbling, moaning and suspiciousness, all of which can feature in **Thyroidinum**. Both are introverted remedies though **Bluebell** is indicated in those who are going through a phase of their lives while **Thyroidinum** is likely to be needed in one whose life is governed by faulty hormones and metabolism. Nevertheless, it is worth considering the use of one if the other has not been as effective as expected.

Esoteric therapeutics

This is a remedy that is for shock to the auric field (see also **Golden Beryl** in *Volume I* which is for the effects of traumatic injury on the auric field). The energy of the chakras most afflicted is of the heart and the throat. It is for this reason that expressing distress on the deepest level is very difficult until this esoteric aspect is taken into account. **Hyacinthoides** is a remedy to consider when there has been emotional trauma in the history of a life force that does not respond fully to the usual, indicated remedies for grief; it is as if the energy body feels it is unsafe to be invested in its physical space. The heart and the throat centres are where it is most difficult to feel comfortable . When such a situation is suspected then it is likely that high potencies would be most useful. The reconnection of these centres into the harmony of the whole should bring about a release from an inner tension that has prevented any true 'still point' being achieved. For this reason it is often a good idea for the patient who is given **Hyacinthoides** in high potency to be referred on to a cranial osteopath or craniosacral therapist for complementary treatment.

Chakras

Crown
The inability to reflect dispassionately on the past due to a partial or complete separation from the events and/or feelings of the time means that the patient goes into retreat emotionally and prefers to avoid having to make the decision to change. They can no longer rely on intuition. There is a break in the communication between crown and brow so everyday practicalities become a chore. Hard to shake off the feelings evoked in dreams; feels as if the dream cannot be shaken off. Dizziness reflects the state of confusion about what the individual needs most to do with their life.

Brow
Very difficult to be decisive; trying to be thoughtful and decisive feels too much like being tied into the present moment. Depressive thoughts with headaches occupy this centre. Cannot make anything of complex discussions; intellectually seems disempowered. Find it hard to make sense of what they have heard or do not want to listen because it is all too much to take in. 'Can't see the wood for the trees' in important subject areas. The sensation of brain expansion that occurs at times is a reflection of how overwhelmed the patient can sometimes

feel. Feels the pull of needing to be in the present and the sense of the past impinging to draw one away from 'now'.

Throat

Difficulty in expressing clearly what they have to say; fears saying too much for fear of evoking any criticism or confrontation. May not feel there is any need to express oneself about hidden depths even though it is clear from the history of the patient that there are things left unresolved. Wants to repulse any kindly intended approach in case difficult emotions are brought up.

Heart and thymus

Hyacinthoides is very much a remedy for the damaged energy of the thymus. It can be indicated if there is any form of corruption in the family history that has in any way influenced the life of the patient. The depressive nature and the 'hanging back' from expression are indicative of one to whom the taint of syphilitic and sycotic ancestry has become adhered. As with almost all patients, there is a considerable element of grief though it is coloured by the buried past. There is a strong awareness of not wanting deceased relatives too close in thought or energy.

Solar plexus

The digestive system is easily upset because it reflects the sensitivity of the throat and heart. Acidity is a measure of the distance they are from the correct diet the individual should really be on. The liver creates heat in the system that con-tributes to the claustrophobic feelings (rather like **Pulsatilla**). The heaviness that is felt generally can also be felt in the abdominal area. Fear is held in the gall bladder causing a lack of courage or a state of anxiety in the process of decision-making.

Sacral

In those with heightened libido there is a susceptibility to venereal diseases which is generated from this centre. The remedy has an affinity for the right kidney. The water balances of the whole system are affected which is manifested in the thickening of fluids in the body to form copious amounts of mucus and, in deeper pathology, pus due to the drying action of excess fire in the liver.

Base

The patient may well be subject to fearfulness. This may manifest in panic attacks or phobias but it can also lead to the extremity of madness. The central nervous system is affected with tension and consequent sensations of tingling. The five senses are affected but most especially hearing and the sense of smell, the sense most associated with the base centre. It may be of service in the healing of damaged nerve tissue.

Case studies

1 'JS. 54-year-old female. Complained of left-sided jaw pain. Pain was driving her mad and no medication from the GP was touching it. Full of anxiety. Also undecided on what to do for the future. **Bluebell** 200/1M/10M given over 24 hours. Pain subsided quickly. One month later she decided to take a course and gain some qualifications.' LS

2 'JB. 74-year-old male. Complained of anxiety: getting very agitated about the forthcoming flight to attend his daughter's wedding. Cannot hold onto thoughts since serious neurological symptoms developed and since becoming very frustrated. **Bluebell** 200/1M/10M given over 24 hours. One month later his wife reported that the flight went well and he enjoyed the wedding. Since then his neurological symptoms are much improved and he is now leading a normal life.' LS

3 'RM. 55-year-old female who complained of suffering from the aftermath of a separation from her husband of 20 plus years. Lots of family tensions involving the husband and teenage children along with huge financial problems. Was due to attend family wedding on her husband's side of the family. **Bluebell** 200/1M/10M was given over 24 hours. The family wedding went well; the family all seemed supportive of her and she managed to have a polite conversation with her husband.' LS

4 'BD. Nine-year-old female. Parents are divorcing; mother has mental health problems. Very anxious; she tried to be the little mother; very

supportive of father. Has developed a facial tic which worsens as she gets more anxious. **Bluebell** 200/1M/10M given over 24 hours. One month later the tic has almost gone and the patient is much more relaxed and is behaving like a normal, happy little girl.' **LS**

5 'Female age 46 years. She came to see me when her dad was diagnosed with cancer of the bladder. She was very upset and worried as he didn't want to have the operation and the rest of the family were all for him to have medical intervention. She was very restless and anxious and so gave her **Lotus** to calm her down.

'She called me a week later to say she was coping well and her dad had agreed to have the operation so she was quite happy and positive at that time and so we just kept on with the **Lotus** as needed.

'She called three weeks later to say he had had the operation and now was in a critical condition. He was still unconscious since the op and they had perforated the bowel during the operation so septicaemia had set in and he was dangerously toxic. She was distraught and so I gave her **Ignatia, Rose Quartz, Lotus** 200s as needed.

'She called two weeks later to say there were some signs of recovery with her dad and he had regained consciousness although he was still septic and incredibly weak. She was exhausted at doing the hospital run every day and feared the future as the doctors had said it might be four to five months before he was out of hospital at best. She had **Phos-ac** 30s.

'She came to see me three weeks later; her dad had now got C difficile and was very poorly again and doctors were not giving anything positive at this point. She was beside herself and couldn't stop crying almost hysterically so she had **Ignatia** 10M. A week later he passed away. He had never recovered properly from the operation. She was terribly low and felt she wanted to run away or be taken away from the situation but knew that wasn't possible. She had to grow up and be responsible and she was so filled with grief and was depressed as she had to organize the funeral as her mother was not coping at all. I gave her **Bluebell** 10M.

'She called me a week later to say when she took the remedy she felt she was lifted out of the situation and felt as if she was in a bubble which felt incredibly safe and comforting. She felt she had recharged and had more strength that wasn't there before. She was able to have space to deal with the funeral and felt that everyone around her gave her space too.

'I remember feeling the same in my own personal situation, and at that time was taken to the bluebell woods where I felt safe and that I had space to just be in an incredibly peaceful environment. In the proving I felt as if I had a thin bubble around me and that I was allowed to deal with my emotions in the bubble, and that it wasn't going to affect anyone else if I got upset in it. **Bluebell** definitely has something to do with the father. My father and grandfather were with me in the proving.'
SEB

14

IVY BERRY

Hedera Helix, the berry

The meditative proving of **Ivy Berry** took place on June 16 2006. The remedy was made from berries that were provided from a churchyard by one of the provers, Jill Wright. They were steeped in ethanol for some 2 months before being taken up to the 30th potency. The provers consisted of 5 men and 7 women, including Janice Micallef, the medium who led the group in meditation.

The Background

The botanical description of ivy tells us that it is the only member of the Araliaceae to grow in Britain, that the flowers are tomentose 5-merous; styles are united; fruit are black globose and that it flowers between October and November. The flowers of the ivy are hermaphrodite, each developing an ovary containing five pendulous ovules which in turn develop into seeds. The seeds may vary in number from two to five and are enveloped in a black globose berry which is fully ripe in spring. It is amongst the favourite food of songbirds, such as thrush and blackbird, and wood pigeon.

The common ivy grows throughout Europe and even as far as Iran. It is a highly adaptable plant being able to grow in clay/acidic, chalky/alkaline or sandy, dry soil. What it does not care for is waterlogged soil or drought for too long a period. It tolerates shade or sun. It is also tolerant of considerable amounts of atmospheric pollution. Its habit is to grow along the ground or to climb up the nearest upright support to which it will cling with tiny suckers. It should not be regarded as a parasite and does not kill off its host tree even if it can cause the canopy of, say, an oak tree to appear to be far denser than usual.

The ivy plant is mildly toxic when consumed in large doses even though it is eaten with impunity by some mammals. People who keep goats know that goats will go for ivy especially when they are feeling off colour. It has also been given to cattle in their feed during the winter. The seeds contain 16 per cent protein and 35 per cent fat.

Ivy has always been regarded as a medicine. The leaves and fruit contain the saponic (soapy) glycoside hederagenin. This can cause breathing difficulties and even coma. (A glycoside is a vegetable substance that yields glucose when it decomposes. A saponin is a glycoside obtained from certain plants that, when combined with alkali, becomes soapy.) The sap of the plant can cause dermatitis, blistering and inflammation in those who are susceptible. (This is effected by polyacetylene compounds.) Ivy is a bitter, aromatic herb with a nauseating taste. It is used to treat rheumatism, swollen tissues, painful joints, burns and suppuration. Leaves contain 'emetine' which is an amoebicidal alkaloid. It also contains chemicals which kill liver flukes, other internal parasites and fungal infections. Excessive doses of the tincture have shown that it causes the destruction of red blood cells, diarrhoea, vomiting and irritability. An infusion of ivy twigs in oil can be used for sunburn. Saponins are shown in animal studies to prevent spasms in the muscles of the bronchial area while emetine increases the secretion and flow of mucus in the lungs themselves.

As a tincture this plant claimed a spectacular cure in the hands of Dr Cooper: a girl of 20 was cured of chronic hydrocephalus with a single drop dose of the mother tincture which needed to be repeated only once after 18 months. The girl was nervous, diffident and unhappy not least as her head was 70 centimetres in circumference and the object of comment and derision. She had had the problem since childhood and it was worsening. One drop of the tincture was placed on her tongue; by the next morning clear fluid began dripping from her nose which continued unabated for three weeks. This fluid was evidently cerebrospinal fluid and as it drained away so the two occipital swellings on either side of her neck began to reduce. When the discharge ceased the swellings were completely gone. The size of the head was reduced to 63 centimetres. Later, some of the symptoms returned but a further dose of the tincture removed them entirely. Dr Clarke says that **Hedera** is a 'sternutatory' (that which causes sneezing) for clearing the sight. Cooper went on to report that he had cured cases of cataract with it.

Keynote effects

An enhanced awareness of the beauties and gifts of Nature: birdsong in particular. A greater awareness of the qualities of light and how that encourages an aesthetic feeling for Nature and art. The remedy fosters the sense that one must let go of emotional 'baggage' in order to follow a more spiritual path. Helps the patient to find ways to make progress from what has been a standing position. Helps in the clearing of toxicity from the body. Calms the mind which is so affected by chuntering thoughts. Relieves fearfulness in children. Eases and resolves fevers which do not respond to indicated remedies. Relieves colds and flu and the resulting symptoms of congestion.

General symptoms

The remedy has healing effects on the sensorium, the heart and circulation, the lymphatic system, the liver and gall bladder, the lungs and, indirectly, the endocrine glands, particularly the thyroid and thymus. In addition it is useful in acute fevers both as reaction to cold viruses and to toxicity. (It may be called for when other apparently well-indicated fever remedies do not act.) Among the most marked effects of the remedy is its ability to encourage liver cleansing when there is heavy toxicity either from long-suppressed emotional issues or from poor nutrition, chemical medication or abuse of the system from alcohol or unwise eating habits. (See other liver drainage remedies such as **Carduus Marianus, Chelidonium, Berberis Vulgaris, Yellow, Tunbridge Wells Water.**) **Ivy Berry** is also capable of encouraging elimination from the blood, the thymus and the lymphatic system. It is useful in eliminating damage to the etheric body from radiation that has gone beyond harming cells and infiltrated the auric field. (**Ivy Berry** follows well after **MRPG 3**, the remedy made from the pulsed microwave emissions from mobile-phone masts, which helps to remove the harmful effects of microwave technology.) In addition, **Ivy Berry** should be considered as a blood purifying remedy, a spleen support remedy and one to influence the bone marrow where new blood cells are produced. (The remedy follows **China Officinalis** very well.) Just as **Ivy Berry** works well at the cellular level so it works at the opposite end of the spectrum of energy, in the etheric body. Here it helps to eliminate the early signs of cancer energy which enters the physical body through the etheric field. It is useful in those who bury the original seed thoughts and emotions of trauma that develop into carcinogenic energy. The characteristic pains of **Ivy Berry** are most evident in the digestive tract: twisting, griping, cramping in the epigastrium and liver area which may extend up into the chest, throat and jaw. Spasms may occur with or without cramps. There is accumulation of phlegm in the throat which is usually the result of toxicity in the liver. Respiration is hampered due to the phlegm or from sensations of tension or constriction in the chest. Susceptible to frequent acute colds which have different symptoms each time. (May start in the nasal passages and descend to the chest or rise from the chest up to the sinuses.) The spine can be painful and cause general restlessness. Twitching on the right side of the body. General tiredness and fatigue.

Miasms

Psora, syphilis, tuberculosis, cancer and radiation.

Mental and emotional symptoms

Mental dullness, lack of awareness and loss of sensitivity especially of one's environment. One may feel locked into an uncongenial routine and be without any means of escape. Loss of creative thought; loss of aspiration or will power to make changes. It becomes very hard to clear the mind of random or jumbled thoughts. Difficult to concentrate on keeping the mind clear of chunter. This may lead to feeling that the environment and material world are too abrasive; sensitivity to external circumstances: noise and speed. Long years of struggle with feelings of resentment. A sense of constant struggle to deal with mundane life. May well be indicated in those who are struggling towards the question: 'What am I supposed to be doing with my life?' There is the knowledge that we live life on a petty materialistic level and that there is something more. Difficulty in expressing emotions that must find a way out; that cannot be buried any longer without causing chronic ill health. There is tearfulness especially accompanied by palpitations or anxiety in the chest. Fixed ideas; fixed patterns of thought and behaviour. Harbours feelings of hatred and deceit especially after emotional trauma that has found no resolution. Insanity: mental imbalance rooted in a dysfunctional thyroid gland or from deep trauma that has affected the thymus. Endless round of old thoughts which means tiredness. A feeling as if one is losing one's mind, one's reason; as if 'I would lose it'. Night terrors in children especially in those who are afraid of going to sleep. The child may say they see monsters in the cupboard or under the bed. Sensitive children who feel vulnerable to the environment.

Physical symptoms

Nose
Coryza with influenza and fever symptoms.

Throat
A sensation of constriction; as if one had swallowed a boiled sweet (especially with digestive pains). A sensation of fluttering. Throat-clearing cough: accumulation of mucus in throat which is chronic. Rough sensation and congestion in the throat.

Chest
Hard to breathe through pains in the abdomen which extend up into the chest. Palpitations. Cramping band around the chest; < during pains from the liver and digestive tract. A feeling of cotton wool in the lungs with cough.

Stomach
Belching. Nausea.

Abdomen
Liver and gall bladder toxicity. Twisting, griping, cramping pains in the liver and gall bladder. Indigestion: trapped wind that causes pains similar to angina. (May prove to be similar to or complementary to **Carbo-veg.**) Sluggish energy in the bowels. Gall bladder discomfort and disease. Toxicity in the liver from chemotherapy, junk food with additives, alcohol and general pollution.

Neck
Stiff and painful; one needs to keep moving it round in circles to release it.

Back
Stiffness and aching which causes restlessness while sitting.

Muscles
Restlessness due to a feeling of stagnant energy in the muscles.

Extremities
Freezing feet.

Sleep
Night terrors in children: they see images of monsters in cupboards or under the bed. Children are fearful of going to bed because they have become aware of psychic forces.

Considerations for the use of the remedy

Ivy Berry is useful both in low 'x' potency and in higher potencies. As a drainage remedy it is invaluable as a liver and gall bladder remedy. It can be used on its own or in combination: **Ivy Berry + Golden Beryl + Hydrastis.** As a drainage and support remedy it works alongside constitutional remedies such as **Thuja, Lycopodium, Natrum-sulph, Nitric Acid, Aloes, China, Chelidonium, Arsenicum Album, Magnesium Carbonicum** and **Carcinosin.** The energy of **Ivy Berry** is dark, like the black globose berry it is made from. In the higher potencies it is useful for revealing the significance and depth of past hidden traumas. It is often indicated in patients who have seemed to need remedies such as **Anacardium, Aurum, Natrum Muriaticum, Lycopodium, Arsenicum Album, Carcinosin, Medorrhinum** and **Syphilinum** but which have not been able to make as much impact as might have been expected. It is also useful when given in relation to new remedies such as **Chalice Well, Emerald, Amethyst, Ruby** and most especially **Oak.**

Esoteric therapeutics

Ivy Berry awakens the creative force within; it encourages fresh starts. It strengthens and highlights links with historical or ancestral events that have left their negative energy on the patient's psyche. Memory of the past, both personal and ancestral, is clarified and, in those who are ready, it will release them from the thrall of negativity but in those who are not it will gently encourage the occurrence of circumstances that will provide further opportunities for understanding. It is a remedy for anyone who is extremely sensitive and fearful of psychic phenomena. It is said to be one of the remedies that can help those incarnated through IVF; it is suggested that such patients need the remedy to be given over many months. It is a useful remedy for those whose auras seem to carry heavy karmic energy that threatens to develop through the physical body as cancer.

Chakras

Crown

Lack of grounding in the base centre profoundly affects the state of this chakra. By encouraging a greater awareness of Nature and its healing powers, there is more sense of peace and tranquillity as well as a better ability to use time for reflection and such activities as meditation that heal the soul. Much of the patient's spiritual connection is hampered by the fixed ideas that clog up the brow centre.

Brow

The chuntering brain is calmed by this remedy when the root cause of the fixed ideas and persistent anxieties lie in the base and solar plexus. Powers of discrimination are weak and there are frequent episodes of being stuck in indecisiveness and confusion. Memory is poor for important past events that hold the key to the present troubles. There is also fear held in this centre: fear of loss of memory; of the mind's power to confuse; of sinking into depression; of dementia; of being left to die alone; of loss of joy. There has been too much conditioning, some of it through years of academic study (education) and a consequent loss of intuitive thought and sheer delight in the unexpected or the unknown.

Throat

Self-expression is limited. Without the sense of oneness with Nature there is great difficulty in linking heart and mind. There is so much useless information in the brain and so little understanding of how to access the emotions of the heart that the voice is underused. The ears are exhausted by listening to one's own internal dialogue as well as having taken in masses of information that has just fed the chunter. The remedy allows the patient to begin to hear anew and to respond afresh. If there is debris in the ears then Hopi candles may be of particular help to this patient. This is one of the very few plant remedies that are recommended for the treatment of radiation toxicity.

Heart and thymus

Though there is hatred and resentment held in the heart, they are due to a sensitive person's response to negative conditioning. The light of Nature has not been allowed to exercise any healing power on the individual. Too much sensory input from the wrong sources such as television, computers and education have taken their toll on the heart centre which was already struggling to find an identity following the emotional impact of lack of empathy or love from those closest. The patient may not even be aware of just how much ground there is to cover in order to heal the emotional desert they experience. Though they may see a beautiful flower, view or creature they do not know how to respond spontaneously and often miss what is around them.

Solar plexus

There is much toxicity in the liver and gall bladder. It chiefly restores integrity to the blood and fortifies the spleen in its jobs of replenishing the blood supply with new cells and maintaining the immune system's adequate response to infection. This is very much a remedy to encourage fresh creative energy so that new ideas arise in the mind and the body is invigorated to be productive.

Sacral

Restores the will to explore and expand consciousness.

Base

With a weak spleen and a mind full of unusable energy, this centre struggles. There may be frequent infections and a history of fevers. There is not enough circulating oxygen in the blood. The musculoskeletal system may feel weak, not least from lack of the physical body being put into use. (The patient does better if recommended to have daily exercise outside in the fresh air.) One is put in touch with earth matters again or for the first time. The five senses are also restored to something of their original integrity: colours become sharper, smells become more acute, sounds are more resonant. Being 'back in touch' with reality takes on both meanings. For those who are exhausted and out of touch with the natural world and have a jaded approach to life as well as toxicity in the blood and liver this remedy restores the vigour needed to start learning again.

Case studies

1 'Boy (four) with a history of night terror. On falling asleep each night, he persistently dreamt of a lady coming to strangle him. He told his mother that the woman had brown hair and a nasty face. He would wake screaming. Once awake from the dream he was unable to go back to sleep. He was given **Ivy Berry** 30 o.d. for one month. Within a few days the dreaming was much less. The **Ivy Berry** was repeated: one twice a week for four further weeks after which he suffered no more bad dreams.' JM

2 'Man (40); an Aries. He complained of a busy mind which prevented him from sleeping properly. He was a typical picture of **Arsenicum** but he had had that remedy as well as a lot of other constitutional treatment over a period of about seven months. In addition he had been given **kali phos** (Aries' tissue salt) and **Passiflora Ø**. He complained that nothing was working. At this point he was given **Ivy Berry** 6 o.n. for 28 days. From the very first dose, he reported, he felt completely better though he did continue to take the remedy as prescribed. He also had an aggravation: he developed a high fever on the first two nights after which he felt completely well.' JM

3 'Nigerian man; a Cancerian. He came complaining of boils all over his body that had appeared after having a course of vaccines for travelling. The boils were all over his body but worse over his legs. His liver pulse showed up how unwell he was. He was given **Pyrogen, Belladonna, Lachesis, Arsenicum** and others all of which made some difference. He kept getting colds with fever which went on for 2½ months. During this time, his symptoms were so bad that his wife threatened to take him to the doctor which he resisted. He was then given **Ivy Berry** 200 in a single collective dose. Within two days he was completely better. The fever-ishness was the first thing to go. He was further **given Ivy Berry** 200: one three times a week. Not only was he completely better but his liver pulse showed up that he was well in himself.' JM

4 'An 80-year-old woman who had had breast cancer and was in remission after chemotherapy came for treatment. Both her liver and spleen

pulses showed up as being in need of attention. She was given **Ivy Berry** 6 twice daily. When she returned she not only felt and looked better in herself but her liver and spleen pulses were both markedly improved and she was able to say, "I really understand why I had to have this cancer. It's made me better before I die". **JM**

5 'A retired music teacher in her early 60s came back after a dose of **Platina** 1M saying that she felt that a sea change was beginning to happen in her life though she felt that she was still struggling to learn to look after herself well. "I don't let myself have those little treats. I don't reward my efforts. I feel that I do so much just to keep the body going. I spend so much time with other people. I am supposed to be retired but it doesn't quite feel like that yet. I'd love to be on my own and not at anyone's beck and call. I am tired and I want to feel that the time left to me can be enriching. I never felt particularly appreciated at the college; I never got any sort of acknowledgement but that's not what bothers me any more. I need to know that there is something worthwhile for me to do out there. Otherwise, what have the last 60 years been about?" She was given **Ivy Berry** 200 – 1M – 10M to be taken at weekly intervals.

'When she returned three months later she related what had been happening in her life. She had begun to turn over in her mind all that had occurred during her marriage. "My endless, something and nothing cough got worse and I realized that it was a grief thing. I realized that I really did go through a lot of stuff with my husband that was never really resolved. He took his own life. He always knew he'd do that when his time came; when he was ill. He knew that's how it would be from the beginning. I did a lot of digging to find out more and it was as if he wanted to leave not even a footprint. I know I feel much more now. Something deep is going on. I have always worn a mask. I cannot stand my own lie any more. I have always tried to fit in and go by the rules and I can't do it any more. I'm afraid of any more resistance in my heart. I don't want to feel I'm fighting off anything in my chest any more. This is my central channel. Nothing is going to stick till I ditch what I'm doing, clear the decks and pay attention to what my inner voice has always been trying to tell me."

'This might have been enough to illustrate the remedy but there was a remarkable follow-up to the remedies she had next: **Syphilinum** 200 (single dose at night) followed by **Purple** 10M (one on waking) and **Blackberry** 30 once a week. She returned some months later and said that she was feeling well and that her energy was very much better. She had been to a craniosacral practitioner who had done work centred on her stomach. This had prompted a memory that at 18 months of age she had swallowed a large quantity of Belladonna berries. Her mother had had a vision of this happening and had rushed to find her. She had taken her off to hospital where she had had her stomach pumped. She was aware of the sense of trauma to her throat, oesophagus and abdomen. "Everything always ends up in and around my throat! This is where I have to do the work!" She said that she was in the middle of clearing and cleaning up her home. She wanted to use new and brighter colours. "I feel joy today. At the moment I'm engaged in earthing. Things are falling into place." Without denying the significance of **Platina** as a positive influence on this woman's progress, it was **Ivy Berry** that initiated her journey back into the past where unresolved problems lay waiting for attention. It opened the way for her to use **Syphilinum** and **Purple** to bring light into what had, up to then, been a dark and rather joyless life.' **CG**

15

JAPANESE WHITE OLEANDER

Hiroshima

The remedy was first proved on 16 January 2006. The proving group consisted of 6 women and 5 men. There was a further short meditative proving on 22 February with just 3 of the original provers present. The reason for this was that Martin Miles felt that there was more information to be gathered. On both occasions the remedy was taken at the 30th potency.

The remedy was made by Martin Miles from a plant growing in Hiroshima, Japan. While on a lecture tour for the Japanese Academy of Homoeopathy he collected samples which provided the remedy. The plant from which the sample was taken was the first to grow after the detonation of the atom bomb in 1946. The following is a quotation from Martin's lecture on **Japanese White Oleander**.

'After the bomb was dropped on Hiroshima the land was scorched beyond recognition. The traditional Japanese architecture is of timber so the city was vaporized within a few moments, leaving only hot, grey ash falling like rain over a large area. Up till that morning of 6 August 1945 the people had considered themselves fortunate as their city had not been attacked from the air like most other Japanese cities. A hundred thousand died in the blast and many more would suffer a slow, painful end over the decades to come from the type of wounds that had never been seen before. Of course, nothing grew in a land so terribly traumatized; it was as if the earth had died. Then, one day, the oleander appeared, a small tree with an exquisitely beautiful flower, some blossoms are red, others white. And so it was that for some years the oleander was the only plant of any kind that would grow in Hiroshima. The oleanders in the city are smaller than those in other areas of Japan and even now the trees and plants that grow there are of less stature than their brothers and sisters that thrive elsewhere. Quite appropriately, the city adopted this lovely flower as an emblem of peace and regeneration.'

The Background

Nerium oleander is a member of the Apocynaceae family. It grows from southern Europe, North and West Africa to western Asia including India, southern China and Japan. It thrives mostly on dry ground, particularly along the dried-out beds of watercourses and in the full sun. It was cultivated by the Romans and features frequently in their wall paintings, notably in those of Pompeii.

The plant is an evergreen shrub that can reach up to two metres in height. The leaves are pale green, lanceolate, thick and leathery; if cut they exude a thick sap that is irritating to the skin. The red or pink flowers are tubular with five lobes which appear in clusters and some are scented. The fruit is composed of a pair of follicles that split open on one side to release the oblong seeds. All parts of the plant are toxic; it carries a fearsome reputation as it has been known to be lethal to both man and beast. Indeed, it has been recorded as a means of suicide in southern India. It is recommended that the smoke of the burning brushwood of oleander should not be inhaled. The toxic effects include nausea, colic, vomiting, low blood pressure, seizures, heart symptoms, drowsiness, tremor, coma and death. Oleander was known to Pliny the Elder who, despite its toxicity, claimed in his *Naturalis Historia* that if taken in wine with rue it could be effective against snake bite.

Hahnemann was the first to prove the plant, the poison of which affects the skin, heart, muscles, nervous system and digestion. Even the scent of the plant can cause symptoms. It also has the effect of paralysing the memory and dulling the intellect; slowing perception and comprehension; causing moroseness and sadness and a powerful sensitivity to slights and being scorned. The Japanese white oleander, taken from such a symbolic place of devastation, must be viewed in a new light despite its obvious connections with Hahnemann's original proving of the unadulterated plant.

Keynote effects

This is a remedy for the profoundest shock; shock that was sustained even years before, that has become a layer of negative energy that saps the constitution of the ability to heal itself. Fearful dread and anticipation of trauma are also allayed in those who have learnt by experience to expect this. In with the shock and trauma is woven deep grief and suffering beyond the reach of familiar remedies. The remedy has the ability to lift into consciousness hidden or buried original causes.

General symptoms

Acts on the emotions, the nervous system, the spinal column, the endocrine glands (particularly the thyroid), the digestion and the skin. Ailments from shock and trauma. Shaking and trembling especially after shock. Post-traumatic syndrome. Injuries to the spine; broken back. Paralysis; Parkinsonism. Numbness, tingling and twitching. Clumsy and awkward in movement. It is useful in the treatment of wounds and burns that do not heal. Predominantly a right-sided remedy. Fever without infection; heat without sweat. Throbbing sensations; in the head, through the body. Herpes with vesicular eruptions. Ulcers that are deep and persist; internal ulceration that defies treatment from indicated remedies. The remedy is deeply syphilitic and complements syphilitic remedies particularly **Syphilinum**. Heals radiation toxicity and radiation miasm. Deformities due to inherited radiation. Burning pains. Contraction and stiffness in muscles and sinews. Cancer diathesis: fast-growing cancers; sudden appearance of terminal cancer; secondary cancers from metastasis; Hodgkin's disease; lymphoma. Swollen, tender glands (especially of the neck). Problems of blood chemistry leaving the patient with allergic reactions with aetiology that is hard to determine. Patients who present with no other symptoms but allergic reactions. Sudden manifestation of pathology; as if it were the chronic of **Aconite**. Eczema and other skin conditions complicated by allergies particularly to environmental hazards and allergens often of an unspecified nature. Sensations of heaviness. A remedy to consider for those who have been through electroconvulsive therapy. Use in conjunction with other radiation remedies with patients who are to go through radiotherapy treatment or for the after-effects.

Miasms

Radiation, cancer, syphilis and psora.

Mental and emotional symptoms

The remedy covers the extremes from hysteria before a crisis or as the result of devastation to passive, unemotional calmness before or after a traumatic event. Helps children who become agitated, tearful and upset before going to school or other events outside the safety of the home environment. Eases tension in those who find it difficult to participate in group activities. The remedy fosters the awareness of the importance of becoming involved with other people in group activities. Shock, trauma and fear. For the results of devastation: the patient is reduced to inactivity, passivity, quiet reflection and lack of awareness of being present; ungrounded. Deep sadness and grief. Useful in those who have suffered from violent cruelty (it can also be given to animals that have suffered in this way). Tearfulness but, in others, emotional numbness. Inability to move from shock and trauma. Passive and ungrounded with no wish to participate or take any responsibility. A state of being beyond fear; as if waiting for no one knows what. Physically present but mentally absent; disconnected as if in limbo. The patient may have a sense of living in the moment before a disaster will happen. Confusion, apprehension, anxiety. Dreading the unexpected.

The other side of the remedy is aggression and selfishness, feeling confrontational and frustrated. Lack of self-confidence. Feels as if 'it's all too much'. Unable to articulate one's needs well; saying one thing but meaning another. Not wanting to bother to socialize; too much effort to talk and be upbeat. It is useful also in those people who hide their true nature beneath a veneer of superficial perfection; they seek to convince the world that their lives are balanced and without difficulties while, in fact, beneath festers a great deal of unhappiness and family trauma.

The remedy fosters calmness, tranquillity and generosity of spirit. It helps patients to feel relaxed after a period of great tension (hence it follows **Oak** well). Like **Chalice Well**, which it follows and precedes well, it will allow those things that are hidden to come to the surface and be identified.

Physical symptoms

Head

Headaches. Tension and tightening in the brain; as if there were pressure built up in the cranium. Wakes with headache which > by evening.

Eyes

Watery eyes especially left. Eyes look glassy. Wakes with red rims. Eyes feel sticky; sticky on waking in the morning. Bloodshot.

Nose

Watery, clear or yellow mucus. Sneezing. Post-nasal drip. Throbbing at the root of the nose during cold.

Face

Sensations of heat with flushing and redness. Twitching.

Mouth

Upper teeth: pain on the right side especially in the molars. Parched. Cracks in the corners of the mouth. Gums feel sore during a cold. Gums feel as if they are decaying. Mouth ulcers.

Throat

Swollen glands with coryza or flu-like symptoms. Glands feel tender in the neck. Tickly cough. Cutting pain across the throat with dry cough. Thyroid conditions especially hypothyroidism.

Respiration and chest

As if one cannot breathe properly; lungs feel constricted. As if breathing in smoke. Feeling as if one were breathing spores into the lungs. Dry cough. Airways feel sore during respiratory tract infection. Cough increases to spasms of dry coughing with bloody and/or profuse sputum. Burning in the oesophagus after eating.

Digestion

Nausea; sickness; vomiting. Burning pains. Stomach ulcers. Duodenal ulcers. Dehydrated. Belching < on rising in the morning. ++ apple and apple juice.

Urinary organs
Frequent urination.

Skin
Burns; wounds; ulceration. Burning pains. Herpes; herpetic eruption in the lumbar/sacral region on the right; vesicular and scabby which takes a long time to heal; dark red stain lingers for considerable time. Warts, verruccae. To be considered for after-effects of radiotherapy scars and lesions.

Neck
Pain in the right side while glands are swollen: burning. Feels as if the muscles and nerves are inflamed. Muscles in the right side of the neck contract.

Back
Sensation as if back were broken. Injuries to the spine; useful after other indicated remedies have dealt with the physical and emotional trauma. This remedy will take the healing into the etheric body. Unable to move from trauma in the spine. Sensation as if the muscles in the lower back on the right side were pulled; twitching of the muscles. Ache in the right shoulder blade < at night.

Extremities
Deformities of bone. Consider in osteomyelitis. Pains in the extremities that are really pains in distant points of the energy meridian of the organ under most stress.

Sleep
Wakeful; < at 4am during throat infection. Feels wretched in the night.

Considerations for the use of the remedy

Compare with all other radiation remedies especially **Plutonium, Rad-brom** and **Rad-iod**. Oak (tension, stoicism); **Chalice Well** (brings up hidden and buried issues that need to be resolved). Precedes and follows well after the new grief remedies: **Aquamarine, Himalayan Crystal Salt, Winchelsea Sea Salt, Emerald, Rose Quartz.** Those who need **Mercury** may well need **JWO** to follow. Works well with **Apple Tree** in those who suffer from persistent allergies of no specific cause. It works alongside **Carcinosin** and **Syphilinum**. A triad remedy to consider would be **JWO + TG + Syphilinum**; JWO and TG may be considered as good partners with any of the following: **Amethyst, Emerald, Rose Quartz, Chalice Well, Aquamarine, Ruby** and **Tuberculinum**. It would also be appropriate to put them with **Arsen-alb, Aurum** or **Baryta-carb**.

Esoteric therapeutics

The remedy is one for engendering calm, peace and balance after a storm of trauma or devastation. It can also be helpful for those who have suffered this in the past and are expecting it again now. The patient is usually ungrounded and unaware of the present moment. The crown centre is either dissociated from the rest of the system or blown wide open: they are unable to reflect on their condition. There is confusion in the brow centre; consecutive thought is well nigh impossible. The throat chakra is blocked and there is no creative expression of the individual. The thymus centre is also of significance: the thymus is almost inevitably damaged in anyone who requires JWO.

The remedy is one of the most important for transformation; transformation from complete negativity and stuck karma to one of movement and in which resolution for past and ancestral trauma can be sought. The remedy addresses the syphilitic miasm at the very deepest level; the patient may require this remedy to be given with **Syphilinum** quite frequently to relinquish the burden of syphilism. A very useful triad remedy would be **JWO + Berlin Wall + Syphilinum**.

Chakras

Crown
Cancer diathesis: < skin, glands, bones; cancer metastasis. Possession: helps to release entities.

Brow
The appearance of perfection which is illusory; looks good on the outside but there is degeneration beneath (**Syph**). Practitioner sees that something is not quite right but cannot identify what; must use the intuition to guide oneself to the choice of remedy or prescription. The remedy fosters greater awareness and consciousness through the experience of suffering and trauma; the patient may be living in denial (hence the image of perfection) but needs to be able

face the deep karmic implications that the remedy can reveal. Refusal to see the truth of the destructiveness of negative forces (whether on a global or local or bodily level). The remedy exposes the faults and negativity of the ego; it fosters the development of the intuition and it encourages people not to live blindly.

Throat
Radiation toxicity: any form that it takes. Loquacity: bubbling chatter with little meaning.

Thymus gland
Syphilitic remedy, which is said to carry the pure energy of Pluto: uncompromising, ruthless agent of transformation; great beauty tempered with destructive power. A remedy that regenerates the protective qualities of this centre. Deep trauma that has its roots in the distant past. Hidden destructive power: creeping, insidious forms of pathological energy.

Heart
Suffering from cruelty. Sadness and depression that has little outward expression though it is the cause of syphilitic disease.

Solar plexus
Corruption of spleen energy (which is often initially indicated by loss of motivation and followed by immune system deficiency). Nausea and vomiting. Blood cancer: leukaemia.

Sacral
Weak kidney energy following harrowing times or severe shock.

Base
Fear especially set off when the base centre is devastated by terrible sudden events (see **Buddleia** which complements). Stunted growth (see **Baryta-carb** which complements). Lack of healing power. Genetic mutation; bone deformities; organ failure. Infiltrating diseases: lymphatic cancers. Burns (like **Moldavite** and **Plutonium**); herpetic eruptions which weep. Old wounds won't heal; ulceration or eruptions; gangrene. Skin: burning pains (like **Arsen-alb**). The keynote of the remedy is transformation; 'a remedy of endings and for new beginnings'. Like the phoenix in its ability to begin again by burning

off all that is no longer of use and keeping that which fosters the renewal of purpose. The auric field of the remedy is calm and beautiful though there is a dark core to it.

Case studies

1 'A patient of mine with long-term ME asked me one day if I had a remedy called **Rhodochrosite** as the word had popped into her head! She didn't know if such a thing existed. Naturally I gave it to her and it helped her levels of energy. She also had a dose of **Japanese White Oleander** later and this was the real turning point in her recovery. She had terrible nightmares and visions after it but, once she emerged from that, it was very transformative.' **PB**

2 'A woman in her late 30s came with extreme nervousness and fear. She was a Scorpio (with the moon strongly represented in her chart). She was obsessive about her health; she was bulimic. She worked very hard; a perfectionist. She was very egotistical and ruthless. She was not a popular person and antagonized everybody she met. Very pushy in business. But she was so sad inside. She was disconnected. She could never keep a relationship and now she didn't want one. She was always frightened that she was not doing enough though her vital energy was really low. She also had very vivid dreams. She had **Platina, Tuberculinum** and then **Lachesis** followed by **Syphilinum**. There was no real change after any of them despite the indications. She then had **Japanese White Oleander** 1M. She suddenly decided to take a month off work; something she had never done before. She returned and had another dose of the remedy after which she took up another relationship and felt hugely better with no panic attacks, bulimia or health obsessions to disturb her.' **JM**

3 'A woman aged 54 came for constitutional treatment. She was a Capricorn, an earth sign that can suffer terribly from being ungrounded as she was. She had a history of electroconvulsive therapy (ECT); she had been subjected to twice the normal amount after she had lost a baby

and gone into what was diagnosed as depression. It was clear that all her chakras were blocked. She never smiled; never showed any sign of joy at all. She couldn't laugh. She functioned like a robot. She had also suffered through a difficult childhood. She had **Phosphorus, Electricitas, Tuberculinum, Phos-ac** and **Pic-ac** with some signs of improvement; there were gradual changes. Each time she had **Electricitas** her glands would react by swelling. It was as if her immune system was trying to unblock something. It was clear that the ECT was responsible for holding her in this blocked state which indicated remedies could only ameliorate for a short while. She was given **Japanese White Oleander** 200 in a single collective dose. Almost immediately she showed signs of improvement. The dose was repeated weekly for six weeks. One of the first signs of recovery was that she started to laugh. She then showed indications for the remedies that she had had before, only this time they did what they were meant to do. She remains well.' JM

4 'A 62-year-old Sagittarian woman wanted constitutional treatment following breast cancer, a lumpectomy and two lots of radiotherapy. Thirty years previously she had been treated with radium for thyrotoxicosis. She was given radiation remedies: **Rad-brom** and **Rad-iod**. These did not make much impression. She had burning symptoms around the area of the scar tissue. All her chakras were spinning in the wrong direction and there were holes in her aura like you always get when there's radiation still attached; grey patches where there's no colour. Her energy leaked away so she was always tired. She was also sad and lacked expressiveness. She had **Japanese White Oleander** 30 daily for four weeks. The effect of this was really positive. All the physical symptoms disappeared; the burning all went. Her energy came back; she felt much happier. And this is how she's stayed.' JM

5 'A very frail woman of 57, a Virgo, came complaining of asthmatic breathing. She was a missionary whose life was concerned with helping others. She had a very sad story to tell of a husband and one son having committed suicide. She had another son but she almost never saw him as he wandered the globe restlessly. He too suffered from asthma. She had a long history of falls and injuries. She had never felt happy and said that she couldn't find peace anywhere. Her aura was dark and heavy.

Every few years she felt an inner calling, a compulsion, to go to Japan to work with people. Her charitable work was unpaid but she would stay helping people for six to twelve months at a time. She had no idea why she felt impelled to do this. She was given **Thuja** and then **Syphilinum** which certainly helped her constitutionally though they did not alter the inner sadness and lack of peace. She then went to see an astrologer who specialized in Kabbalistic astrology,[20] a system which concentrates on the past rather than the future. She was told, without any prior information from her, that she had had several past lives in Japan, that she had suffered there and that she had died in one of the atomic explosions of 1946. She was given Japanese White Oleander 200: one twice each week for four weeks. (She did not know what she had taken.) When she returned she sat down and said, "I don't need to go back to Japan any more. I'm done. I'm free." In the following months she had the remedy twice more. She no longer feels the need to wander anywhere. She feels happy and contented and her breathing is normal. What is more, her son returned to this country and got married and settled down.' JM

6 'A 74-year-old man, born in Aries, came for constitutional treatment. He appeared very carcinogenic. He had had radiation treatment for a thyroid condition many years ago and then the thyroid had been removed. There was, as there so often is in cases like this, a family history of thyroid-related problems. He was never happy. He was always suppressed. His throat chakra was completely blocked. He had **Carcinosin, Nat-mur, Arsenicum, Rad-brom** and **Rad-iod**; all the remedies you might expect. He also had **Thymus Gland** and **Syphilinum** as well as the combination of **Rad-brom + X-ray + Plutonium** up to the LM VI. There was some amelioration but nothing that was convincing. He then had **Japanese White Oleander** 30: twice daily for three weeks. The effect was very rapid. He just got much better very quickly. He needed it repeated a couple of times a while later when the carcinogenic state seemed to be returning but JWO 200 cleared it each time.' JM

20 My research has shown that Kabbalistic astrology concentrates on looking into the origins of karmic connections. Rather than looking predictively at a subject's life, it looks back at astrological links with parents and recent past lives in order to highlight aspects in the chart that offer explanations for karmic difficulties. CG

16

LAPIS LAZULI

The transcript for the proving of this remedy is lost. The remedy's materia medica is taken from the lecture notes of Martin Miles and of the author which were based on the transcript. The proving took place in late 1998. It was proved by the original group of the Guild of Homoeopaths. The proving was based on the 30th potency. The piece of lapis that was used to make the essence remedy was one that contained a seam of iron pyrites.

The Background

Lapis crystallizes in masses, cubes and dodecahedral crystals. Its chemical formula is complex: $(Na,Ca)_8 (Al,Si)_{12}O_{24}FeS\ CaCO_3Al_2O_3$ (Sodium calcium aluminosilicate). It is a combination of minerals, primarily lazurite and calcite. Where iron is present there will be seams of pyrite. Other minerals present are silica and aluminium with sodium, lime, iron, sulphuric acid, sulphur and chlorine. It is of a deep blue with flecks or seams of golden iron pyrites.

Historically it was the 11th stone of the breastplate of the high priest of the temple of Jerusalem. It forges the link between the material and spiritual realms. This is because the flecks of 'gold' (iron pyrites or fool's gold), which represent the energy of the material world, are embedded in the blue stone which represents the energy of the higher vibration of the heavens. Lapis was known in ancient times as the stone of heaven. In some traditions, the Ten Commandments were written on tablets of lapis. The Greeks and Romans bestowed lapis on those who were to be honoured for their bravery. It was also regarded as a stone of friendship. Ancient physicians regarded lapis as a healing stone of great potency; they saw it as a major remedy for the eyes. They would place a lapis stone in a bowl of warm water and then use the water to bathe affected eyes. It was also used on swellings and on sites of pains especially if the stone was warmed first. It was known as a remedy for ague (malaria), melancholia, neuralgia, spasms, cramps and blood disorders. Lapis is deemed to be ruled by Aquarius. Painters used to use crushed and powdered lapis lazuli to create the deep blue seen today in depictions of the vestments of the Virgin Mary.

Keynote effects

By helping to clear the brow centre lapis facilitates grounding, awareness of necessary mundane practicalities, expansion and the ability to seize opportunities that would otherwise be missed. It balances the idealistic with reality.

General symptoms

Though virtually no physical symptoms were registered in the meditative proving, exhaustion, stagnation and low immunity would be key general symptoms to consider. With the main components being silica and aluminium there might be trembling with fatigue; growing pains in young children especially in those who have a tendency to constipation; loss of stamina and inability to put on weight accompanied by pastiness with dark rings under the eyes. (These may also denote potential pathology of the thyroid.) Nervousness and agitation from insecurity or loss of self-confidence are also highly likely. The presence of sulphuric acid suggests that patients might also suffer from blood disorders including haemorrhaging, ecchymosis, hot flushes and a tendency to boils as well as tremulous weakness and a failure to heal quickly. The presence of chlorine might suggest that the patient would suffer from respiratory problems of the naso-pharyngeal tract, the larynx and the upper lobes of the lungs as well as soreness and dryness of the eyes or inflammation and lachrymation.

Miasms

Psora, tuberculosis and sycosis.

Mental and emotional symptoms

The absence of physical symptoms in the proving seems to mirror this remedy's striking state of being above the physical body. It is highly unlikely that such a universally well-known crystal would be without a complement of physical symptoms and it may be a leading symptom that the patient takes little or no notice of the pathology that actually ails them. Paradoxically, it is a remedy for 'seeing' though seeing through perception. Intuitive and sensitive but has trouble with practical matters. 'In the world but not of it.' Far-seeing but blind to close reality. Idealists who have altruistic motives. (This links them into the Aquarian energy of those who are strongly humanitarian and always seeking the common good, yet paradoxically can be detached, as if one step beyond everyone else.) Can appear to be either haughty or out of reach emotionally or intellectually. If rejected and betrayed deeply enough they can become like **Platina**. They reject the mundane; can be very dismissive. In the negative state they can become haughty and judgemental; bigotry. They prefer to join organizations with a strong structure as they are too impractical to create their own structure. Spaciness, light-headedness; 'head in the clouds'. Very intuitive; perceptive; clear-thinking but all on a limited range of subjects. Intellectuals who get stuck in their minds and who do not feel free enough to use intuition. Feelings of being 'stuck' and as if the world is closing in on them. Feel restricted by outside structures, regimes and influences around them. (So they often seek to escape the structures – such as in a religious group that they belong to or have joined as the organization or group proves too restrictive.) They need and like to be part of a group or family but they must have freedom as well. Claustrophobia. Perfectionist due to their desire for control. The degree of control can shut off the emotions as well. Everything has to be perfect to reflect the perfection of their mental and spiritual aspirations. They tend not to listen to good advice. Others say of them, 'They don't seem to hear what I said.'

Strongly idealistic which can drag them into a tubercular state. Then they seek to expand their boundaries beyond their capabilities and live in a fantasy world in which they imagine great success. Little transpires of this as they become bogged down in the thinking and not in the doing. (This links in with the Sagittarian energy that goes off at tangents into exciting new thought vistas without securing any solid foundation.) They seek perfection before they have dealt with their miasmatic inheritance and karma. (This is a particularly sycotic/syphilitic trait.) Are transported by their enthusiasms so that they forget to complete everyday tasks; get carried away before making certain that they have all the necessary basic information. Poor memory. Fear of the future with guilt about the past which they find hard to deal with because none of it matches up to their spiritual aspirations. Depression < for difficult relationship. Can feel restricted by a partner who isn't giving them enough space though the partner is << by the lack of grounded practicality and inability to live in the here and now. (This can be typically Sagittarian.) They feel better if they can write down their ideas (brow activity); they feel better if they can speak of their ideas (throat centre activity). Nervous anxiety; anticipation; excitability. The remedy is generally calming and uplifting. Eases everyday stresses and strains. Assists the ability to talk on important issues and helps the articulation of ideas. (Works well with **Turquoise** in this aspect.) Restores objectivity in those who are too emotionally involved to see clearly.

Physical symptoms

Almost no physical symptoms were evident from the meditational proving. However, it has been recorded that **Lapis** can be used in the treatment of disorders of:

- the throat and thyroid gland
- the thymus gland
- bone marrow
- the immune system.

It is said to have an affinity to the Eustachian tubes and hearing loss. Can be considered in treating miasmatic inheritance; **Lapis** works well as a support to the nosodes. As the stone is composed of the minerals silica, calcium, aluminium, iron, sodium and sulphur it would seem to follow that **Lapis** is a remedy that has affinities for all the major constitutional types.

Considerations for the use of the remedy

Lapis may not be easy to see in a patient particularly if there is physical pathology present which might sway one's ideas towards using therapeutically chosen remedies or polychrests that would appear to cover the whole picture more. However, **Lapis** is compatible with most remedies and may well be of value as an opening prescription or as one that goes deeper into the finer vibrations of the psyche in cases where the indicated remedies do not seem to penetrate far enough to make lasting change. It is worth considering the following remedies as complementary.

- **Lycopodium** shares many of the characteristic mental and emotional aspects of **Lapis**. Even if there are all the usual **Lycopodium** symptoms of < 4 – 8, disgruntled liver with < sugar, wheat and dairy, hypoglycaemia and so on this does not discount a dose of **Lapis** to encourage mining into a deeper seam of mental and emotional disturbance.
- **Sulphur** may only be differentiated by the usual modalities of heat and thirst as well as its tendency to be dishevelled but, as with **Lycopodium**, these typical symptoms would not preclude a prescription of **Lapis**.
- **Arsenicum Album** may occasionally be found to need a dose of **Lapis** when the patient is not perfectionist about everything but is inclined to be entirely devoted to a particular activity or discipline about which there is the expected fastidiousness.
- **Tuberculinum** shares the **Lapis** idealistic nature.
- **Sepia** in the menopause whose distemper may look similar to **Lapis Lazuli**.
- **Psorinum** is complementary to **Lapis** because it mirrors in the worldly what **Lapis** shows us in the finer vibrations of the spirit. In this regard, **Iron Pyrites,** not yet a well-known or proved remedy, is also complementary.
- **Stonehenge** which helps to bring aspirations to fruition. It is complementary in that it follows well being a remedy to construct or reconstruct a vision of purpose; it galvanizes the will to complete a mission or realize a creative intention.
- **Thuja** (which often precedes **Lapis**) is differentiated by the sense of doubt and anxiety that the patient may do their best to hide.
- **Copper Beech** (another remedy that has trouble sorting out the significance of past experiences) has the fear of not being able to achieve fulfilment before their allotted time and is far more restless and anxious.

Lapis is closely associated with **Pineal Gland** (and its function). Also linked to other crystal remedies: **Fluorite** (both green and purple) as this stone is generally for clarifying the brain so that it can assimilate and understand and store information which is held in such a way that the intuitive process is enhanced.

Esoteric therapeutics

Affects the crown, brow, thyroid, thymus and base chakras. It particularly forges a link between the base and the brow centres. Hence it is often useful to precede it with a complementary base-chakra remedy such as **Psorinum**, **Sulphur** or **Morgan Pure**.

Finds it difficult to reconcile or balance the spiritual element with the physical. Cannot bring spiritual ideas down to earth and process them. For those who aspire (crown and brow centres) but who cannot make their aspirations into a reality (weak spleen energy). The spiritual and the worldly are so far divorced that there is a sense of duality. This makes them easily possessed. Promotes access to and understanding in the esoteric sciences. In this regard it can be used in conjunction with Saturnian, grounding remedies like **Oak** or the other tree remedies. Invaluable for clarifying the clouded vision of the intuitive mind.

Lapis is influenced by the planets Mercury and Jupiter. Mercury may cause considerable confusion and disillusionment. Jupiter may bring on fantasies that are unrealizable. Lapis is the colour of the throat chakra and it is a remedy that heals the energy of this centre. It is excellent for singers who have difficulty with their voices. **Lapis** is preceded well by **Turquoise** which will clear any stuck grief from this centre so that the **Lapis** will help the patient direct the voice in a musical sense.

In crystal healing lapis has a venerable tradition. According to Hall[21] lapis is a royal stone. It was revered in ancient Egypt as a stone to open the heart to love and to lead the soul to immortality. 'A metaphysical stone par excellence, lapis is a key to spiritual attainment.' She goes on to tell us: 'Harmonizing body, emotions, mind and spirit, it brings deep inner self-knowledge and multi-dimensional cellular healing. A powerful thought amplifier, [it] stimulates higher mental faculties and encourages creativity. This stone teaches the value of active listening and helps you to confront truth wherever you find it and to accept its teaching. Facilitating expressing your own opinions and harmonizing conflict, Lapis aids in taking charge of life. This stone brings honesty, compassion and uprightness to the personality.'

21 *Encyclopaedia of Crystals*, Hall

Chakras

Crown

There is difficulty in finding the link between the spiritual, emotional and physical bodies. Though they aspire to the world of their spirit and they may find it easy to inhabit it, they cannot ground any of it. Though they can reflect deeply, they are unable to put any of their insights into practice as the physical world never seems to live up to their high ideals. They may fly in dreams but then not be able to return to waking with anything like an experience.

Brow

There is no true focus in this centre as there is so little ability to discriminate between the real and the unreal, what is illusion and what is fact. Their keen intellect helps to keep them at arm's length emotionally so that detachment is maintained; this is how they prefer it. If they are obliged to make judgements that reflect on the worldly aspect of things then they can be harsh and unfair. Yet at other times they appear to be dreamy and 'not able to see the wood for the trees'. They may have strong intuition but it works chiefly, it seems to them, to keep trouble at bay whereas, in fact, it merely prevents them from learning more about the people and circumstances that are around them. They are alert to psychic attack, sometimes so much so that others might say that they are paranoid or at least oversensitive to criticism. It is also for those who prefer to live in an intellectual bubble and rely on the brain to provide all important information. This is a remedy of missed opportunity due to the brow centre's habit of raising its sights too high for anything mundane to be wholly acceptable.

Throat

The ears hear but are deaf to the ordinary; the voice speaks but the words are carefully measured in case they encourage too much closeness. Self-expression is difficult as there is little apparent warmth for anything but the closest relationships such as with spouse and children. This is a person who is described as distant while those who know him or her well realize that there is difficulty in expressing the inner world. There can be thyroid insufficiency as a result of this situation.

Heart

The heart seems closed though this conceals much soul-searching that goes unnoticed by others. The heart energy wants to reach upwards into the realm of spirit and does not want to deal with much that is earthly. In the extremity of symptomatic distress or in old age, this patient is inclined to declare that they do not want to be here. Hidden in this picture is a certain amount of disappointment in their sense of achievement. High blood pressure is a likely manifestation of physical trouble.

Solar plexus

Earthly challenges are uncomfortable; conflicts are anathema. This is not a competitive soul. Their main earthly challenge is to do with securing a congenial atmosphere that is conducive to harmony and calm. If this is not possible then they will have a difficult time with their digestion and their eliminative processes. Constipation should be expected.

Sacral

This chakra is affected at the level of the kidneys. Emotions are not strongly in evidence, not because they are not there but because they are deeply held and heavily guarded. The water balances of the body therefore may be upset and cause difficulties with urinating or with retention of water. In women there are hormonal difficulties which manifest in a way to illustrate retreat and a search for simplicity which is unrealizable. In aspects of earthly love, the **Lapis** patient will be inclined to idealize the partner or, if in a tubercular phase, to be overindulgent in sexual activity.

Base

Anxiety and fear undermine this chakra. It is to run away from facing the harsh lessons enforced by Saturn that a person arrives at the point of needing this remedy. Among those Saturnian lessons are those of the miasms: the patient does not want to deal with the forms of elimination that are dictated by deeply held miasmatic influences, especially those of the psoric and syphilitic states. For this reason it is not unusual for a patient to come for treatment when they are displaying typical signs of the tubercular miasm, that is in a state of wanting to break away and find new ground. **Lapis** often causes a patient to 'come down to earth'.

Case studies

1 'Female 42: homoeopath and single mother. A regular patient of homoeopathy who had suffered severe back pain with right-sided sciatica (for which she had successfully taken **Kali-carb** 200) and residual but debilitating aching in the lower right leg (which had been removed with **Lachesis** 6 once a day for three days). She returned feeling more positive and wanting to make decisions about moving home and completing her studies. "I've got slightly more focus but I want to be in touch with my higher self. I need to be in fullest command of my third-eye centre so I can continue with my decisions."

'Apart from low energy from time to time, she was otherwise well. She is a sensitive person who relies a lot on her sense of intuition yet she still felt stuck. There has been much in the last few years that has obliged her to concentrate on domestic and family issues and the health of her young daughter. She has given the impression of being someone trapped in a domestic situation from which she sees little relief. She has seemed frustrated by not being able to use her training and her intuitive gifts for practising. She was given **Lapis Lazuli** 1M (one at night and one in the morning) followed by **Clear Quartz** 30 (one 2x per week for six weeks). The **Lapis** was prescribed on the constitutional picture and the **Clear Quartz** was used to amplify its effect and to establish a greater balance between left and right sides of her body, something which she herself acknowledged was a problem.

When she had finished the six weeks of the **Clear Quartz** she rang the clinic to ask for some more of the whole prescription as she had felt so well since taking the first lot. "Fantastic remedy! I really liked it! I found huge, positive aspects straight away. I've got lots done. I had this shooting of energy up into here (brow). There was no putting up with any rubbish! I've had a different head-fill. It's really shifted things. I've concentrated on school issues for one thing. I'm much more flexible about things. That chitter-chatter mind stuff is just not there. I've had a really clear two months. I haven't felt so heavy. I've just felt more positive. I've looked into courses; I've put my house on the market. I've looked at one or two properties and feel it's the right thing to move; I've started doing some life-coaching. I've faced up to this whole procrastination thing. I've felt more like my old self than I have for the last three years." (It is worth noting that this patient felt that the degree of focus she attained was unusually clear and almost like wearing blinkers. She felt that her field of intellectual vision when dealing with whatever her mind was set on was narrowed to a point, very much as if she were aiming her sights at something. This is in line with the way others have experienced the effects of **Clear Quartz**. [See **Clear Quartz**, case 1.])' **CG**

2 'Male patient, 62, cartoonist. His work as a cartoonist had been very successful but the work had always been erratic. He came feeling very depressed and creatively blocked; something that he had never previously experienced. I gave **Lapis Lazuli** 1M as I felt that he somehow had never fully expressed his potential despite his enormous success. Within two weeks of taking the remedy he had written a full musical – lyrics and music. He hadn't realized he had any musical talent but had picked up a keyboard in his daughter's room and begun playing!' **HJ**

17

LIMONIUM SINUATUM

Statice

Limonium or statice first came to attention as a potential remedy when gathered by Martin Miles and the author with Janice Micallef in May 2005 during a Guild of Homoeopaths seminar week on the island of Paros, Greece. The plant grows plentifully along the shores of the island and it was in flower during May. Though the students had come together to do meditative provings of **Senecio + Tyria Jacobeae** and **Aquamarine**, **Statice** called our attention with its colour; it appeared to create a mauve or amethyst haze along the beach. Despite the delicacy of the colour, the energy of the plant seemed to be very strong and had a deeply relaxing quality. (It was interesting to note that the swath of statice plants from which the sample was taken was bulldozed into the sand at the end of the week's stay in preparation for the summer season of tourists.) A spontaneous proving of the plant occurred on the evening of its collection when Janice, Martin and the author were sitting in conversation with the bunch of statice on the table in front of us. (See page 236 for the details.)

The full meditative proving did not take place until 9 November 2007. This was during the period of Scorpio ('the month of the ancestors' which marks the start of the passing of the year) and two months after Martin had died. This was the first meditative proving of the group that had convened without Martin's presence in almost seventeen years.

The Background

Limonium is a member of the Plumbaginaceae family (leadwort). It has various common names, such as sea lavender and marsh rosemary but is best known as statice or (when used in dried flower arrangements) everlasting; it is not related to lavender or rosemary. The remedy is made from one of some 125 species; it is the commonest variety that grows vigorously in Greece from where the specimen was taken. It is mostly a perennial herbaceous plant that inhabits salt marshes and seashore sites or cliffs; other varieties prefer alkaline or gypsum soil and grow in the interior of continental masses.

The plant is rough to the touch as its curiously four-winged stem is covered in tiny stiff hairs. Each of the abundant corymbs (panicles) is three-winged and bears papery, violet-blue calyxes with tiny white flowers. It can grow up to 40 cm in height from a basal rosette of pinnately-lobed leaves. The plant is apomictic: it reproduces without fertilization which means that its seeds are genetically identical to the parent plant. Apomixis is nature's own cloning device. Limonium has been cultivated in Britain since 1791. It is often used for floral decorations and dried to create flower arrangements.

It is worth quoting from *A Modern Herbal* by Mrs M Grieve who writes about the American sea lavender:

> It has long been in use as a domestic remedy for diarrhoea, dysentery, etc. but is only used as an astringent tonic after the acute stage has passed. It is also very useful as a gargle or wash in ulcerations of mouth and throat, scarlatina, anguinosa, etc. The powdered root is applied to old ulcers or made with a soothing ointment for piles. As an injection the decoction is very useful in chronic gonorrhoea, gleet, leucorrhoea, prolapsus of womb and anus and in some ophthalmic affections.

(A decoction is one ounce of powdered root to one pint in wineglassful doses.)

Keynote effects

This is one of a number of remedies for healing the long-continued effects of ancestral energy: the unresolved issues that have become a maintaining cause for the patient even if it seems to have little to do with the presenting complaint (which is particularly true when other, better-indicated remedies have been given and have failed to relieve). It releases patients from being stuck on the deepest levels of the psyche and spirit. It also works on the level of the miasms which have become ever more firmly entrenched in patients' vital forces. It affords a patient greater awareness of his or her physical body, of the relationship between the psyche and the body and of ways in which the patient can take responsibility for the internal cleansing and healing of that body. It is said to be one of the most useful remedies for alignment of the spine. A key word in the understanding of the remedy is 'entanglement'; the patient is afforded the opportunity to undo the knots tied in all the threads of history that make up his or her past.

General symptoms

Statice works on nerves, the heart and circulation, the endocrine and digestive systems and the skin. It has an affinity for the throat and the thyroid, the spinal column, the coccyx and the digestion.

Paralysis and conditions of the nerve fibres. Restores integrity to the endocrine system especially when the pituitary gland has been compromised; the body clock is out of sync. Has an effect on the cerebrospinal fluid and restores the connection between the hypothalamus and the pituitary. This may result from the harmful effects of the many types of pollution that can disturb endocrine function: medical drugs, vaccination, radiation. Heart conditions including angina. To be considered in cases of thyroid pathology when indicated remedies do not complete their action. Dryness of mucous membranes: lungs dry out; emphysema. Joints dry out: arthritis, ankylosing spondylitis. Encourages the drying up of mother's milk. Re-establishes the water balance in the body. Breakdown (psoric) of tissue: osteoporosis; repair of necrosed tissue: after myocardial infarction. Breakdown of body's defences from artificial substances in diet. Restores the integrity of cycles: menses. Doziness and sleepiness or insomnia. Eczema and psoriasis: of use as an intercurrent for indicated remedies that do not complete their action. Digestion: used in low potency it is helpful in improving assimilation and absorption. It helps to restore to consciousness the connection between the patient and their digestive system, so easily disturbed by poor routine, pollution, speedy lifestyle and bad habit.

A dose of **Statice** before birth is said to limit the strength of influence of the ancestral themes of trauma in the baby's family. As **Statice** is complementary to many remedies called for by the birth process, it is worth considering as an intercurrent at this stage of life.

Miasms

Psora, syphilis, sycosis, tuberculosis, leprosy and radiation.

Mental and emotional symptoms

Statice restores conscious awareness where it has been lost through persistent familial patterns of behaviour, grief, bad habit, pollution, orthodox medication, or unresolved relationships or events that hold the patient as a victim of birth and circumstance. Patients who have been conditioned not to be able to see their own reality; they view life through the filter of another's influence. It may seem that the patient's emotional responses are stunted. There is some loss of the individual's identity. This is very much a remedy for the 21st century in that **Statice** awakens a patient to becoming a self-determining individual capable of making choices that set him or her on the appropriate life path after he or she has been subjected to years of suppressive relationships, education, etc. Such patients may seem to be willing to set out on the road of self-healing through alternative means but sooner or later they falter, finding the going too difficult. When this is suspected, it is often the moment to consider the use of Statice. Part of the picture is that the patient is either unclear about or uninterested in what is best for him or her especially regarding diet and nutrition. There is a blind spot about health issues, about who to see for medical help or about the need for fresh air and exercise and looking after the physical body. The patient may even be doing well with homoeopathic remedies but then choose to see the doctor or a specialist. There is a sensitivity due to heightened sensory response to environment, atmosphere, colour and touch.

A fear of disease, of death, of change; the fear of change is very strong. This fear of change leads to a feeling of insecurity as indicated remedies begin to make changes in the patient's life. It is as if he or she does not want to give responsibility to Nature to bring about evolutionary change. It is as if the patient is habitually stuck in the state of disjunct physical, emotional and spiritual bodies. (Hence the wish to see doctors who take over the responsibility for the healing of the physical body.) Of use in treating men with confidence and adequacy problems in relation to women.

Poor memory especially for names. Mind feels either blank or thick and 'difficult to move' < for a sense of congestion in the frontal lobe. The patient may give the impression of being 'entangled' in some way or express themselves as being locked into a family pattern. The story that is unfolded (possibly over several appointments) is complex, convoluted and often confusing. It is usual for the life history to be a tapestry of connective threads stretching back into the lives of the parents and grandparents particularly on the mother's side. In this history there is a lot of unresolved trauma and grief that may not actually be anything directly to do with the patient. Nevertheless, the energy of all this past history is what is blocking the patient's progress beyond the mundane, routine and habitual. Statice has been suggested as a remedy that may become useful in the treatment of people with learning difficulties.

Physical symptoms

Head
Intense pressure in the brow area. A sense of being blocked in the front of the brain. Intense throbbing in the frontal area at times. A feeling of congestion in the head which interferes with thinking. Pressure in the frontal area < over the right eye and extending down the nose.

Eyes
Changes in vision that cause the patient concern. Fear of blindness. Dryness of the eyes (possibly < menopause).

Nose and sinuses
Stuffy sensation as if a cold were about to start though it comes to nothing. Stuffy nose that feels dried out. Sensitivity in the right nostril as if a sneeze were coming on or even as if a nose bleed were about to happen.

Face
Sharp pain that extends from right upper jaw vertically up the cheek.

Throat
Sore throat that seems to herald a cold. Dry throat; feels parched but without thirst. Throat is tickly with 'claggy' mucus with a slimy mouth. Pathology of

the thyroid gland < for spinal misalignment. Throat can feel as if shaped like a funnel.

Chest
Tired feeling in the lungs and chest with discomfort around the lower ribs.

Heart and circulation
Palpitations. Sensation of blood coursing through the body. Angina. Reynaud's syndrome.

Stomach
Nausea; nausea and pain when dealing with the stress of change. Appetite for the wrong food and drink. Digestive system feels tired and overtaxed.

Abdomen
Tension and discomfort in the intestinal tract. Sensation of sagging.

Back and nervous system
Stiffness of the spine. Paralysis, creeping. Tingling and numbness. The remedy has an affinity for all nerve fibres. Of use in treating patients with MS. Also after acute injuries where **Hypericum** has been of service. Twitching of the nerves. May be of use in treating patients suffering from scoliosis or kyphosis. Indicated in those whose posture has altered to accommodate pain after acute or traumatic pain. Follows **Emerald** after operations when the patient's body may have been forced out of alignment. Also to be considered after a patient has been mistreated osteopathically. Neck is stiff. Coccyx is chronically painful: dragging, aching and sensitive.

Limbs
Jerking of the legs.

Fever
NBWS feverish infection. Patient feels out of sorts since flu, cold, fever.

Skin
Eczema. Psoriasis.

Considerations for the use of the remedy

Statice can be compared with and contrasted to several other remedies including **Ayahuasca, Emerald, Sycamore Seed, Plutonium, Moldavite, Rose Quartz** and **Rosebay Willowherb**. It is also helpful to consider it in the light of other remedies such as **Aconite, Arsen-alb, Thuja** and **Syphilinum**.

- **Ayahuasca** is just as much a remedy for tangled history especially where there is a connection with the maternal line. However, **Ayahuasca** is often easier to see early on in a case and there is always some degree of chronic fear that is more apparent than with **Statice**. **Statice's** fear is more to do with change and the state of the physical body's relation with the circumstances and environment on one hand and with the emotions and spirit on the other. **Ayahuasca** is far less concerned with the outside world and, even though not articulated, more aware of the dangers to the mind and spirit.

- **Emerald** is a remedy to do with the state of the ego; it has been called the 'wounded ego'. **Statice** is much less easily defined; the ego has been less wounded than emasculated or suppressed so that individuality is threatened. In **Emerald** there is little sense of the ego being subsumed by the weight of family history.

- **Sycamore Seed** should be considered as a remedy close to **Statice** in that it precedes it and follows it well in the treatment of those who have spinal misalignment. It is also often called for in the treatment of the pituitary, the hypothalamus and for realigning the body clock through its affinity for and work on the sphenoid bone – a part that can so easily be compromised when the spine has been traumatized or has lost alignment.

- **Plutonium** and **Moldavite** are both remedies that can create profound life changes that a patient needing **Statice** would find not only difficult but potentially threatening. Preceding either of these remedies with **Statice** may encourage the patient to trust the process of healing at this level.

- **Rose Quartz** is a remedy of inestimable value in treating patients with heart and circulation pathology. It is entirely complementary with **Statice**.

- **Rosebay Willowherb** has in common with **Statice** the core theme of separation between the body, mind and spirit. However, in **RBWH** the patient is very likely to be struggling with the cancer miasm while **Statice** patients are seeking to become unencumbered of ancestral energy. Patients who do not deal with their **Statice** state are likely to reach a condition in which they need **RBWH**.

- **Aconite**: in moments of crisis when **Aconite** might be indicated, **Statice** may well be called for to follow.
- **Arsen-alb**: can feel just as insecure about change especially when the underlying constitution is **Calc-carb**. The **Arsen-alb** patient (especially in heart conditions) is just as likely to consult both alternative practitioner and doctor and thus confuse the healing outcome.
- **Thuja** may be required to unblock the brow centre to ensure clearer perception of the patient's predicament. **Statice** may become more obviously indicated after a dose of **Thuja** in a high potency. **Statice** may well turn out to be a remedy commonly used after **Thuja** and **Arsen-alb** have been prescribed for conditions such as asthma.
- **Syphilinum** is one to follow or precede **Statice** as the latter is regarded as a profoundly syphilitic remedy. Though **Statice** may not seem particularly syphilitic in its physical symptoms (at least, the symptoms as we know them to date), it is so, by dint of the slow but sure progress to self-destruction by means of wrong choices and neglect of the correct nurture of the body.

Another remedy that should be considered along with **Statice** is **Thymus Gland**. In cases where the ancestral connection is strong and the patient is unaware of how to become a purposeful individual, broken free from the influence of the past, then **Thymus Gland** needs to be considered as a potential partner in a combination with Statice. An example would be **TG + Ayahuasca + Statice**. Another might be **TG + Statice + Syphilinum**. A third might be **TG + Aquamarine + Statice**. Aconite + Statice + Rose Quartz is a combination to consider in acute angina cases. It is safe to use this in the 200, 1M or the 10M before giving the indicated remedy (i.e. **Cactus, Latrodectus, Arsen-alb** or **Naja**) as it can take the fear out of the situation.

Statice + Plutonium + Syphilinum is a combination for cases of an extremely stubborn nature where the patients are completely unenlightened as to their potential for individuality. They are completely locked into illusion and delusion about how the world is and have no idea of the concept of mental and emotional autonomy, their lives being governed by the strongest bonds of familial conditioning. Their judgement is clouded and they are always led to make wrong choices, often the same choices they made before or that were made before by others. **Statice** patients are as if conditioned to follow blindly where others, usually of the female family line, went before.

Esoteric therapeutics

This is a remedy for the loosening and gradual release of ancestral karmic energy that is acting as a maintaining cause for pathology in the patient. For those who find it impossible to shift away from chronic illness or firmly held emotional troubles despite the best intentions and perfectly adequate prescribing. In this context it is best given with a preliminary dose of the miasmatic nosode that most illustrates the condition. It may also be given in combination with the nosode of choice plus **Thymus Gland** in an LM potency for the prescription to reach the deepest level. Alternatively, **Statice** with the nosode and a complementary crystal remedy will form a deep-acting combination that can be prescribed either as a single dose or as a repeated weekly dose. The crystal remedies that most complement **Statice** are **Amethyst**, **Aquamarine**, **Rose Quartz**, **Lapis Lazuli**, **Moonstone** and **Rhodochrosite**. In those cases where the practitioner perceives a degree of darkness about the aura then **Moldavite** can be of service. **Ayahuasca** is also a remedy that has an affinity for **Statice** as it has such a lot to do with connections to forebears. Where the effects of **Statice** need to be amplified in order to effect the necessary reaction towards healing then **Clear Quartz** will be of most value.

Statice is a remedy to consider in clearing houses of negative ancestral energy. It can be used for spraying the house to be treated by putting the remedy into the water of a new house plant spray.

Chakras

Crown
Enhances spiritual awareness and reception; facilitates meditative practice; clarifies spiritual issues. All the work done on the other chakras up to the prescription of **Statice** would have been having the effect of clearing the path for eventual spiritual awakening. The whole process may be likened to spiritual evolution; a spiritual metamorphosis.

Brow

One of the great remedies to unblock the clouded or blinded brow centre. It is comparable with **Calendula, Calc-carb, Moonstone, Lapis Lazuli** and **Sycamore Seed**. There is a sense in all these remedies of not being able to see what needs to be done to make progress. The patient is not in control of hormone output; the body clock is not functioning properly. The cerebrospinal fluid is as if in need of cleansing; it is sluggish and torpid.

Throat

Lack of ability to express at this fundamental level. The remedy fosters the link between base and heart while opening the brow so that the throat may express the need to choose a different direction in life.

Parathyroid

Helps with difficulty in stabilizing when caught between illusion/delusion and reasonable normality.

Heart

All the excessive sensitivity of the physical body is a form of expression for the suppressed heart. The remedy opens the heart chakra up to the possibility of change. It is said to bring the sense of joy back into the heart centre.

Solar plexus

The nutritional problems of this remedy are also an expression of the closed heart and brow centres. Low potency (6x or 9x) doses given over a long period may help the patient to become aware of how he or she is not attending to his or her own personal needs. This is a patient who needs to be taught to re-evaluate his or her diet. They become aware of nutrition as part of the healing process.

Sacral

The kidney energy is not strong in **Statice** patients. They do not drink enough pure fluids. They need to be encouraged to school themselves to drink more water and to avoid tea, coffee and alcohol. Some may need to stop drinking too much fruit juice. Men may feel downtrodden and unable to own their masculinity fully. Others may be heavily macho and prefer to disown their feminine side. The remedy helps these men to achieve a balance. (See **Ash**.)

Base

Out of touch with essentials; poor sense of boundaries; loss of connection with Nature. Enables one to overcome fear especially of the unknown and of the future. Encourages one to put experience to good use. Enables one to receive from and connect with ancestral roots. One of the main remedies for those whose spirit or emotional energy is not in alignment with the physical body. This is one of the great realigning remedies. Often useful for those with constantly relapsing skin conditions. The remedy affords basic protection for the aura. The constitution is strengthened so that the five senses do not react in a way that is disturbing to the economy of the body.

Unofficial proving on Paros

On the evening of the first day of the week on the island, while we were relaxing over a hot drink, the conversation between Martin Miles, Janice Micallef and myself turned to personal history. Within a few minutes Janice got up to fetch a notebook, saying that we had gone into a spontaneous proving of **Statice** (which we only knew as 'everlasting' at that time), a bunch of which was lying in front of us on the table. Martin spoke openly about his difficult past with his mother and how her life story had indelibly marked his own. He felt that her life had been the result of family karma especially held in the female line. As he spoke he was visibly moved and clearly felt his connection with his mother very strongly, something that he had not felt for a long time. In my turn, I was reminded of the strength of personality of my own mother and her extraordinary resilience in the face of considerable hardship throughout her life. Through this I, too, was brought to consider the fault lines of female energy running through my ancestors and spoke of their powerful influence on me. However, we all subsequently forgot about the notebook in which Janice had been jotting down the details of the conversation. It was only when it came to writing up the proving from the transcripts of the meditations that we remembered it, though at first Janice thought she had lost it. We found that most of those early thoughts were germane to the proving.

Case studies

1 'A 34-year-old Cancerian woman came following a break-up with her husband. She has had two children, now teenagers. There is a family history of syphilis on her mother's side and of sycosis on her father's side. She feels devastated by her husband's decision; he left her saying that he was gay and he blamed her for the failure of the marriage and his need to break free. She is fearful of becoming ill and is terrified of death. Her digestion is bad: she has problems with assimilation and absorption. Her heart centre and solar plexus are closed down. Over time she was given **Nat-mur, Carcinosin, Syphilinum, Opium, Ignatia, Lycopodium** and **Arsen-alb** all of which had some influence if only for her to slip back. She was given **Statice** 10M, single collective dose. Within two days she said that she felt completely calmed down. She went to her solicitor for advice about the breakdown of her marriage. She had an aggravation of the symptoms in her digestion for which she sought her doctor's advice but never took the prescription given to her. After a further dose of **Statice** 10M she returned feeling completely well.' JM

2 'A nine-year-old boy who was a Virgo was brought for treatment. He had been rejected by his mother at birth. His mother had wanted a girl and when she found out that she had a boy she had a fit of screaming in the ward, so much so that the midwife had had to remonstrate with her. At the moment that the mother started her tirade the baby had turned blue. He had never been well since. His brow and throat chakras were blocked. The boy's attitude and behaviour were not pleasant. He was rude, surly and truculent. He was nasty to his friends. He never spoke in the consultations. He was given **Statice** 10M. He became a very nice boy after this and it held.' JM

Janice Micallef writes: 'I use **Statice** in clearing houses of difficult energies especially when the problem is of ancestral origin. I also always like to give **Statice** to a mother in her third trimester. I give it one each week for three weeks before the baby is born as it seems to facilitate the birth. [See 'Case studies' in **Blue**.] Two women who suffered from Parkinson's who both had dysfunctional parents were given **Statice** with excellent results on relieving the shaking.'

18

MALUS DOMESTICA

Orchard Apple Tree

The proving was carried out on 30 April 1999 by 9 members of the regular proving circle with the medium. It was later proved again by the second group of 7 women and 3 men.

The remedy was made from an old apple tree whose bark was covered in oak moss and lichen, whose form was twisted and gnarled and which, in spite of not having been pruned for many years still produced abundant quantities of fruit. The tree grew in an untouched orchard in Hampshire in the UK and had not been sprayed at any time with any chemicals. The parts taken were the bark, the twig and the leaf. The remedy became known as **Apple Tree** before the correct nomenclature was established. Therefore, it is likely that it will continue to be commonly referred to in the vernacular.

The Background

The remedy comes from an indeterminate sweet orchard apple. *The Illustrated Encyclopaedia of Trees* tells us that 'The Orchard Apple is not a true species in the strict botanical or horticultural sense. It has no wild predecessor but is wholly man-made by selection and breeding. It is thought that *Malus sylvestris*, *Malus dasphylla* and *Malus praecox* were used as parents but other Asiatic species such as *Malus sieversii* may also have been involved. Centuries of development and a few happy accidents have resulted in sweet eating apples and sharp fruit for cooking and for cider. It is reckoned that over 1000 species have been named. However, modern legislation and mass-production have reduced diversity. Just a handful of good-looking cultivars now dominate the market and many fine-tasting varieties have become very rare. The ordinary garden with an old named apple tree in it is increasingly important for the future conservation of obscure threatened cultivars. The British countryside in particular is littered with "apple core progeny" – trees that have grown from discarded cores of apples eaten many years ago. Abandoned rural railway lines and country lanes are common locations and even urban roadsides still support a few trees. Most are of little consequence but some bear very acceptable fruit.'

This remedy is not to be confused with **Malus Sylvestris**, which comes from a small tree, native to Europe, Scandinavia and parts of Asia Minor. The *Encyclopaedia* also tells us that 'Everywhere it is confused with the domestic apple trees which have escaped from cultivation and become naturalised. The fruit of the true Crab Apple is 2 – 3 cm across, yellow-green, flushed with light red and often speckled with tiny white spots . . . Crab Apple was one of several species used in the development of hybrid domestic apples and seedlings were cultivated for use as under-stocks on which to graft orchard apples . . . It is often a shapeless tree with several stems and a bushy top. Some branches, especially towards the base, develop short pointed spur shoots. Trees of up to 200 years old are known.'

Many species of apple tree are quite hardy, surviving relatively low temperatures, some trees managing well below freezing. Most species provide wood that is excellent for veneers and decoration. Craftsmen delight in using apple for its beautiful grain and warm colour though it is a wood that is tricky to season as it tends to split if dried too quickly. It is much sought after by sculptors as it is a very hard wood that carves well. It is commonly used by woodturners for carving into small pieces such as fruit or figurines.

Mrs Grieve tells us that the chief dietary value of the apple lies in the malic and tartaric acids which are of most benefit to people of sedentary habit, liable to liver disorders (such as gout) and whose systems are hyperacidic. These acids in the fruit help the body to digest other foods. It was one of the reasons for people in previous centuries being so keen on apple sauce with rich foods such as pork and goose. It has been noted that people who have drunk sugar-free cider have been virtually free from calculi (stone formation). Apple cider vinegar is an invaluable digestive aid in those who are over-acidic as it assists in creating the correct balance between acid and alkali in the body.

It has long had a medicinal reputation for rheumatic and arthritic aches and pains. Mary Thorne Quelch, in *Herbal Remedies and Recipes* (1945), says 'The belief that eating apples will keep old age at bay is very, very ancient. In Norse mythology, when the gods realized they were growing old, they adopted a diet of apples, convinced their youth and energy would be restored. That apples could possess any such power would be scoffed at in the last century but now the pendulum is swinging the other way and modern analysis has shown that apples contain a larger proportion of phosphorus than any other fruit and phosphorus renews and strengthens the nerves of body and brain.' Stewed or very ripe apple has been known as an agent of relief in constipation. However, Mrs Quelch warns that the old adage 'An apple a day keeps the doctor away' may not be entirely reliable: it was 'probably intended to convey the information that eating apples will prevent or cure constipation. That is not true invariably. There are people who suffer from acute indigestion after eating apples either raw or cooked and in some extreme cases declare the fruit actually causes constipation.'

In ancient times the apple also played a significant role. The Trojan Wars were the result of a competition between the goddesses, Hera, Aphrodite and Athena as to who was the most beautiful. Hermes gave an apple to the Trojan prince, Paris, to award to the one he thought most lovely. On being bribed by Aphrodite with the love of Helen, he chose her to the fury of the other two deities who promptly initiated the downfall of Troy. Pomona, the Roman goddess of fruitful orchards, was regarded as the protector of apple trees. Her feast fell on 1 November, after the harvest, when games would be played, apple bobbing among them, cider would be drunk and baked apples eaten. This feast was later associated with Halloween or Samhain, a Druidic festival in ancient Britain coinciding with that time in the year when the veil between the living and the spirit world is considered at its thinnest and when celebrants would be able to go on shamanic journeys in search of understanding, knowledge and healing by connecting with the spirit home of ancestors. This is the month of Scorpio, the sign of greatest hypersensitivity and anxiety about the processes of destruction and the one that is directly opposite Taurus, the sign most associated with the fecund spring.

Some writers have thought it unfortunate that it was the apple that was hijacked by the translators of the Bible to be the tree of the knowledge of good and evil when fruitfulness and abundance are what it signifies so strongly. Yet this is to confuse the tree with the serpent that tempted Eve. The Eden metaphor makes more sense when the apple tree is seen as providing Adam the opportunity to understand himself; to become aware of his relationship with his world; to feel confident enough to go out of the Garden to make his own way. Ancient Celtic legends, among which there is a garden and tree myth, tell us that there was a magical silver apple branch, the silver bough, that represented a link with the unseen world, the world of spirit. Thus the tree of the knowledge of good and evil becomes rather less threatening and more benign. Perhaps there is no surprise in the fact that Venus is said to rule this tree.

Keynote effects

The gradual reduction of hypersensitivity on any or all levels. It affords the patient more time and space to seek calm and quiet in order to allow natural processes to be re-established in those whose lives have become affected by anxiety and excessive thinking and in those who feel that they have 'lost their way'. A remedy to foster a sense of stillness after agitation and restlessness. Following this there is a greater sense of knowing one's direction. More than anything, this is a remedy of self-knowledge.

General symptoms

Sensitivity on all levels of the mental, the emotional and the physical body. Allergies: any type of allergic reaction or physical intolerance may call for this remedy. Weaknesses, dizziness and impaired functioning of the vital organs from multiple allergic reactions. The remedy works on the oversensitivity and over-reactivity of body chemistry; where cellular activity is chaotic or difficult to assess. Assimilation and digestion are improved. It purifies the blood and balances and organizes the endocrine system where these are disturbed by excessive sensitivity. Where the digestion and the blood chemistry is broken down; on the point of physical collapse. Patient might appear to be reasonably well but might actually be very unwell. Helps to rebuild the constitution of those suffering from wheat, dairy and sugar intolerance. If this proves to be so then the patient should follow a very strict dietary regime. Affects the spine especially in those who have symptoms < by poor nerve conduction through the coeliac plexus which is common in wheat and gluten allergies. Cleanses the cerebrospinal fluid: refines and balances it so that hormonal output is optimized.

Inoculation damage. Helpful during the menopause. ME and chronic fatigue syndrome. Tendency to develop cancers and tumours. The remedy is said to help the body to shrink cancerous tumours especially those of the brain. Restores the integrity of the cranial rhythm by affecting the pituitary, the sphenoid and the ventricles of the brain. (Follows and works well with **Sycamore Seed**.) Soothes and aids the mucous membranes in the alimentary canal: restores proper digestion. Eases constipation (see **Black Obsidian** below). Emphysema or blocked energy in the lungs. Another remedy to encourage purification of the liver. It profoundly and positively affects the spleen and in so doing encourages a renewal of creative spirit energy. A remedy to consider in terminal cases where the patient is uncomfortable and distressed; they are stuck in a limbo of medication and fear and have little peace of mind to order their thoughts and feelings (see **Dolphin Sonar**).

Miasms

Psora, tuberculosis, sycosis, cancer and leprosy.

Mental and emotional symptoms

The patient may have been engaged in chuntering thoughts about just who they really are: 'Who am I and what am I doing here?' A desire to be swallowed up into 'nothingness'; desire not to have to think and react. Mental exhaustion. Slowness. Feels locked into the brain; trapped in the head. Feelings of being lost. Unable to find the right terms to express themselves so they remain silent though much still goes on inside the head. Feels like a prisoner. Determined and stubborn. A desire to shout or scream from all the emotions that are bottled up. Violent thoughts which are never voiced but that feel like an inner expression of anger. Has been suggested as a remedy for autistic tendencies. Feelings of confusion. Oversensitivity especially in the fearful. Sensitive to criticism; to slights; to humiliation; to 'atmospheres'. > Children who become excessively sensitive especially after inoculation; children who are afraid of school. There is fearfulness of the ageing process (see **Fagus-purp** in *Volume I*). Fear of dying. Feels alone and lonely. Patient might not be aware that he or she is lonely. The remedy helps people to feel the need to seek a link with others. Feeling blank; wants to sit and drift in and out of thoughts. Sense of not being able to get back to where one was. Oversensitivity of the psyche. Speaks quickly; more quickly than usual. Mental instability and hysteria. Helps to alert sensitive people to the truth about relationships that are built on false premises; that are manipulative rather than unconditional.

Physical symptoms

Head

Pressure in the head; a sense of great activity in the head. Heaviness; from containing too much thinking. Head is generally sensitive. Strong desire to have peace in the head. A sense of everything passing to and fro through the head. Brain chunter. A sense of having feelings held in the head. Pressure on the right side of the head. A possible choice for brain tumours where other remedies may not be indicated or do not fulfil expectations. Sensation of a blockage in the forehead.

Eyes

Right eye waters. Has been suggested as a remedy for optical illusions.

Face

Heat in the face; in the cheeks.

Throat

Fear of choking. Sensation of lump in the throat. Throat feels blocked.

Heart

Raised heartbeat with sense of pressure in the head especially in the forehead. Oppression about the heart area.

Male and Female

Sense of blockage in the uterine region. Menopausal symptoms including hot flushes which manifest particularly in the head, face and hands though are felt all over. Revitalizes sexual energy.

Skin

Roughness of the skin; dermatitis; allergic or reactive eczema.

Back

Lower back ache < the sacrum and lumber regions especially in those with scoliosis. Pain in the left scapula. Pain at the bottom of the neck. Spasms in the neck < right.

Sleep

Restless and wakeful with anxious dreams.

Considerations for the use of the remedy

The patient manifesting symptoms similar to **Apple Tree** is likely to feel uncomfortable in terms of allergies in the spring months (though this is not incontrovertible) while in the opposite time of year, as the autumn leads into winter, they are likely to feel more insecure emotionally. This swing between the physical and the emotional is not always part of the picture but if it is evident it can be a pointer to prescribing **Apple Tree**.

Comparisons with other remedies include the following:

- There is much in **Apple Tree** that might remind us of **Arsen-alb** with the restlessness, anxiety and feeling worse for not being in control. In a patient with allergies prominent in the case whose symptoms seem to indicate **Arsen-alb** but who does not respond thoroughly, **Apple Tree** may complete the process of improvement or make it possible for the more familiar remedy to work more deeply.
- There are similarities with **Nat-mur** in the mental and emotional sphere: resentment and withdrawal being the most obvious ones. **Apple Tree** is complementary to **Nat-mur** though an intercurrent dose may well initiate changes that seem to move away from the latter remedy in favour of brow and crown chakra remedies such as **Rainbow** or **Purple**; even **Moldavite**.
- **Baryta-carb** is also an obvious comparison to make given that both remedies cover mental exhaustion, anxiety and the desire to avoid conflict. Yet **Apple Tree** is more potentially volatile and hypersensitive.

Works well with the nosodes, **Psorinum**, **Tuberculinum** and **Medorrhinum**; also **Carcinosin** before the cancerous state becomes physically manifested. Can appear like a cross between **Baryta-carb**, **Silica** and **Arsen-alb**. Works well and supports the action of **Emerald** and is supported well by **Green**. The same is true in relation to the bowel nosodes, **Proteus** and **Gaertner**. Follows **Sycamore Seed** well.

Esoteric therapeutics

Gives the subject (either in meditation or through intuition) the sensitivity to receive only the correct information. It allows the subject to discern what is true and what is false – which means that it sifts out of the subconscious any receiving of the intuition that is fostered by the sycotic miasm. > Spiritual discernment. It helps to illuminate what is illusory and delusional. It balances the chakras. Is said to help subjects to process karma. Protects those who are subject to the manipulative or evil thoughts and wishes of others (see **Olive**). Encourages the generation of wisdom rather than cleverness. Apples are associated with worldly knowledge. Links the past with the future to afford the patient a sense of continuity and of their place in the procession of their ancestry. Being such a hard wood the apple is associated with earth and grounding.

Chakras

Crown
Sets the patient back on their true spiritual path after a time of sensing that they have lost their way.

Brow
Opens the brow centre after a period of confusion and feelings of being prey to fears and anxieties. Brain chunter gives way to more measured thought and an ability to judge what is of real benefit.

Throat
Loss of the ability to express what is felt in the heart has created a lot of the suffering that indicates the need for **Apple Tree**. The remedy opens up the link between heart and brow and encourages the use of the throat as the means of expression of what lies locked in both. With this goes a greater ability to cope with the environment which may be harbouring the allergens that have been causing so much physical and mental slowness and sensitivity.

Heart

The patient feels held back by the past though they may not be able to see it as clearly as this. The past may include others who belong to the patient's past who are holding them back through old associations and emotional ties. The more loaded in the heart area the patient is by people and events from the past, the more likely they are to be sensitive to allergens of any sort.

Solar plexus

Poor assimilation and absorption in the gut in those who have heavy hearts.

Sacral

Suppressed emotions held in the sacral area lead to repressed sexual energy. Weak kidney qi due to anxiety and having denied the need to deal with emotional difficulties, either inherited or otherwise. The water element is strongly associated with **Apple Tree** especially through the fruit.

Base

Ungrounded and blocked from moving forward; threat of stagnation. Allergic reactions on any level; often multiple allergies.

Case studies

1   'An Aquarian woman who had been coming for treatment for about eight years suffering from chronic arthritis and thyroid problems, returned for her regular appointment. She was on thyroxin and had been for many years. She was also on an immunosuppressant. Though her arthritic symptoms had improved beyond any expectation, her fear of coming off the drugs was too strong for her to risk. It was apparent that there was a lot of fear stuck around her throat (chakra) causing the thyroid to swing and produce obsessive compulsive symptoms. She tended towards passive/aggressive behaviour though this too had improved on previous treatment.

   'She had helped nurse her mother to her death as a child and [felt it was then that she had] lost her trust in life. Fear and anxiety as to what might happen and a fear that anyone [close] should die underpinned this case. She lived in a flat in a retirement block which she had moved into because of the arthritis but she had realized that, having improved in her physical condition, she had moved too early in her life. She watched various people around her deteriorate and this aggravated the situation.

She came with inflammation in her eye as well as the feeling that the anxiety was deeper and that she had a lot of anger "over the stupidest of things". Her sleep was always a problem, made worse by her anxiety which was still about all the things that she couldn't control in her life or in the life of others around her. She was given **Apple Tree** 1M weekly for six weeks.

'She returned with the eye symptoms 80 per cent better. Her anxiety and sleep patterns had become worse initially but had then improved considerably. She was now able to express her anger in a way she had not been before; she was really clear about the cause of the anger. She felt easily insulted by the injustice of being surrounded by people who were dependent on her but who were not as mentally agile or intellectually gifted as herself. Though she realized that she had in some way more control over her neighbours, she was cross with herself for being in this situation. Though she wanted to move away from them, she felt that she couldn't turn her back on them, not least as they were company she'd miss. She felt that **Apple Tree** had brought her far more clarity in her mind.' **GM**

2 'In the late autumn of 2003 a woman of 41, a jeweller who owned her own shop, a long-term patient who had a very sensitive system that chiefly manifested symptoms in the digestive tract and the bladder, came complaining of being chilly, bloated and craving all the wrong things to eat including chocolate, sugar and bread. (She usually did well on **Lycopodium**.) Her periods were not satisfactory and she felt that her womb was tight. "I swing from feeling fat and comfortable to being quiet and snappy. I'm very judgemental." She wanted warm and comforting food. She was restless and anxious. "I keep needing to do things." She also suffered from tinnitus: a ringing sound. She found it difficult to balance her roles as a shopkeeper and an artist. She was given **Arsen-alb** LM1. She reported that she felt calmer and less agitated but the physical symptoms had not abated at all. Her chief concern was that her

bladder now felt as if she were starting cystitis and her right kidney ached. She was given **Berberis** 3x daily which removed the urinary tract symptoms though the bowel symptoms continued and she was as disgruntled with her situation as before. At this point she was given **Apple Tree** 30 to be taken 3x per week.

'She returned almost four months later feeling much better in general though she still tended to feel cystitis symptoms whenever she went away from home. (She always carries **Berberis** 3x with her.) She feels more positive and is enjoying her work. Her digestion is back to normal and she now has the strength to avoid all the comfort foods. "I know that I am just so sensitive to chocolate and sweet things and they always get to me. I am so much better if I avoid them and if I remember to drink plenty of water."' **CG**

3 'A mother of four, married to a city businessman, had been treated for several years for a whole range of problems that included hormonal difficulties including hypothyroidism (not severe enough for medication). She was overweight, overanxious and over-adrenalized. She wanted the very best for her children and drove them purposefully towards their academic goals to ensure their places at the desired schools and eventually at university. She had been brought up in a household where the men were given all the attention and the women were left to fend for themselves. She was highly articulate and gave the impression of sharp intelligence. She had had many prescriptions; not all of them by any means proved effective. She was a diligent patient in that she always took the remedies exactly as prescribed but she always felt that they fell short of her expectations. She complained.

'She was sensitive to wheat, dairy and sweet foods. These always gave her trouble in her digestive system or disturbed her sleep or interrupted her periods or gave her a great dip in energy . . . or a combination of these or all of them. Nevertheless, she was as remarkably consistent in keeping her appointments as she was in seeing cranial osteopaths, kinesiologists, nutritionists, healers and acupuncturists. At one point she came to report that she had been to Spain and had indulged heavily in all the foods that she knew were bad for her. She was sent off with **Malus** 1M: one every two hours for three doses. When she returned some three months later she said, for the very first time, "I've think that I've been doing pretty well!"

'This improvement lasted for quite a while but she succumbed to more bread and pasta: "It was inevitable really!" When it happened again she was given a repeat prescription of **Malus** 1M with exactly the same result.' **CG**

19

MICROWAVE RADIATION PULSED G3

The remedy was made by Janice Micallef from brandy exposed to microwaves from a G3 mobile phone mast for a period of six weeks. A bottle of brandy was suspended from a branch of a tree within 100 yards of a mobile phone mast and left for six weeks. Before this version was made, there had been two unsuccessful attempts to prepare it; both times it was sabotaged. On the first occasion the brandy had been stolen and on the second the bottle had smashed after a squirrel had gnawed through the suspending string. The remedy was also made using ethanol as well as brandy. By studying the etheric or auric field, Janice found that the remedy made from brandy was the more active. The remedy was potentized to 30c. Participants took one dose of 30c daily for three to four days before and one dose of the 30c at the start of the meditation; further to this a 'cross' of the liquid potency of the 30c was marked on each one's forehead. The remedy was continued for a further seven days after the meditation.

There were two provings done on separate occasions from which these notes were taken. In the first session there were 11 women and 4 men; in the second there were 5 women and 4 men. In the meditation the provers were asked to visualize a sphere of white light, 7 lamps, a circle of angels, 4 guardians and a doorkeeper with a staff in his left hand standing by a door through which the provers were invited to go to sit in a room filled with candles where they would receive information on the remedy.

The Background

Microwave Radiation Pulsed G3 became a remedy as the result of an acute awareness that mobile phone masts were fast becoming a serious threat to health owing to the low frequency emissions they send out. A mast was erected within 150 metres of Janice Micallef's house; her family began to experience symptoms within a short time: malaise, nausea, fatigue, etc. It was also noticed by various people that mobile phones were a potential hazard for remedies. People who left mobile phones within two metres of remedies risked destroying the energy of the medicines. Furthermore, it was realized through anecdotal evidence that many people who use mobile phones with any frequency are putting themselves at risk of dangerous changes to their body's energy. This was borne out by articles published in various publications showing the infiltrating effects of radiation emitted by mobiles.

A patient who wondered whether mobile phone mast emissions were harmful and might be causing her symptomatic reactions mentioned that a friend of hers, otherwise a healthy woman in her mid forties, had been taken into hospital suffering from pains in the right side of her abdomen. The doctors at first thought that she was suffering from either appendicitis or from ovarian cysts. Scans and the remainder of the symptom picture ruled out the former though there was speculation about the cloudy mass that appeared on the subsequent X-ray. An operation disclosed that there was a large area of scar tissue in the abdominal cavity in the region of the right hypochondria. This was removed; the histology report subsequently found no cancerous changes. The doctors were unable to find an explanation. However, on leaving the hospital, the woman's husband handed her a car coat she particularly liked to wear. On putting it on she automatically put her hand in the right-hand pocket and found her mobile phone. She at once felt certain that her activated phone, which she always kept in this right-hand pocket, had been responsible for her condition.

A patient, a fireman, spoke of his alarm after having, in an idle moment with colleagues at the fire station, aimed his thermographic camera at a friend who had been talking on his mobile phone to his partner for half an hour. What so appalled him was that the camera highlighted a 'hot spot' (usually associated with the hot epicentre of a fire) in the friend's head.

Microwave technology and other forms of radiation have similar effects on people who are susceptible. Those who complain about symptoms as a result of mobile phones echo others who complain about the effects on them of what are known as non-thermal electromagnetic fields, mostly from their computers connected to broadband or Wi-Fi. Many patients report that they suffer from eye strain when working with a computer. Others say that they can sense the radiation that is emitted from their machines and that 'it gets to me' after a short while. The author has the same sense and is unable to use a computer for more than 20 minutes at a time without an unpleasant tingling sensation creeping up the hands, into the wrists and into the forearms with a general sense of lassitude overcoming him. One patient, a bookkeeper who worked for a firm of accountants and who used computers all day long, asked what she might do to protect herself from the harmful effects of the radiation. She purchased a large clear quartz which she placed very close to the computer she used in the office. Within seven days this crystal had crazed throughout its inner structure. She returned to the shop and showed it to the geologist from whom she bought it. He was astounded and exclaimed that what had happened to the crystal was 'not possible'; while it might be crushed or broken into smaller pieces, internal crazing was the work of something extraordinary and outside his understanding. She was quite clear that the stone had not been crazed when she purchased it.

The adverse effects of radiation are not news. Only two years after electrical brain signals were first discovered in 1875, a study was made of reactions to electromagnetic fields in a dog's central nervous system. By the 1920s alpha brain waves were discovered and within ten years tests on plants, animals and humans showed how EMFs affect living tissue. G. M. Beard, in an article in the *Boston Medical and Surgical Journal* (80) of 1869 called 'Neurasthenia or nervous exhaustion', noted that this condition was suffered by telegraph workers in the USA. In 1928 complaints were made of ill health among workers building an experimental radio transmitter at the General Electrical plant in New York. According to 'Overloading of Towns and Cities with Radio Transmitters (Cellular Transmitter)' the main effect was a rise in body temperature. However, dizziness, nausea, weakness and sweating all became familiar symptoms of radiotherapy that was developed not long after.[22] These

22 Hecht, Karl and Savoley, Elena N published by International Research Centre of Healthy and Ecological Technology, Berlin, 2007

same symptoms are still recognized effects of radiotherapy today. The US military documented a variety of side effects from the use of and exposure to radar: male sterility, testicular degeneration (in dogs), cataracts and blindness, leukaemia, brain tumours and unprovoked haemorrhage.[23] In the 1950s Russia began using pulsed microwaves to monitor activities in the US embassy in Moscow. Though there was a diplomatic cover-up, two US ambassadors died from cancer and a third developed a disease akin to leukaemia.[24] Almost all research into microwave technology reports similar findings: that in those who are susceptible microwaves tend to cause enervation, burning (sometimes on the skin as would occur with ordinary radiation), headaches, disturbed sleep patterns, nausea, depression, cataract and deterioration of sight, carcinogenic changes in cell reaction and function and changes to blood cells that may lead to leukaemia. According to one source,[25] though acid rain is regarded as the chief culprit in deforestation, EMFs are also responsible for damage to plant life as well as to bee and bird colonies.[26] Certain viruses are also said to be influenced by microwaves; unfortunately for us, positively. What has prevented so much information against microwave technology from reaching the public includes financial implications for vested interests, military research and the refusal to accept that anything so apparently convenient might be undermining to health.[27] Some of the provers were delighted with the results of the meditation as they experienced real curative changes particularly in the areas of energy, libido, communication, sleep, perception and arthritic pain. Others felt an awareness of how the remedy might be useful, whether or not there was actual harm from electromagnetic fields, in the treatment of specific disease states: MS and locomotor ataxia;

23 'A Clinical Study of the Results of Exposure of Laboratory Personnel to Radar and High Frequency Radiation' Daily, LE; US Naval Bulletin 41 1943

24 Becker, Robert O, *Cross Currents: The Perils of Electropollution, the Promise of Electromedicine,* Tarcher/Penguin, 2004

25 'The Effects of Microwaves on the Trees and Other Plants', Martinez, AB, December 2003

26 'Cell Tower: Wireless Convenience? Or Environmental Problem?' Levitt, B Blake, New Century Publishing, 2000

27 For the information in this paragraph I am entirely indebted to an article, 'Attitudes to the Health Dangers of Non-Thermal EMFs' by Michael Bevington (Jan 2008 – revised edition). For further information on the significance of microwaves, the politicization and the scale of the cover-ups see http://www.es-uk.info/docs/ 20080117_bevington_emfs.pdf where the full list of references may also be found.

Parkinsonism; schizophrenia, epilepsy, dementia, ME, Alzheimer's, AIDS, some cancers and chronic fatigue as all these conditions show similarities to the effects of the remedy.

Keynote effects

The restoration of the integrity and improved functioning of the central nervous system. There is a relief from what some describe as 'bone tiredness', a sense of utter lassitude and exhaustion felt in the limbs but also affecting the mind. There is also a return of both emotional and physical feelings where these had been dulled or suppressed.

General symptoms

The central nervous system is affected; there are pins and needles, numbness, tingling and dyspraxic tendencies. Paralysis can set in. Spatial awareness is impaired. Inertia. All the electrical impulses of the body are affected adversely. Mental degeneration. Sensations of pressure and heaviness are experienced. The whole body or just the head can feel heavy. There is an exaggerated awareness of the difference between the two sides of the body: left and right; also of a dislocation between the top and bottom half, above and below the pelvic area. Sensation as if the body is dying. Sensations of both heat and cold; heat is mostly internal and cold is external. Waves of icy coldness creeping up the back. The endocrine glands are impaired; the thyroid and the thymus take up the radiation and become infiltrated and damaged. Kidney energy becomes exhausted quickly which means the filtration system of the water in the body is affected. The calcium/magnesium balance is disrupted. Spleen energy is affected making it harder to maintain the integrity of the immune system; there is a greater tendency to succumb to infection, especially viral (patients can feel as if they are 'coming down with something' all the time). Schizophrenia is aggravated; Alzheimer's is initiated. Epileptic seizures are <. Headaches and head pains; migraine. Carcinoma particularly of the head; may cause tumours to be incurable by any means. The body's structure is weakened so that old injuries become worse in their effects; old injury patterns return if they have not been completely dealt with. Arthritic tendencies were observed with pains in joints especially of the hands and fingers. Fleeting, darting pains (especially in the head). Rashes on the skin. Deeply syphilitic and carcinogenic but also disrupts the water balance of the body (sycotic). Accident proneness. Tendency to suffer burns through carelessness. Burning sensations generally. The remedy can be used to remove the effects of geopathic stress.

Miasms

Radiation, psora, syphilis and sycosis.

Mental and emotional symptoms

Profound lack of emotion; inability to access emotions. Sense of lost volition; wants to curl up in the foetal position. Has a sense of going round and round in circles but stuck at a very slow speed. Yet also has the opposite: sense of going too fast. Sense of shrinking; several provers had the feeling of 'Alice in Wonderland' shrinking. Fearfulness but not extreme: more a sense of wariness; watchfulness, anticipation. Sense of complete blankness; inability to register anything: cold, quiet and confused. Sense of being completely stuck; unable to move forward. Sense of feeling hollow and inadequate. Desolation with a desperate need to protect the body from harm. Cannot find a way to fulfil any wishes; balked ambition; feels thwarted. Always feel that they are being undermined; cannot make any progress. Depressed and weak-minded. Cannot concentrate and stay focused. Deluded about what they need to do: spends lots of time frittering away valuable time. Too tired to think; too tired to act. Mind goes blank. Hard to put thoughts into words. Sense of unreality; 'floaty' and detached. Feels as if there are no boundaries. Hyperactivity and restlessness of the brain; can't switch off. Anxiety and excitement alternate: switches from one to the other randomly. Uncontrollable anger. Fearfulness yet does not know of what. Aversion to anything old; only wants new things. Has been suggested as a remedy for social misfits: for those who can't organize themselves properly and who are ultrasensitive and have hyperactive minds that don't switch off; they also swing between being excited and electrically charged and anxious, fearful and exhausted.

Many of the provers became sensitive to different colours: orange, yellow, red, blue. They also reported that they had difficulties with their electrical machinery.

MRPG3 is likely to be of signal use among children with behavioural problems who have learning difficulties and who find the computer draws their attention. These children can seem to be addicted to the screen; they are also given to keeping their mobile phones on them at all times. It will be noted that the level of their communications with others while using the mobile phones suggests a stunting of the intellect.

Physical symptoms

Head

Fleeting, darting pains in the middle of the head. Pains in the temple. Sensation of nail driven into the left side of the head but without pain. Head feels as if it is expanding. Pressure on both temples. Sensations of uncomfortable radiating and penetrative heat going into the brain. Head feels heavy; 'stuffed up with cotton wool' sensation. Sensation as if the brain is shrinking within the skull, leaving a hollow space. Hyperactivity of the brain bad enough to cause the sense that there is no peace or rest. Temporal arteritis (much relieved in one of the provers: the pains moved from the temples to the chin and then >>).

Eyes

'Jiggling' sensation in the left of the eye socket. Nystagmus.

Ears

Earache in the left ear. Pain penetrates into the left temple. Heightened sensitivity to high-pitched sound; loud noises felt invasive – sense that it was not possible to shut out extraneous noises. Meniere's disease. Burning sensation extending into the head after use of mobile phone (see 'Case studies' below).

Nose

Profuse nosebleeds.

Throat

Thyroid malfunction leading to chronic fatigue. Tight sensation around the thyroid.

Respiration

Hard to take a full, deep breath. Shallow breathing. Heat and constriction in the chest. Lungs feel congested.

Chest

Breast cancer (especially of the right it was suggested). Discomfort around the heart. Aching in the chest. Poor posture with rounded shoulders and 'caved in' chest which makes it difficult to take in a deep breath. Tight band around the heart. Agitation in the heart: a feeling of excitement but involving the urgency of wanting to communicate though in a driven, jumbled manner. Discomfort around and in the mediastinal region. Tension in chest. Arrhythmia and tachycardia.

Solar plexus

Nausea. Sensations of heat rising up from the solar plexus and into the breasts (especially the right). Pain in the gall bladder; ++ chocolate and no appetite for savoury things; + alcohol. (One patient reported being able to eat food to which she was normally intolerant such as wheat and dairy.)

Abdomen

Constipation. Aching in the liver.

Female

Pain in right ovary. Lowered libido: too tired. Increased libido with a greater sense of freedom reported by one patient.

Male

Libido increased 'more animalistic, aggressive and dirty' but aware of the negativity of this. Atrophy of the testes.

Skin

Itching. Rashes: red with no spots < under arms and on right breast. Small red eruption on side of chest and on the back. Increased perspiration.

Neck and back

Sensations of cold running up the back. Pain in the sacral region. Pain in the neck.

Extremities

Vibrations running through the hands and up into the arms as if there were something alive in there shifting things; likened to the effects of moxa and the sensation of heat that this can create. Dyspraxia and clumsiness. Unable to coordinate limbs properly. Nervous tremors. Jerking of lower limbs in bed at night; violent in left leg. Buzzing sensations in the limbs. Muscle pains and stiffness (greatly relieved in one patient).

Sleep

Wakes suddenly in the night with sense that someone else is present. Delusions on waking of hearing sounds and seeing lights. Hard to fall asleep or to stay asleep. Dreams of parasites, cats, water (sea). Also libidinous dreams. Of cooked sausages, clearing menstrual debris, electrical equipment and earthquakes.

Considerations for the use of the remedy

Strong relationship with **Syphilinum**, **Thymus Gland** and **Ayahuasca**. Can be put into combination with these remedies: **TG** + **MRPG3** + **Syph** 10M or **TG** + **MRPG3** + **Ayahuasca** 10M or **Syphilinum** + **Ayahuasca** + **MRPG3**. Has similar energy to **Mercury** and might be considered if **Mercury** fails despite being indicated. (Giving **MRPG3** before a dose of **Mercury** in a patient living within the range of microwave radiation can encourage the main remedy to work more thoroughly.) Also complementary with **Carcinosin**. **Phosphorus** follows well and antidotes.

Esoteric therapeutics

The remedy was viewed by the provers as one that heals the aura, the etheric body and a fragmented chakra system. Despite the fact that mobile phone masts are human constructions and emit harmful radiation, the energy that is produced can be turned to advantage to deal with problems that occur in the age that created it. At a time when materialism is so fuelled by the need for high-speed electronic communication, we are most in need of healing in areas that are increasingly viewed as no longer significant or necessary for our well-being: the intuition, a spiritual pathway, esoteric understanding. By potentizing the energy it is possible to apply its remedial action either to those who are unable to cope with, or those so damaged by, the increased speed and demands of the age. Through the action of the remedy it thus becomes likely that the results of the remedy will include opening up the channels of discovery of spiritual pathways and the honing of intuition.

Radiation borrows the body's own energy, uses it, depletes it without allowing for its replenishment and destroys the life force from within.

Chakras

Crown

Blocks the chakra from receiving on a spiritual level. In general it was apparent that the negative energy of mobile phones and their masts works to block spiritual growth and positive, creative intuition and it does this through the typically insidious, infiltrating manner that is common to all radioactive energy.

Brow

Blocks this centre from perceiving. This can result in the subject living in a permanent state of delusion; this is greatly exaggerated if the patient has a history of (or is indulging in) hallucinogenic drugs. It may become significant in the understanding of this remedy that for almost the entire history of microwave technology there has been a parallel history of false information, dissembling and cover-up. This may lead to our use of the remedy for those who are lulled into a false sense of security or deprived of a voice by vested interests. Another aspect is of significance to this chakra partly due to the connection of Mercury to the brow centre: those who have amalgam fillings in their mouths and who use mobile phones are likely to be far more affected by the radiation emissions. Mercury discharging into the system can carry the radiation quite quickly into distant organs such as the brain, liver, gonads and kidneys. This may well be trigger enough for the carcinogenic state to become physically manifest in the form of tumours. These may be inoperable and resistant to all treatment.

Throat

This centre is blocked because the thyroid gland acts as a sponge in the presence of any form of radiation. This puts at risk the metabolism of the body and the way the body clock works. Communication becomes increasingly difficult partly because of the blocking of this centre and partly because of the break in the link between head and heart.

Thymus gland

The body's ability to set up the immune system properly is affected so that one is increasingly susceptible to viral infection. As the thymus is also damaged by vaccines this centre is doubly at risk when children use mobile phones.

Sacral

The kidneys are unbalanced and weakened thus putting into jeopardy the ability to deal with ancestral, karmic issues as it is the kidneys that are most involved in this.

Base

Anyone suffering in the way that indicates the need for this remedy is not 'in' their base centre; they are not grounded and are in danger of becoming unbalanced in their whole energy body.

Provers' experiences

1   Grahame Martin, one of the provers, wrote of his experience of lecturing on this remedy.

'Presented the remedy **Microwave** to a group. Prior to this I had spent some time preparing the presentation and also reading through and highlighting official documentation outlining the effects that microwaves have on the human body. Almost immediately I found myself in a fog of confusion. This also manifested as a separation between me and the group to whom I was presenting the proving information. I [also] became disconnected from the information in front of me that I had written about . . . [I was unable] to tie that information together and explain what I felt was the meaning of individual aspects of the proving.

'There was also a very significant feeling that came over me and that was to continue regardless. This was as if I had been taken over by the desire to appear normal or to appear to remain completely in control when it was obvious I wasn't. When it came to presenting official findings of how microwaves act on the human condition I found I could barely hold onto the information on the page, let alone read it out in a cohesive fashion.

'The presentation of radiation remedies is always difficult as the mind tends to go blank. However, what was significant here was the need to continue regardless. [I speculated later] that the addictive need to communicate that comes with the use of mobile phones, had somehow been picked up in the proving; it was as if I couldn't put the phone down.

'Although this was quite an embarrassing hour or so for me, with me appearing as if I could neither read nor think, what came from it was an invaluable side of the proving of the remedy. We have patients that come to us with all forms of addiction but how often do we think to look at the insecurity that is produced by the addiction to having to have and carry a mobile phone wherever the person goes? . . . there seems to be something within the nature of this radioactive energy that is addictive.'

2 'At the end of a lecture at the Centre for Homoeopathic Education when I had presented the remedy to a fourth-year group, one of the students related the following anecdote. He said that his wife worked for a businessman who was normally a fit and healthy individual. He developed a pain in his shoulder and neck which was severe enough for his assistant to advise that he should take time off and see a doctor. He consulted a doctor in Harley Street who, after some ordinary questioning, asked the man if he used a mobile phone. The businessman admitted that he did and that he used it all the time for his work. The doctor told him to come back and see him after a few weeks but only to use an analogue phone from now on. The businessman complied and was delighted to find that the symptoms completely disappeared after a short while. Intrigued, he went back to the doctor and told him that he was well but that he was keen to know how the doctor had diagnosed the problem. The doctor told him that he was familiar with the risks involved with the use of mobile phones as he was part of an official body funded by the government looking into the effects of using such equipment' CG

Case studies

1 'A woman came to the drop-in clinic feeling "tired and spaced out". She complained of a headache that affected the whole of the side of her head; that it made her feel "muzzy" and "not with it". Her speech was slower than usual and she gave the impression of not wanting to be bothered with anything which she agreed was exactly how she felt. Despite close questioning there seemed to be no defining picture in the case so she was asked what she had been doing that day. She explained that she had been on the motorway all day and had been using her mobile phone for much of the time. She was given a dose of **MRPG3** 30 there and then. Within 30 seconds she said "What on earth was that remedy; it's amazing! I can feel my head lifting, my headache is almost gone and I can think straight. I had this burning in my ear and that's gone too!" Her complexion had also changed; she was no longer rather grey skinned and she clearly had far more animation. When told the name of the remedy she swore loudly and dug in her handbag for her mobile phone. "Are you seriously saying that this caused me to feel so dreadful?" The question was obviously rhetorical as she hurled the phone against the far wall.

'Within half an hour of this patient's experience another patient came in with very similar symptoms. The only difference was that the second patient had burning in the opposite ear. When asked if she held her mobile phone to the affected ear she agreed that she did and that she had spent the previous half-hour talking to a friend. She too was given **MRPG3** 30 which had a very similar effect though the recovery time was about ten minutes.' **CG**

2 'A young lady in her mid 30s who had been treated for chronic fatigue syndrome, originally came after trying many forms of treatment without success. She and her husband manufacture and sell specialist clothing; it is a very demanding job but she had been unable to work consistently for a long time. This had put pressure on her husband and, although he was quite understanding of her condition, it caused many arguments. She was very tiny in build and had a very spiritual nature; she talked to her angels frequently. She loved children and wanted to be a nursery school teacher or childminder but felt she could not because she didn't

have the energy to train and also her husband felt she should put all her energy into their business. They both wanted children but so far she had felt she was too weak to sustain a pregnancy and her husband thought they didn't earn enough to bring a child into the world.

'She had very little energy at any time and was very nervous and anxious most of the time. She had very little self-confidence. She could only manage to do anything physical in short bursts and had to rest most of the day. She had very little appetite. She would feel hungry but get full and bloated very quickly. Her husband also had digestive problems and suffered with hives. She had several remedies over the following year: **Gelsemium**, **Pulsatilla** and **Lycopodium** all made a difference but were not holding.

'On one particular visit her relationship with her husband was particularly bad and on the drive from the North, where they lived, they had not spoken and she felt that although they loved one another, the pressure was too much and they might split up. I felt there was something I was missing so on this day I expressed this thought and during the consultation asked her to describe where she lived. She told me they lived over a shop and had their business downstairs and in the yard. It was situated in a small high street. I then asked her to describe the feeling she got in each room and if she felt more tired in some rooms than others. She said she couldn't work at her sewing machine in the shop for more than half an hour before getting exhausted. I then asked her to describe the area outside the shop. She told me there was a fire station opposite the shop, set back from the road. I had an "ah ha" moment and asked her if there was a G3 Mobile phone mast on the top of the fire station; she confirmed that there was.

'I gave both her and her husband **MRPG3** 30c: a single dose before they left me. I also gave her more **Lycopodium** in the same potency as previously given. A few hours later she rang me and asked what they had been given because on the journey back they had both experienced a feeling of a huge weight being taken off them and feeling much lighter. She felt she had more energy than for a long time. They had also resolved some of their differences. By the next consultation she was feeling back to normal and this held. They have since had the flat and business cleared of geopathic stress and I periodically give them a single dose each of **MRPG3** 30c.

'She has since then trained as a childminder and had a baby who is now three years old. They have a much more harmonious relationship and their business is going from strength to strength. **MRPG3** was definitely the breakthrough for sorting out a lot of the problem and enabling other remedies to hold.' JL

20

NATRUM BICARBONICUM

Sodium bicarbonate

The remedy was proved during the meditation circle held on 20 November 2009. Nine women and four men were present including the leader of the group. The remedy was taken in the 30th potency. One dose was given orally and the liquid was dropped on each wrist. Only the leader and the supplier of the remedy were aware of what the substance being proved was. The remedy was prepared from a level teaspoonful of sodium bicarbonate from Boots, the chemists, in 99 drops of ethanol. The liquid was not heated to melting point but vigorously succussed; the single drop of this original 'mother tincture' added to make the first dilution therefore contained undissolved powder. As a result it may be that this remedy should be regarded as an essence remedy.

The Background

Sodium bicarbonate is otherwise known as baking soda, bicarbonate of soda or sodium hydrogen carbonate. Its chemical formula is $NaHCO_3$. It is found in mineral deposits almost anywhere in the world. It was first investigated scientifically as recently as the first half of the 19th century.

Sodium Bicarbonate is a white crystalline powder that is stable with a specific gravity of 2.16 and a melting point of 50°C. It is an alkalizing agent that is vital to the body's biochemistry in reducing acidity in muscle tissue after exertion. It is also used as a medicine and as a cleaning agent. In medicine it is prescribed for metabolic acidosis, alkalization of urine, urinary tract disorders (cystitis) and in drops for softening ear wax. It is a primary constituent of domestic cleaning fluids and is used in products such as toothpaste. It is combined with acetylsalicylic acid and citric acid in the production of aspirin which is used for pain relief and blood thinning. It is known to reduce acid in the system and to raise blood pH levels. Though sodium bicarbonate is regarded as harmless to the body there are several characteristic side effects: flatulence, flatus, abdominal cramping and breathlessness; the chemical affects or has an affinity for the digestive tract and the lungs. Long-term excessive use can give rise to raised blood pressure and swollen ankles and feet. Athletes have long thought of sodium bicarbonate, when taken before exercise, as having the potential to reduce lactic acid in the muscles after exertion which in turn reduces characteristic burning pains in overused muscles and provides greater staying power. Tests undertaken by various groups have concluded that it is likely that taking a supplement of sodium bicarbonate before intense exertion can enhance physical performance when the amount consumed is in the region of 0.3g per kilo of body mass. However, this practice does not suit all athletes as some taking this restricted dosage have complained of abdominal cramps and diarrhoea. Perhaps there is no surprise here when we consider that not all athletes have the same constitutional biochemical make-up.

Traditional home use of sodium bicarbonate includes applying a dilute solution to skin problems such as acne, sunburn, insect bites and stings and as a mouthwash to ease the pains of aphthous ulcers. Rather more extravagant claims are made for the chemical by those promoting it in the treatment of cancer. It has been used both orally and intravenously to combat the growth and metastasis of cancer cells even in those suffering from terminal cancer. The thinking behind this is that alkalizing the body thoroughly makes it an inhospitable environment for the development of cancers and that the use of sodium bicarbonate as one of the most readily assimilated alkalizing agents can effect the necessary changes.[28] According to some, combining sodium bicarbonate with either maple syrup or blackstrap molasses enhances the Trojan horse effect that comes with it.[29] Despite some anecdotal evidence that such

28 One highly controversial theory suggests that cancer is triggered by candidiasis,
   a yeast condition that can affect the whole body, which is best eliminated by
   using sodium bicarbonate to change the fungus's ideal environment. See
   www.regenerativenutrition.com/content.asp?id=490 (Feb. 2010) for a fuller report.
29 Ibid.

treatment has benefited some patients, medical science disputes such claims and suggests that the concentrated use of sodium bicarbonate may be harmful.

It is instructive to compare sodium bicarbonate with its close relative, sodium carbonate (the homoeopath's **Natrum Carbonicum**). Sodium carbonate is otherwise known as washing soda, soda ash or soda crystals. Its chemical formula is Na_2Co_3. Its melting point is 851°C, considerably higher than sodium bicarbonate's. It is mass-produced synthetically from rock salt (**Natrum Muriaticum**). It is a natural cleanser and forms the basis of many scouring, deodorizing cleaning products. It is an irritant to the lungs and the eyes. See below under 'Considerations for the use of the remedy' for a more direct comparison between the two remedies.

Keynote effects

The two main effects on the physical body are to correct the water balance in a system that is dehydrated and to foster a less acidic internal environment. It benefits the central nervous system that is lacking sufficient water for its efficient functioning and it cools an overheated body or vital part. It can cause an increased thirst in those who are chronically disinclined to drink water to their own detriment and it is of considerable benefit to those whose bodies are over-acidic. Just as importantly, though less obviously symptomatically evident is the fact that the remedy facilitates the flow of esoteric energy throughout the body via the meridians. As such it can benefit those undergoing acupuncture, shiatsu or craniosacral treatment as it maintains changes effected by those treatments. (See page 11 in relation to the acid/alkali balance.)

General symptoms

The remedy reduces irritability within the system from hyperacidity and lack of water. Dehydration is one of the strong themes of this remedy. In those whose systems are like a car deprived of enough water and oil, **Sodium Bicarbonate** is indicated by lack of thirst (or a strong desire for water), a desire for sweet foods, a tendency to sluggishness and candidiasis and stiffness and/or aching in muscles and joints. Excessive amounts of lactic acid in the muscles. Either the whole body tends to overheating or a part shows symptoms of heat or even inflammation. The brain may be included in this description; there is irritability in the tissues of the brain (which may not be diagnosed until cranial osteo-pathic or craniosacral treatment highlights it) which can result in headaches, hot head, flashes of irritable moods or mental symptoms (see below). Muscles feel tired, stiff and achy; joints lose their range of articulation. There is a tendency to injury from slight causes: strains and sprains. Chronic sprain injuries that do not recover under the influence of indicated remedies such as **Rhus-tox, Bryonia** and **Ruta**. Acidic indigestion with heartburn. Hiatus hernia with acid reflux. Intestinal borborygmi (rumbling and bubbling); regurgita-tion. Abdominal cramping. Diarrhoea and the consequences of loss of fluid from the body. Nausea with breathlessness especially in those with heart, lung and digestive symptoms. Metabolic acidosis[30] and acidosis in children where there is nausea, vomiting and weight loss accompanied by headache and lethargy. Breathlessness especially after exertion. Poor nutritional assimilation especially in those with a tendency to excessive weight and shallow breathing. Obesity with overheating of the body. Poor elimination through the bowels and kidneys. Alternation of constipation and diarrhoea is possible. Unwell since the loss of fluids during an acute bout of gastro-enteritis. Dehydration from loss of fluids or from lack of thirst. Skin is dry, lacks tone and frequently produces eruptions; acne. Sweat: profuse and/or odorous and with heat not necessarily due to exertion. Feeling heavy in the body. The right and left sides of the body do not feel integrated or the disparity is evident from pulse reading. Malignancy of chronic conditions especially of those areas already mentioned. The ingestion of sugar will compromise the healing initiated by this remedy; it is necessary to put the patient on a sugar and alcohol-free diet, an instruction likely to be resisted or transgressed by the patient (see below in the 'Mental and emotional symptoms'). The biochemistry of the body may be in need of thorough assessment. The patient may present a history of having been given multiple supplements for nutritional imbalance but with little result or of being in need of nutritional support. The fundamental block to naturopathic supplementation being effective may be found in the lack of water

---

30 To date there is only one homoeopathic remedy listed in the repertories for
   acidosis: **Natrum Phosphoricum**. This is surely an anomaly that needs to be
   redressed. **Arsen-alb, Nat-mur, Nux Vomica, Mag-mur** and others all have
   symptom pictures that cover hyperacidity levels. Now **Sodium Bicarbonate** joins
   this list. However, whether or not homoeopaths will gain experience in using any
   of these remedies for this condition, a very serious and potentially fatal illness in
   the chronically sick requiring regular conventional monitoring, is a moot point.
   Nevertheless, any of these remedies may well be of significant preventative value.

balance and the lack of adequate conductivity of the central nervous system. Another aspect is that of slow healing. The remedy is one for the liver, gall bladder, kidneys and spleen. It can be prescribed on the meridians that are connected with these organs as well as the triple heater meridian in order to act as a drainage and support.

Miasms

Psora and tuberculosis.

Mental and emotional symptoms

Concern about material circumstances; worries and anxiety about day-to-day life. Confusion and lack of clarity. Feels distant, vague and not with it. Concerned about physical health but unable to find ways of improving it. Reluctant to change eating habits even when on a diet that is harmful. Lives a life of two halves: on one hand he or she is active in the material world with all the stresses and strains which result in harboured physical and emotional toxicity, and on the other hand feeling rather adrift and lacking in focus which has much to do with vagueness about spiritual orientation. There is an awareness of the disjunction between having to operate in the material world and wanting to become acquainted with deeper or higher aspects of the self. Feelings of loneliness; history of lonely childhood. Feels that something remains left undone, incomplete; unable to make progress as a result. May start to express this dichotomy haltingly and then say, 'I've no idea what I'm talking about' or 'Am I making any sense at all?' Feel they are in a contradictory state and one that has no obvious historical starting point. Regret and disappointment about past choices made without full knowledge of circumstances; for those who have leapt before looking in major decisions of life. Dullness of the mind with doubts about motivation. Often 'in two minds' about this or that. In a contradictory state. Fearful of not being clever enough; of not being able to learn sufficiently well; self-esteem further reduced by making comparisons with other people. Feels that other people are able to go quicker and that one is left behind. Feels hurried. Is aware that the mental and physical bodies are not entirely in harmony.

Physical symptoms

Head

Sensation of heaviness in the head. Brain feels overloaded. Heat in the head. Pressure in the head. Head feels both full and empty at the same time.

Face

Eruptions that appear with continued stress. Acne. Dryness of the facial skin.

Throat

Acid rising into the throat from heartburn. Dryness of the mucous membranes.

Chest

Shallow breathing. Short of breath. Coughing: continuous from a dry throat and chest. Hot from coughing. A feeling of weakness in the chest.

Digestion and stomach

Fluttering as of butterflies in the stomach: excitement felt in the intestines. Stomach may feel both full and yet empty at the same time. High dependency on sugar; a strong desire for sweet food, dairy products, carbohydrates such as pasta, acid fruit and coffee. Diet may be mostly fast food or a preponderance of bread: sandwiches and toast. Regurgitation; rumbling and gurgling in the abdomen. Poor nutrition; malnourishment. Lack of thirst: the patient may not drink much or any water and only drink fruit juice, tea, coffee and alcohol. The remedy encourages the patient to drink more water. Some patients have a very strong thirst for cold water but it does not satisfy them and may contribute to the symptom picture by causing a noisy gut and fullness in the abdomen. These patients are usually liable to feel overheated and sweaty. Nausea that comes on in a wave. Vomiting with burning sensation. Chronic indigestion. Malignant stomach conditions.

Skin

Sweating: watery, odorous, profuse. < coughing. Heat in the skin. Eruptions of pimples or pustules. Acne. Painful stiffness of the limbs < after exercise. Weakness of the arms. Limbs on the left do not coordinate well with those on the right.

Neck
Pressure at the back of the neck from tension.

Considerations for the use of the remedy

The remedy may be considered as both a constitutional remedy and a drainage and support remedy. As the latter it should be used in low potency over a long period. It can be given in the 12x or 6c daily for up to three months and raised in potency step by step, each potency achieving a deeper effect of detoxification and alkalization. As an LM potency it should work on the subtlest levels of the being. As a drainage remedy it will be called for in acid constitutions; often those who lead a contemporary version of the 'hunter-gatherer' existence though by no means exclusively such people. (Such patients are often blood type O and have contributed to their condition by eating an improper balance of protein foods and heavy carbohydrates such as bread and pasta, neither of which are suitable for this blood group but which can become an addiction.) It will also be indicated in those who are dehydrated; lack of thirst is commonly a paradoxical symptom of this condition. Sustained use of the remedy in those in whom it is indicated should encourage a stronger thirst and a keener sense of appetite for the correct food for the individual. The patient will do better if they manage to cut down on sugar and sweet foods though this will be difficult as it is an addiction. This is also true if they cut out coffee. Many patients who find themselves in need of a remedy such as **Sodium Bicarbonate** do well when they take organic cider vinegar in warm water as a supplement; one dessertspoonful is usually sufficient.

The remedies with which **Sodium Bicarbonate** is most associated include the liver remedies: **Arsen-alb, Calc-carb, Chelidonium, China, Lachesis, Lycopodium, Mag-mur, Merc-sol, Nux Vomica, Nat-mur, Nat-sulph, Phos, Sepia** and **Sulphur**. It is also compatible with the bowel nosodes. If any of the miasmatic nosodes become indicated while a patient is on a course of low potency **Sodium Bicarbonate,** it will not interfere with its action and will continue to support the afflicted digestive system. In the tissue salt range, **Sodium Bicarbonate** in high potency is well supported by **Nat-sulph** 6x, **Nat-phos** 6x or **Ferr-phos** 6x.

It is probably important to compare **Natrum Carbonicum** with this remedy as they are so very close and share many physical symptoms. To date, **Sodium Bicarbonate** is mostly seen as a remedy of cleansing and neutralizing excessive acidity in the body. This aspect was disproportionately evident during the proving. However, the mental and emotional picture, though doubtless incomplete as yet, suggests that this remedy has a breadth and depth equal to the other salts. **Sodium Bicarbonate** is likely to share with **Nat-carb** the high degree of sensitivity not only of the skin, mucous membranes and the nervous system but also of the mind, manners and emotions. The true differentiation is to be found in the duality of the bicarbonate. While **Nat-carb** is a remedy of irritability, introversion and reserve, **Sodium Bicarbonate** is one of being stuck in confusion, dilemma and indecision even though this may not be what has brought the patient for treatment. Both remedies are indicated in acidulated people (who often have the tempers to go with it) but **Sodium Bicarbonate** is less shut down emotionally than it is anxious to find a meaning to their life. There is a spark of questing spirit in it that keeps the patient from completely shutting down like **Nat-mur** or fending off the world like **Nat-carb**. The problem for the **Sodium Bicarbonate** patient is how to make the connection between the spirit and emotional and physical bodies. If a patient has been given **Nat-carb** based on the aggregate of physical general and particular symptoms but without success, it would make sense to consider the use of **Sodium Bicarbonate**.

Esoteric therapeutics

Crown
The confusion and lack of clarity in the brow centre cause a sense of being unconnected or a disconnection with spiritual awareness which the remedy can reverse when there is a willingness to engage on this level. If the patient is too earthbound with toxicity in the lower chakras then the energy of the crown centre can be fostered by using low potencies over a long period.

Brow
Confusion, blankness, a feeling of being stupid; of being prone to making mistakes and being indecisive all belong in this chakra. A balance is struck by this remedy in this centre between material and emotional needs with the emphasis on knowing intuitively that the status quo cannot continue with any degree of security in health; the status quo being one of worldly demands overwhelming emotional needs.

Throat

This centre is 'underused' in the sense that the patient has been unable to articulate clearly what is felt and thought with the result that he or she has allowed the 'muscle' of expression to atrophy or has spoken with feeling that, once released, is regretted; the patient says things that 'come out' wrong or that don't match the reality of their creative mind.

Heart

The patient is often too preoccupied by their health (either physical or mental) to be able to see how the heart centre may be in distress. The causation of the general state often lies buried in this centre. The originating causes of symp-tomatology may, to outsiders, be obviously here but the physical state may need to be worked on first for full opening of this chakra. Detoxing the lower chakras should lead to greater clarity of heart-purpose.

Solar plexus

Toxicity in this centre is a very necessary focus of attention, with acidity of the whole system stemming from imbalance between the various organs of digestion – all as a result of faulty eating habits, lack of water and emotional disturbance held in the organs of the lower chakras. The fire element is powerfully in play here; stomach energy, which should descend, is being interfered with by liver energy so that fire in the stomach now rises, variously causing uncomfortable heat in the upper body, heartburn, dehydration with stiffness in the limbs and even pain in joints. Creative motivation is weak because the spleen is so occupied with maintaining the immune system in the face of the increased susceptibility to minor infection that there is little energy left in this organ for the raising of fresh 'food energy' to rise into the heart and lungs. The stomach lacks water; it has become dehydrated and needs plenty of liquid sustenance.

Sacral

The kidneys are dehydrated, the bladder is usually weak and the ligamentous tissue of the area is susceptible to loss of elasticity. Libido is low. There is a tendency to emotional turmoil especially in crises and this can bring on bladder troubles. There is a tendency to thrush; candidiasis alters the patient's awareness of their relationship with this centre: it becomes one of worry, even hypochondriasis. Weak kidney.

Base

As a salt remedy, this is one that serves the base chakra well. In being used to detoxify the system, the remedy is inevitably drawing the patient towards becoming more and more grounded. If the system as a whole is able to eliminate, all the structural areas that are stiff, painful or inflamed should be relieved of symptoms.

A Prover's experiences

1 'Sodium Bicarbonate ... not my favourite remedy to start with but now it's settled down. It started cleansing my bowels the morning of the proving, several times before we sat down and I was quite worried about having to leave the circle but it was such a great proving I don't think I even mentioned it at the time! Definitely cleared the bowels very well especially if I had sugar, rich food or alcohol over Christmas; I knew I would need to be near the loo the next day. Would start off almost constipated then get looser each time. Also quite a lot of wind and burping, really noisy and gurgling. (Quite a task to cover up with a houseful of people!)

'Felt very hot in the proving even before we started but my temperature has been better since and not sweating as I was although my face flushes very easily still. Skin has been doing a lot of detoxing; a few spots, dry skin all over. I felt very calm during the proving and have mainly been so since and much more connected spiritually. During the meditation I felt I couldn't get the knowledge I needed and there was too much to learn and I couldn't absorb it all. I felt stupid.[31] Since then I feel it doesn't matter! Also that I do have the knowledge and that it is there to tap into without trying so hard. I feel like I have slowed down and can see how others are on the hamster-wheel and I am watching them thinking how ridiculous they are achieving nothing but more stress. [I have] better energy in the mornings.'

31 The subject has, in the past, done so well on **Baryta-carb** that she claims that it is one of her favourite remedies. It is likely that **Sodium Bicarbonate** has an affinity with the carbon-related remedies.

2 'After the proving I was exhausted. On arriving home I fell asleep from 6.30 to 8 o'clock and was in bed by 9pm. I spent four days in bed! Coughing (a lot) with the cough slowly becoming more productive with small amounts of green sputum. I had a sensation of a lump in my throat, my head felt about to explode and my ears felt blocked. There was copious egg white mucus from the nose. The catarrh turned yellow then green – yards of it. It went on for days. I had an insatiable thirst for cold water: pints and pints of it – three pints in one night, six or eight pints in the day. No appetite. I was feverish; kept going hot and cold. [I wanted] sleep. I slept most of the four days. On day five I got up but had no energy; felt very spacy – everything was a huge effort. Once I was up and about the cough continued dry and tickly for over four weeks. I wanted to sing but couldn't as I immediately started coughing again. Mentally and emotionally [I feel] much lighter and happier; I just wanted to sing all the time.'

Case studies

1 'A man in his mid fifties, easily susceptible to stress, with a history of bowel problems (tendency to constipation, bloating, wind and heartburn), returned for treatment after having had various remedies over at least two years. He felt that most of his prescriptions had helped though he remained worried in case any new remedy might exacerbate his piles which tended to bleed when he strained to pass a motion. He was given **Sodium Bicarbonate** 12c to take each day for six weeks. He wrote halfway through this period to say that he was doing well on the new remedy; that he had not suffered any aggravation of the piles; that his libido had unexpectedly returned and that he no longer needed coffee to keep him going and that he now had no interest in sweet foods.' CG

2 'A woman of 72, of strong physique and constitution, complained of heartburn and other digestive problems. She was intolerant of dairy food; raw vegetables caused diarrhoea. She was unable to eat anything that tasted acidic. If she ate anything that aggravated the acid level in her system she would suffer headaches of a migraine character. She also had

sinus trouble with a continual post-nasal drip. She mentioned that she was only otherwise troubled by the stress of constantly worrying about things she was unable to do anything about. This not unusual picture was only qualified by a history of TB in the family (her paternal grandfather). She was given **Tuberculinum** 100 followed by **Morgan Gaertner** 30 (several times a week). On this she felt that she made some progress: her energy was better and her digestion was less of a problem though there were occasions when the motions were loose or constipated. She next had **Lycopodium** 100 while the bowel nosode maintained continuity. Her energy continued to improve; the bowel also felt better and more reliable. She still had flatulence at times and she still felt the acidity problem was there; she had had a headache recently for the first time in a long time. At this point she was given **Sodium Bicarbonate** 30. After the first dose she had a sudden bout of severe heartburn some hours after eating. She avoided anything to eat that might cause further acidity and found that the heartburn gradually eased off. Her energy levels improved considerably again, the flatulence eased off completely and her motions were normal.' **CG**

3 'A woman in her 60s who had chronic digestive problems despite years of homoeopathic treatment came with symptoms of acidity and anxiety. She had always found that **Arsen-alb** alleviated the worst of her suffering but that it was not now doing much for her. She had nausea once she was lying down in bed and she could not bear anything to touch her abdomen, even the bedclothes. She battled with excessive mucus in her throat. She avoided wheat and dairy as they exaggerated her indigestion. She was given **Sodium Bicarbonate** 12 daily. She became so attached to this remedy that she asked to be able to continue with it. She felt that it not only removed the acidity but that it also cleared away much of her anxiety. She now takes the remedy only if she feels she needs it which happens if she is stressed or if she has eaten something she should not have eaten.' **CG**

21

OLEA EUROPAEA

Olive

The remedy was proved by means of meditation on 23 July 1999. There were 6 provers, 2 men and 4 women, and the medium. The remedy, which was made from the leaf, twig and bark of the tree, was taken in the 30th potency.

The Background

Olea oleaster, *Olea lancifolia*, *Olea gallica*, Queen olive and Manzanillo are all kinds of Olive. The wild olive originated from Asia Minor and spread to Europe, Africa, Japan, China and Australia. Today there are some 750 million trees, 95 per cent of which are growing in the Mediterranean. The olive is hardy to minus 4°C. It grows abundantly, particularly in the iron-rich soil of Spain and in Greece and Italy. It tolerates virtually any kind of soil though it is known to do best as a crop plant when grown in calcareous soil. It prefers well-drained ground and thrives in full sunlight or semi-shade. It is evergreen with opposite, lanceolate leaves that are a little over five centimetres long, pale green above and silvery beneath. The bark is pale grey, deeply fissured as it ages and with an increasingly gnarled appearance. Old trees assume extraordinary contorted shapes. It can grow up to six to nine metres and has a ball-like canopy. There are small creamy-white flowers which are fragrant and hermaphrodite; the tree is self-pollinating. The flowers are followed by the oval-shaped, oil-rich fruit which contains the thick, bony seed. There are green and black varieties, the latter of a dark purple hue. It takes 10 to 20 years for the tree to mature. Some specimens have survived to reach a venerable age of up to 1,000 years.

The olive has a complex chemical constitution. Its constituents include oleic, palmitic, stearic and linoleic acids among others; it also contains squalene. It is unique in the plant kingdom in that its seeds contain albumen, normally associated with eggs. Calcareous soil produces plants that provide the oil with the smoothest and subtlest flavour and the least acidic effects.

Cold-pressed virgin olive oil is the result of crushing the green olives between mill stones (traditional) or spinning them at high speed in metal drums (centrifugation – a modern method). It is unadulterated by chemicals while refined oil is treated chemically to remove strong tastes and to neutralize the oleic acid content. Over 50 per cent of the Mediterranean oil is of too poor quality for the table and is not marketed for consumption until it is chemically refined and filtered through charcoal. Virgin olive oil contains no carbohydrates and no protein. It is rich in saturated and unsaturated fats, the bulk being monounsaturated fats. It is also a source of vitamins E and K.

The uses of the olive are numerous. The oil from the crushed fruit has always been an essential ingredient of salad dressings, for example. It is perhaps the best of all cooking oils (usually in its refined state) as it is chemically stable even at high temperatures and of superior taste with vital health-giving properties. It has also been used as a dessert fruit when the unripe olives are steeped in water to reduce their naturally bitter taste.

In the warmth of the Mediterranean its bark exudes what is known as *gomme d'olivier* which was employed as a vulnerary. Modern science has endorsed ancient wisdom: because of the polyphenol antioxidants in the fruit, olive oil is beneficial in maintaining arterial elasticity and lowering the susceptibility to heart disease and stroke. It is also considered a natural method of lowering 'bad' cholesterol (LDL) in the blood as well as reducing blood sugars and con-tributing to the lowering of blood pressure. (Laboratory tests on mice have shown that applying olive oil to skin damaged by UVB rays is protective.) It has also been used as a liniment to aid wound healing. It is antifungal, antipru-ritic, antiseptic, astringent, emollient, mildly laxative and demulcent; it is a cholagogue and a febrifuge. Consuming the oil reduces gastric secretions which makes it useful in combating hyperacidity and easing the symptoms of peptic ulceration. As a decoction it is used to treat fevers and as a tranquillizer. It has been used as a hair tonic and a dye and to combat dandruff. The oil has been used since the earliest times for lamps and in temples and churches during religious ceremonies. It is exclusively used in the lamps burning during some Jewish festivals and rituals.

Apart from the oil, the olive tree provides wood for furniture. It is of value to cabinetmakers for fine-grained pieces that take a deep polish. The wood has a faintly discernible fragrance. It has also been used for statuary since the most ancient times not least because the contortions into which the bowl of the tree tends to twist often suggest figures. Many old churches in Spain and Italy have gnarled statues of saints and the Virgin Mary tucked away in odd corners which are redolent of the trust their makers had in the natural energy invested in the tree to hold the spiritual essence of their fervent belief.

The olive was recorded as being of benefit to man by the Minoans of Crete 3000 years ago but has been known for far longer as the first olive presses date back to 1600 BC. It was regarded as sacred to ancient Greece and to Athens. Athena, Zeus's daughter, won her father's contest among her fellow gods to provide the capital of Greece with something the people would most treasure; she struck the soil with her spear and caused an olive to grow. The people were so delighted and so much more appreciative of it than of any of the other gods' ideas that Zeus gave her the honour. She gave her name to the city and stood as its patron and mentor from then on. Champions at the Olympic Games were always given crowns of olive leaves cut from a wild tree by a gold-handled blade in the belief that the tree's vitality and longevity would be transferred to the victor. Great battle heroes were given the same coronets of olive for bravery. The olive is still regarded as a symbol of peace, goodwill and wisdom hence the phrase 'to offer an olive branch'. There is also the Biblical story of Noah and the dove he sent out at the end of 40 days of rain to go in search of dry land. The bird brought back an olive twig. Mrs Grieve, in her *Modern Herbal*, reminds us that Moses exempted from military service all the men who worked on olive cultivation. Universally the olive has always been regarded as a symbol of purity and goodness and it also represents happiness.

Keynote effects

It is a calming remedy for the hurt mind; a tranquillizing influence on those who carry shock and trauma in the psyche and are unable to release them. It slows down an agitated system. This is most especially true of those who are in some way affected by others who would wish them either harm or to be easily manipulated; being in another person's thrall. It affects those who have been involved in emotional feuding and have been subject to psychic attack by the other party or those who have inherited bad feeling from previous generations involved in family or community ill feeling. It calms agitation, restlessness and anxiety in those whose energy field is darkened by or heavy with emotional turmoil.

General symptoms

Olive works on heart and circulation: it improves oxidation in the blood, encourages the lungs to open when they have been restricted by diaphragmatic tension and pressure due to stuck emotions. It improves the quality of the tissues of the cardiovascular system; it improves elasticity in the arteries (especially in low 'x' potency) and may prove to be of value in the treatment of patients with high cholesterol. Atherosclerosis. It also may prove to be of particular value in one whose cardiovascular system is such that open-heart surgery has been mooted (always bearing in mind the rest of the remedy picture). The physical agitation and anxiety that are present in this remedy are often characteristic of those with potentially serious heart pathology: restlessness, irritability, anxiety and even a dry, irritating cough. Mucous membranes become ulcerated especially in one who is subject to resentment and fearfulness. Inflammation of the digestive tract: intestinal mucous membranes become raw or even ulcerated. Affects the spleen and pancreas though the pathology reported may well only appear to affect the spleen meridian. The same is true of the gall bladder: symptoms may only manifest on points of the gall bladder meridian distant from the organ but the remedy will affect the whole system as it tries to demonstrate typical 'gall bladder' distress. Joints also come under the influence of **Olive**: inflammation, pain and degenerative changes may all indicate its use. To be considered in polymyalgia when other symptoms agree. It helps to prevent the onset of osteoporosis and may still be indicated if the process has already started. Both the discs of the spinal column and cartilage are affected as are the growth and strength of hair and nails. **Olive** acts as if it were a skin balm: it is useful in all skin conditions marked by irritability, sensitivity and agitation. It is useful both in potency and as a cream.

Miasms

Psora, syphilis, sycosis and tuberculosis.

Mental and emotional symptoms

Panic, confusion and turmoil; much agitation and anxiety. May be used in the acute as well as the chronic state. Unable to think clearly or to articulate well; in extremis acts as if disorientated. Cannot express feelings through the throat centre. Irritable and unable to let go of interfering emotions. Resentful, bitter thoughts about things that have happened or words that have been said. Offended by judgements that have been made. A strong sense of injustice but feelings of impotence to do much about it. Stuck in feelings of anger and unable to forgive. Distressed to be in an antagonistic state and to be unable 'to forgive and move on'. Despair of ever moving out of the negativity. Wants strongly to forgive and accept but holds the energy of the negativity deep in the tissues: of the heart, the diaphragm, the bowels, the gall bladder and the chest. The weight of past events (either distant or more recent) is too heavy to be able to enjoy the experience of the moment. Feels shocked and traumatized but does not know why. For those who hold onto their trauma despite well-indicated remedies. (If a patient is prescribed this remedy for a long-held trauma that other seemingly well-indicated remedies have been unable to influence, the result may be an episode of agitation. If this is the case and the period of agitation takes a long interval to develop then the aggravation should not be interfered with on any account. It must be allowed to work through the system thoroughly as it may herald an aspect of the carcinogenic miasm which would require attention next. **Carcinosin** is a remedy that follows **Olive** very well.) Fearful of their mental and emotional state in case it is harming them. Fearful of dealing with emotional issues. Sighing with a sense of not being able to take a deep enough breath when emotions are running strong. Indecisive especially when emotional strife is acute. It is useful when otherwise indicated for those who are attempting to reduce their prescribed antidepressants: the agitation and fear that can result are potentially reduced. For the effects of emotional shock when the subject is left with the burden of fear, humiliation, hurt and/or injustice; there may even be a sense of disbelief that anyone could have behaved towards them in such a manner. In contemporary jargon: the patient's sense of personal space has been invaded. Useful in those who have a fear of public speaking; self-conscious before an audience.

Physical symptoms

Head
Pressure on the vertex.

Eyes

Dry and sore. Poor vision; worsening through emotional crisis.

Mouth

Bitter taste.

Throat

Sensation as if swollen; thyroid feels larger. Irritating persistent cough. Cannot shift the persistent mucus in the larynx which is sticky.

Respiration

Wants to take a deep breath but cannot; as if one cannot take in enough air. Sighs. Feels the burden of emotions in the chest cavity.

Digestion

Hyperacidity. Inflamed stomach, sphincters (cardiac and pyloric). Acid indigestion. Peptic ulcer. Tension held and felt in the diaphragm.

Back, neck and shoulders

Tension and pain. Polymyalgia. Osteoporotic changes.

Extremities

Painful joints: aching. Inflammation of joints not through traumatic injury. Stiffness and rigidity of muscles.

Considerations for the use of the remedy

Olive may be compared with a number of other remedies:

- **Peridot** which is a remedy for the heart centre where forgiveness and acceptance of past trauma are also featured; Peridot is far less agitated, irritable and anxious. Both remedies may be indicated in those who suffer psychic attack or are under the negative influence of another person. However, in the case of **Peridot**, the influence may not come from such historical roots; it may come from the result of one incident.

- **Carcinosin** is often the remedy that follows **Olive** or it may have been given intercurrently when other indicated remedies have failed; the carcinogenic state usually offers us the reason for the patient's susceptibility to harbouring emotional trauma.

• **Staphysagria** has obvious parallels with **Olive**: the sense of impotence in the face of aggression; the inability to deal with the effects of abuse. **Staphysagria** does not have the physical agitation, restlessness and anxiety of **Olive** except when exploding into rage; it has a unique picture of physical concomitants and in **Olive** there is more the sense of being under psychic attack from another. **Staphysagria** is more prone to physical and emotional abuse; **Olive** to mental abuse which hurts the emotions.

• **Buddleia** also covers the tendency to draw emotional trauma into the digestive tract and threaten ulceration of the mucous membranes; this remedy shows less physical agitation though may be more demonstrative of emotional pain with tears and anxiety; it is less concerned about 'me' than **Olive** and more worried about the state of the family, community, planet; there is in **Buddleia** a far more clear element of disaster rather than being the subject of psychic attack.

• **Tiger's Eye** also has physical agitation and restlessness, anxiety and irritability but the underlying negative energy stems from damage to the generative organs and, to a lesser extent, those of the solar plexus or to hysteria.

The underlying causation for the use of **Olive** can lie deep in the past. It may not even originate in the patient but in the patient's family dynamic. Amongst the peoples of the Mediterranean bitter family quarrels have never been uncommon and enmity between protagonists of emotional dramas has led to fearful degrees of hatred and what amounts to psychic attack: evil thinking directed at another. Nearer home, Celts have also contributed to a slipstream of bitterness that following generations have had to contend with. Despite the more closed emotional heart of the Anglo-Saxon psychology, such negative energy also plays a part in undermining the health of many though it is much more likely that the bitterness would be between members of the same family or team of colleagues. It is also more likely that the originating causation is of more recent time: warring siblings, for example, who are in bitter dispute over the estate of a dead relative or feuding office workers involved in deadly competition, but where one side is threatening, intentionally destructive and manipulative. However, such high drama may be far from the story of any other patient in need of **Olive**; it might well be indicated, say, in one of a couple, both of whom have been unable to come to terms with separation and visiting rights for their children, who feels maligned and slandered by the other. There are some patients who actually say that they feel that their lives have in some way been blighted by the behaviour and attitude of another or of others. If the rest of the **Olive** picture is there then the remedy will surely bring them to a point of understanding and acceptance so that they feel they can let go of the tensions of the past.

Both **Emerald** and **Green** are associated remedies: they precede and follow **Olive** well. **Green** is particularly useful when the sense of trauma is characterized by any shock that is sustained from an unexpected source: an erstwhile friend who suddenly shows up in a new and negative light, for example. **Nitric Acid** is well supported by **Olive** as is **Anacardium**. As a combination tincture to support the heart centre in a case of potential heart pathology **Crataegus** Ø + **Arnica** 6 + **Olive** 6 is useful. Martin Miles recommended the use of **Olive** + **Buddleia** with another of choice from among remedies with an affinity for the digestive tract for those with inflammatory and ulcerative activity in the stomach or intestines following a history of shock and trauma that has gone to this part of the system.

It is worth mentioning that dreams may play a significant part in witnessing the action of this remedy: trauma and shock from the past may be released or relieved during dreams. It might be of benefit for the patient to record the dream or dreams that occur after taking the remedy.

Esoteric therapeutics

Olive works on all chakras but has an affinity for the clearing of shock and trauma from the tissues of the heart, lungs, blood and digestive tract. As it is a remedy that fosters understanding, forgiveness and acceptance it is very much a remedy to purify stuck and toxic negative energy and particularly that stemming from being transfixed in a condition of bitterness or from psychic attack.

Like **Buddleia**, **Olive** is indicated in those whose boundaries have been breached. **Buddleia**'s principle activity is on the crown centre, heart and base; **Olive** works on the brow, heart and solar plexus. They are complementary remedies and support each other in one who feels the devastation typical of **Buddleia** as well as the characteristics of **Olive**.

Chakras

Brow
The remedy restores equilibrium where there has been panic, disorientation and a lack of consecutive thought. It helps protect the delicate balance of the mind in one who is subjected to the untoward influence of others when there is no paranoia in the picture. It fosters a necessary sense of detachment so that decisions can be made with greater confidence.

Throat
The ability to express emotion is restored to this centre which is often blocked with catarrh or restricted by a persistent cough.

Thymus gland
If there is ancestral trauma and shock in the picture then this centre will need attention. If the elements are typical of **Olive** then it can be given in combination with **Thymus Gland** and **Syphilinum** as an LM or in high potency. An alternative that might also be indicated when there is fearfulness as well as a history of trouble descending through the female line would be **Thymus Gland + Ayahuasca + Olive**.

Heart
When the tissues of the heart centre, whether in the heart itself or in the lung field, are compromised by held-in emotion and trauma **Olive** will work to release these. It may have to be given for a considerable time especially if the LM option is chosen. (Bear in mind that **Carcinosin** is a heart centre remedy and is well supported by **Olive** especially in the LM.) Much tension in this centre may be derived from a taut and tense diaphragm which is redolent of stuck emotions.

Solar plexus
The organs of the solar plexus are particularly susceptible to the toxic emotions characterized by **Olive**. Liver and gall bladder may both manifest distress either as headaches or muscular pains and rigidity (either shoulder, right neck and occiput, right forehead) and the spleen may show weakness as lack of motivation and loss of drive. The stomach may produce excess acidity.

Base

Lack of confidence and of self-worth. Feels undermined by the attitude and activity of others. Skin symptoms manifest as part of the irritability that this brings up.

Case studies

1 The following is the experience of a homoeopath who had difficulties with a patient over a few months.

'I've always had a problem with boundaries with patients but never in my wildest dreams thought I would get involved in something as deeply as I did. A patient of mine who was a very complex lady started to get far too involved with me and my life and I was hearing from her several times a day. I realized after a while that a lot of the things she told me were not the same as those she was telling another professional colleague of mine (whom she was consulting at the same time for osteopathy). Nothing was adding up and it seemed more and more that she was very manipulative and deceitful and I found I was increasingly uncomfortable in her company. We decided, after a lot of advice, to both stop treating her as she was not being honest with either of us, which of course was a very difficult decision. She was not happy and I was having a lot of homoeopathy for protection and was coping with the backlash from her on a daily basis.

'One day I received an email from the patient which quoted every text and email I had sent her over months of treatment and it shocked me to the core. I felt deeply distressed and quite frightened by her persistence of contact. I remember when I read the email that I took a deep, sharp intake of breath and I felt I could not let it out. It was almost trapped in my chest and was very painful. I felt I was being stalked and I was scared. I felt I was a subject of her obsession. I felt violated and completely exhausted and traumatized but was really restless at the same time and couldn't sit still or sleep. I was very agitated and I couldn't think straight and felt I could not continue to do my job and didn't want to either. I just wanted to stop her connection and felt that I was almost being possessed.

'I was given **Olive** 30, 200, 1M over 3 days. My first physical symptom was that I could breathe again. It was very exaggerated like a 'first breath' and I cried and cried which was very cleansing. We went on holiday a few days later and my husband commented that I had come back! He said I had been very withdrawn and vacant before our holiday but was back to my old self again. I was very calm and restful on holiday but once home I had a really high temperature for almost a week and really detoxed in every way! It felt like I had cleansed mentally and physically and things really improved from that point.'

2   The following was from a patient who had been coping with grief and anger over the behaviour and malice she felt was directed towards her by a relative.

'**Olive** 1M – I was given this remedy when I was having some terrible problems with my mum's husband's son! My dear mum had just passed away and her stepson was withholding possessions from me which she had left to me in her will. They were not expensive but of enormous sentimental value. I was so angry+++. I wanted to kill him which was not a good emotion to have and there was nothing I could do. After several heated arguments, the frustration and upset was too much to bear especially as I had just lost the dearest person in the whole world to me. I took this remedy and the feelings of anger ebbed away and within a couple of days I was much more chilled about the situation. Now, some five weeks on I still do not have these things, even solicitors have not made it possible yet. But I know that one day I will, hopefully, get them back and if I don't, I don't; I'm not going to lose my health over it. The anger has diminished a lot. I am just trying to deal with one day at a time.'

3   'A girl of 11, a Pisces, was brought by her mother for treatment for a "nervous stomach". She was very pale, almost white. She was very easily chilled. She was shy and timid and, her mother said, a very fussy eater. Any stress gave her pains in her solar plexus: exams, going to school even. I noticed that the energy of her solar plexus chakra was spinning the wrong way. She had **Arsenicum**, **Arg-nit** and **Lycopodium**, all of which did something good but they couldn't hold. She had **Thuja** as well. **Arsenicum** did the best and gave her some relief for about six weeks. The second time I gave it to her it lasted for three weeks. **Arg-nit** held

for not much more than a week. Then she had **Olive** 30: one daily for seven days. She had a bad aggravation for three days after the first or second dose; the mother rang up in an anxious state and was on the point of taking her daughter to the doctor but was persuaded to let the remedy take its course. Then the symptoms all subsided very quickly. She needed the remedy repeated later on when she took it for another seven days, this time with no aggravation. She has needed nothing since.' JM

4   A woman of 36 came with severe panic attacks; she was brought by a relative. She was a Scorpio; Scorpio people find it very hard to shift out of anxiety once they are in it. This woman's parents were both killed in a car accident when she was four years old. She had fear of the police; of fire engines; of going out alone; of not having any company. She had to be with someone all the time. The aura of her solar plexus was black; it looked completely blocked. The fear she held in her lower body was almost palpable; she was full of shock, layers and layers of shock. She had several remedies including **Arsenicum**, **Nat-mur**, **Ignatia** and then **Tuberculinum**. She did better on the **Tub** and she had some relief for about six weeks. Then she had **Lachesis** which is a good remedy for Scorpios. The surprising thing was that the blackness of the solar plexus got bigger. It was then that she had **Olive** 30: one three times a week for four weeks. All the blackness disappeared; her solar plexus was much better. After this all the remedies that had been indicated before and now came up again, really worked well. She gradually reached the stage where she had no further panic attacks. Each time they began to creep back she had a further dose of **Olive** 30 and more layers of shock would be released.' JM

5   'A man of 65 who had severe eczema wanted help to relieve the skin symptoms. The eczema was cracked and weepy. He did well in himself on **Thuja** and **Medorrhinum Americana**. He found that the greatest relief was from **Olive** cream that he bought off the Internet. All the aggravating symptoms calmed right down every time he applied it.' JM

6   'An Indian girl of 18 came with Hodgkin's disease with a particularly swollen thyroid gland. She was a Libran. She was in deep shock having suffered from trauma including a difficult birth. She appeared weak,

fragile and confused. Her mother, who accompanied her, also had a similar picture though there was no major physical pathology in her case. There was a story attached to the case: the mother said that during her pregnancy with her daughter she had been subjected to evil thoughts from another member of the family and that it had probably affected the child. Then her husband had died when the girl was six years old. She said that he had gone to work one day, in perfect health, but had become ill during the morning. He developed a violent red rash on his legs, came home at lunchtime, felt unwell with breathing difficulties and then suddenly died of an asthma attack. She said that her father-in-law was being particularly malicious towards his son at the time.

'The girl was given quite a series of remedies, all of which had reasonable indications though none of them did anything like enough and did not hold. They included **Nat-mur, Tuberculinum** (which improved her constitutionally for a good period; it is often a very useful remedy in Hodgkin's), **Syphilinum, Phytolacca** (which certainly eased the glandular swelling for a short while), **Ayahuasca, Berlin Wall** and **Holly Berry**.[32] She was then given **Olive** 200 once a week for three weeks. The effect was remarkable. The Hodgkin's symptoms all began to abate and her feeling of being under attack all the time faded to being manageable. After the **Olive** the remedies that had been indicated before and that came up again now all worked much deeper. They held. She needed several more intercurrent doses of **Olive** periodically and it always did the same thing: it calmed her nervous symptoms completely and eased the thyroid and glandular symptoms and the mainstay remedies of **Phytolacca** and **Syphilinum** worked really well. The case is ongoing but the pathology is now no longer stopping her from living a normal life.' JM

---

[32] **Holly Berry** is a deep-acting remedy that is one of the most frequently indicated for auric protection. It is useful in a case where the patient has been a witness of traumatic situations, has suffered acutely and is emotionally over-sensitized as a result. One of the keynotes is that the patient cannot take any more suffering. It has been successfully used in acute situations as well as in chronic cases. A patient who had been raped and had decided to prosecute her attacker went into sudden acute kidney pathology with severe, paralysing pain and urethral stricture and tenesmus. **Holly Berry** 10M relieved all symptoms before the ambulance arrived.

22

ORANGE

The remedy was proved by two circles of 6 women and 3 men on 3 April and the 17 April 1998. Each participant was given a single dose of the 30th potency to take. The remedy had been made up by Katherine Boulderstone at the Helios Pharmacy in the same manner as she developed the other colour remedies of the spectrum.

The Background

Orange is the mixture of red and yellow. Its complementary colour is blue. It is thought of as a 'warm' colour (thanks to the yellow) and is regarded by many as the colour of energy, action and strength; all attributes of the fiery sun. Yet, in the vibrant shade of the fruit it is named after, it is the colour that most people, at least in Western countries, shy away from wearing as it attracts too much attention to itself. Nevertheless, colour therapists agree that those who do wear it (and wear it well) are likely to be thoughtful and serious people at heart however extravagant they might be in manner.

Of the colour spectrum orange is the least popular and least understood and is interesting for the paradox it presents. While it is said to be the colour of the sacral chakra in the Hindu 'rainbow' system, it appears to have as much to do with the mental sphere as the sexual centre. It represents balance and reason; it is the colour of measured thought that leads to true wisdom. The orange robes of Buddhist priests signify the search for this attainment. The balance between justice and mercy, order and chaos, thought and feeling, truth and lies, reality and illusion are all held in orange. It is the colour required to influence the search for this wisdom and it is the colour that governs those things that present sufficient challenge to ensure that the journey is worthwhile. Energy, strength and action are pitted against ambition, pride and exhibitionism.

Colour healers use orange to engender joyousness, enthusiasm, self-confidence and creativity and to dispel despondency, dependency and antisocial feelings. Crystal therapists work with carnelian, orange calcite and tangerine quartz, among others, for the same purpose. It is orange that is used to stimulate the mental body and to increase the power of logic and the power to conceptualize. It speeds up the brain's ability to make connections by increasing the oxygen supply. It is what we need to open up the mind to allow creative ideas to flow freely. Small wonder that so many businesses use either the name or the colour or both in their publicity.

The intensity of the colour can be a mixed blessing. It is well known that enhanced creativity can increase libido and appetite but it can also lead to excess and cravings: overindulgence can sometimes be the result of too much 'orangeness'.

Other cultures see orange differently. North American Indians see orange as the colour of kinship; in a tribal society this is of immense importance as regards mutual recognition and stable relationships. In China and Japan orange is the colour of happiness and unconditional love. In ancient times orange was symbolic of courage. In Elizabethan England, when sumptuary laws were in force to dictate just what colours were permitted for the different classes, orange was worn by the poor because the rose madder dye that made the orange was not fast and would fade quickly with washing. It was in the early 1500s, in Tudor days, when the word 'orange' was first used to denote the colour.

It is worth quoting the painter, Wassily Kandinsky, who said, 'Orange is red brought nearer to humanity by yellow.' Van Gogh said, 'There is no blue without yellow and without orange.'

Keynote effects

Peace of mind is brought about by stilling its chattering and relaxing the faculty of harsh critical judgement. This leads to sufficient balance to be able to reason with the aid of intuition rather than relying solely on the overworked intellect. This in turn leads to less fearfulness because of the enhanced ability to recognize what the self most needs; the negative attribute of yellow, cowardice, is tempered by the positive fiery quality of red. However, in some there can be a sense of elation and positive excitement at the anticipation of clearing the mind and expanding the emotions. There is the discovery that it is no longer necessary to force the pace of things; all that is needed is to let the process take care of itself.

General symptoms

This is, above all, a remedy for distressed mental faculties and the relationship between the mind and body. It is indicated in one whose excessive mental activity threatens to overwhelm the physical body's ability to sustain perfectly balanced functioning. Where there is no peace of mind there is no peace in the body. Particularly affected are the endocrine system and the vital organs and their relationship to each other. The organ most vulnerable to the lack of sympathy between mind and body is the heart. Pathology is likely to be first manifest in the lungs and chest though any part of the organism may respond well to the remedy when it is indicated. Of the endocrine glands it is the pituitary gland that is likely to be the most obviously out of sync. The remedy has a strong affinity for both lobes of the pituitary and the cerebrospinal fluid that flows past them. What makes the pituitary vulnerable to stagnation is over-adrenalized activity: the patient thinks too much, too fast and too intensely for the system to maintain its integrity. Sensations of blockage arise: in the lungs, the throat, the stomach and the sexual organs. Cramp may seize the muscles of the extremities. Visual acuity can be impaired. The kidneys and spleen respond to the remedy especially if there has been any pathology of these organs that has left the constitution weakened. Early signs of heart pathology are likely to be centred on the right side of the organ. A general state of congestion in mucous membranes, bowels or any hollow organ may be indicative. For those who have responded well to radiation remedies, **Orange** should be considered as a follow-up remedy as it has qualities that afford deep protection against this most insidious form of toxicity. It should also be considered in cases of persistent headaches that may or may not seem to be associated with any other concomitant symptoms. It is reputed to be one of a group of remedies most useful for rites of passage, particularly of birth and death (cf. **Blue, Sandalwood, Ayahuasca**). **Orange** is also a remedy that should be considered to unlock a stuck case where well-indicated remedies do not create the expected and necessary curative changes. In such cases the patient is likely to manifest mental symptoms that, in the patient's own estimation, appear to take priority over physical symptoms that, in themselves, would be significant enough to cause considerable distress. It has been said that **Orange** should not be a remedy to be given as a first prescription (see Case 1 below). Like so many of the caveats in homoeopathy, this caution may turn out to be unnecessary in cases where the remedy is obviously the similimum.

Miasms

Psora, sycosis, tuberculosis and radiation.

Mental and emotional symptoms

Sensitivity, anxiety and restless mindedness. Brain chunter that disturbs sleep and working patterns. A profound sense of the lack of peace. Inability to 'see the wood for the trees'; stuck in the minutiae of the mind's troubles and unable to see the big picture. Lack of clarity; the mind's eye is unable to visualize anything entirely positive. Egotism; the strong ego overrides common-sense solutions where pride might be dented. Too much calculation stunts the imagination; the left brain overwhelms the right. Excessive activity in the mind with tiredness of the physical body; the adrenal energy is all focused in the mental sphere while the body struggles. Poor memory, blank mind, confusion and feelings of disconnection in one who has had a long but unsuccessful struggle in the mind to cope or to work problems out. This is true even for one who appears to be mentally alert. A sense of mental compression may arise as if the walls are closing in. Seeks solace for mental distress in comfort food or in sexual activity. These become ways of feeling more connected. There can be a profound sense of dislocation or disconnection; of being 'outside' looking in. The inner person can feel outside and disconnected from the physical self. There is difficulty in staying grounded and in focus. The head and feet seem to be travelling in different directions. They know what needs to be done but either do nothing about it or do the other thing. There is often a feeling of too little space. This can be an entirely mental sense or it can be physical. A disinclination to participate; does not want to talk or hold a conversation. Prefers to sit in silence. Alternates brooding with bursts of enthusiasm for new thoughts that may lead to a solution (which is seldom acted upon).

Physical symptoms

As with a few other new remedies such as **Lotus** and **Rainbow,** there is a paucity of physical symptoms as so few were actually manifest in the proving. In the case of **Orange** it is worth noting that it can influence any part of the system and may do so to a relatively deep degree. What will determine its likeness to the pathology is the state of the mind in relation to the physical body.

Head
Headache in the frontal region; mid-brow. Intense pressure in the centre of the forehead. Compression or expansion sensations within the cranium.

Eyes
Aching of the eyes. Ability to focus varies: poor acuity. Aching and fading focus alternate.

Ears
Sensitivity to sound. Excessive irritability due to loud music or sudden intrusive sounds.

Throat
Sensation of compression or blockage.

Respiration and chest
Congestion in the lungs and mucous membranes. Asthmatic breathing. Thick mucus in the bronchioles which causes compression in the chest.

Heart
Awareness of the heart within the chest. Compression or expansion sensations in the heart area. Excitability affects the heart's beat.

Abdomen
Very sharp pain in the inguinal ligament on the right side.

Male and female
Sensations of blockage in the uterus. Weakness after sex in both men and women.

Urinary organs

Discomfort and feeling of strain in the kidney area; possible inflammation. History of kidney problems which is not completely resolved. Passes less water than is drunk.

Extremities

Cramp especially in the right foot; all the toes curl under.

Sleep

Restless and anxious sleep.

Considerations for the use of the remedy

This can be a frustrating remedy for the prescriber as it is hard to assess its indications. It is often intuition that is the main guide to its use; we are left to understand why it was necessary after the event when the patient returns and relates how they have fared. Partly this is due to the apparent lack of strong definition among the physical symptoms and partly to the fact that the patient may, paradoxically, complain about physical symptoms and not give much time to the mental and emotional ones. We have to see beyond the limitations of the patient's words to gauge the level of distress the mind is at in relation to the physical body, particularly in relation to heart energy or, sometimes, sexual energy (which is more commonly seen among men). What we do see is that there is a store of constitutional energy that exists and that is drawn on by the patient even if it is misspent or misdirected or simply waiting to be put into gear. It has been described as a 'doorway' remedy; when it is opened then the patient is able to continue more purposefully.

It is worth noting its affinity to other brow chakra remedies as it precedes them very well (though it is likely that they will be given afterwards, in support, as **Orange** was not 'seen' before). Chief among these are **Calc-carb, Calc-iod, Baryta-carb, Lycopodium, Merc-sol, Sulph** and **Tuberculinum.** Of the new remedies we should consider that the following have a strong affinity: **Blue, Clear Quartz, Copper Beech, Ivy Berry, Oak, Pomegranate, Rainbow, Sandalwood** and **Sycamore Seed. Thymus Gland** also has strong associations. It is another 'doorway' remedy; where there is a need 'to get to the other side' of a block to cure that is not specifically miasmatic. In **Orange** the block is the lack of real connection between the mind and the physical body and the disparity between intellect and intuition. In **Thymus Gland** there is traumatic history to be dealt with. The different aspects of the two remedies can be strongly interlinked. Both remedies have one aspect in common even though for different reasons: they both help the patient not to keep trying to force the natural pace of things. While **Thymus Gland** is mostly to do with the pacing of development (physical, mental or emotional), **Orange** is more connected with forging links between the mind and the heart; getting the mind to be in harmony with what the heart most needs and wishes in reality, which it is often unable to do until the thymus gland is unburdened.

Another thing to be mentioned about this odd remedy is that it is contraindicated in one who is purposefully but negatively manipulating the lives of others for their own and selfish ends. This brings up an anomaly: **Merc-sol** is just such a remedy state that can do this most particularly in a patient who is strongly syphilitic. (This caveat may not be of importance in those who need **Merc-sol** influenced by either the sycotic or tubercular miasms.)

Esoteric therapeutics

Orange, the remedy, is most closely associated with the brow centre, the chakra of wisdom. It is the centre governed by Mercury, the planet associated with the winged messenger of the gods, the carrier of the caduceus that variously symbolizes trades and the undertakings of the gods, astrology and later, commerce.[33] The 'metaphor' of this chakra is exemplified by Hermes Trismegistus, the ancient divine who was melded with the Egyptian god, Thoth, by the Greeks who occupied Upper Egypt following Cleopatra's demise. These two deities and the later Roman version, Mercury, were all worshipped as one. Thoth and Hermes were gods of communication, writing, astrology and alchemy. Thoth, the ancient Egyptian god of time, wisdom and writing had the head of an ibis, the bird that symbolizes wisdom and learning as it spends its life sifting through mud with its long curved beak much as a pen's nib would scratch away at a paper. Writing of those times was in glyphs, symbols of sound energy that can be used for creating positive change, much as are the Aramaic and Hebrew written languages.

---

33 The caduceus, with its two entwined snakes, the double helix, is often confused with the rod of Asclepius, a rod with a single snake. The mistake arose when the US army adopted the caduceus as the symbol for the Army Corps in 1902. It is the rod of Asclepius, the asklepion, that represents healing and the practice of medicine.

Thoth was a mediator and a peace-keeper. He and his wife Ma'at, the goddess of justice, were always present at embalming rituals. Thoth would weigh the dead person's soul, to assess its merits, against the ostrich feather of righteousness that Ma'at wore in her hair. Ma'at would sit atop the scales to ensure that the procedure was correctly carried out. In the Book of Thoth there were two spells written down: one was to understand all creatures on earth and the other was to be able to raise the dead. Such aspirations were closely connected with the origins of alchemy and the Kabbalah, not the search for turning base metal into gold but the search for spiritual union with the universal source of energy for which gold was no more than a metaphor. Hermes Trismegistus was also associated with the biblical prophet Enoch, grandfather of Noah. Enoch was credited with teaching the ancient peoples writing and the art of building cities with the necessary laws and moral guidance that maintained them. This composite figure of Hermes, Thoth and Mercury was also the man of legend who, surviving the destruction of Atlantis, carried the wisdom and learning of the lost continent to the civilization of ancient Egypt where it was buried in metaphor and obscured by mythology to await a time when it might be understood by all.

The imaginative extravagance of mythology, whether it is Egyptian, Greek, Roman or Biblical, may seem a long way from the remedy, **Orange**. However, the brow centre (and thus the whole) is so often in trouble when we become waylaid by left-brain reality; when we persist in looking at things exclusively with the scrutiny of logic. We fail to see or hear what Hermes, the messenger of intuition, would tell us. We forget how to weigh things in the balance of our individual minds; heart and mind become gradually separated. We have grown distant from the metaphysical meaning of Thoth and Hermes. We live in a time when all that is left to us is mercurial materialism that must be explained by reason. What we lose, apart from a sense of personal security (which can only come from within and not from without), is the creative 'at one-ness' with the universe.

Chakras

Crown
A remedy that encourages spiritual awareness without losing grounding. Eases sleep that is unrefreshing due to anxieties.

Brow

Nurtures the ability to use intuitive thought where it tempers excessive rational thinking that threatens to distort reality into anxiety. Opens the channel between the mind and the heart so that judgement is softened by charitable thought. Fosters self-discipline where once one would rush into doing things hastily. Affords time and space in order to organize difficult worldly matters without panic. Mental breathing space.

Throat

Dispels the compression that often impedes the energy of this centre due to unresolved emotions. Unlike other remedies that affect this centre deeply (like **Blue**, **Emerald**, **Rhodochrosite**, **Sea Salt** and **Turquoise**), it enables the patient to understand how less needs to be said rather than the more of pent-up emotional turmoil.

Heart

Stillness and peace become possible where there has been doubt and anxiety.

Solar plexus

Challenges and conflicts assume smaller proportions. A cooler mind is able to minimize what seemed insurmountable.

Sacral

Kidney qi is better conserved. Water is more evenly distributed in the body. Sexual energy is better harmonized with heart energy.

Base

Better judgement skills give greater assurance in one's grounding; one feels surer-footed in dealing with worldly matters.

Case studies

1 'A mother of two in her early 50s sat down at her appointment and said "I feel challenged". She had a history of alcoholism and it had been 25 years since she had left the clinic that had turned her life round. She ran

her own business for which she had been given awards in her industry. Her last prescription had been **Calc-carb** 10M; she had been doing well but was concerned about a colleague on whom she had been relying but who had made some dubious decisions that bothered the patient. She had decided to go on a silent retreat in order to "take stock". Then, having returned from the retreat she felt a sense of "arrival". She hugely benefited from the meditation practice and thought it a "revelation".

'"Everything since coming out of those nightmare years was about trying to find balance, equanimity. I've come to understand what happened to me. Everything was based on my father's approval. As long as I could have his approval I knew who I was. When he died I didn't know who I was. When I was told he had died there was a 'boom' in my head. I began to bang my head on the wall and after that there was this complete blank. When I went into that clinic I was back in the same place as I had been when my father died. Then when I was on retreat I felt I found my place. You know, I recognized myself in a past life: I saw myself as an orange-robed Buddhist monk, old, wizened and bent forward."

'Nevertheless, she now felt very challenged by the acute crisis that her colleague had thrown her into. "The stuff that's hit me in the last few days is amazing! A real struggle!" she was given **Orange** 1M (one at night and one in the morning). Two months later she returned for a follow-up: "I feel much better!" She had had to dispense with her colleague but did so without provoking any recrimination or antipathy. "It was amazing! The power of the blockage and all that created. [Once I had done it] bookings have been coming in and everything has been so easy. It was like swimming through treacle before. I've had a real feeling of letting it all unfold. I know I'm seeing with my third eye. I'm on earth but in my brow. I've really been learning from meditation that all these hooligan thoughts are only temporary. Eventually you reach stillness. Recently I've found that I've been finding solutions to the thought problems. The solutions all seem to be just underneath all the chuntering thoughts. I'm really calm; there's no tension or stress."' CG

2 'An Aquarian woman in her mid 40s came for treatment though she was, by and large, physically well. She had complained of being ratty with the children; of being in too much of a rush; of trying to cut out all the unnecessary things in life; of being in need of meditation. She had already had

a series of appointments up to this time covering some six years when she had done well on **Lycopodium, Sepia, Tuberculinum, Hornbeam, Oak** and other remedies. She had divorced in this time and had found another relationship. She was becoming interested in yoga and felt the need to become proficient in its study so that she could teach it. "I don't quite feel that my mind is associated with what I am feeling. I want to encourage my female side. I'm not a joiner of things. I prefer to be on the edges. I want to meditate but I know I have to be grounded to make that work."

'She had been thinking about the prospect of having another child and had also considered moving abroad and taking up Ayurvedic massage. She already had three children and horses and dogs. She was given **Moonstone 10M** (single dose) which she found calming. After it she did not mention again the desire for a fourth child or any move abroad. She began to have her amalgam fillings removed as she felt that they were a likely hazard to her health. When she returned three months later she said, "What I'm working on is my third-eye centre. For some time now I've been stuck here. It's not moving. I feel that meditation is beginning to work, something's happening. I notice the connection between the brow and the sacral chakra. It's as if I hold all my tension in my sacral area."

'She also noticed that whenever she felt tense or nervous she felt the tightness in her upper chest and was aware of how her voice would lose any resonance; she could not use it to project herself. "I can hold my own in a political debate but when I want to talk about anything to do with my needs or wishes I seize up. I always accommodate others before myself. It's a childhood pattern."

She was given **Orange** 1M: collective single dose. When she returned she was complaining of having a lot of mucus in her frontal and ethmoid sinuses which she was trying to drain away. She wondered if paint fumes had been the cause. She then reported, "What I had last time was fantastic! It felt like flying! I got such clarity. There was all this clearing. It was all part of the movement of where I know I'm meant to be going. Everything is opening up in the heart centre. I am now very happy to observe things rather than try and analyse everything and get all tied up."

'She trained as a Yoga instructor and developed a teaching practice and has remained well and content.' JM

23

ORYZA SATIVA

Organic Brown Rice

The remedy was proved on 6 February 1998 by the meditation group consisting of 5 women and 3 men and the medium. Each person was given the 30th potency. It was also proved separately by the students on the Guild of Homoeopaths postgraduate course on 25 April 1998 when 11 women and a medium took part.

The Background

Brown rice (*Oryza sativa*) belongs to the grass family: *Graminaceae* or *Poaceae*. It is an annual plant with several jointed stems which reach 60 centimetres to 3 metres in length; the lower part floats underwater while the upright stems emerge erect. The seeds are produced in panicles which droop with the weight of the rice grains. It is the endosperm of the grain that is the part eaten.

Rice is descended from wild grasses. It has been cultivated for thousands of years beginning in South-East Asia. There is archaeological evidence that the Chinese were growing rice some 10,000 years ago. There are many varieties of rice; some 50 or 60 are grown in India alone. It has been exported to southern Europe, the Middle East, East Africa and the Americas. Most types of rice require irrigation though there are some that can be grown on dry ground. News of the value of rice as a foodstuff was brought to Western countries by early travellers from Greece, Portugal and France. They noted that not only was rice used for cooking but also for ritual purposes; it was part of the cultural heritage of South-East Asia.

There are three main types of rice: 'indica' which is fluffy once cooked and easily eaten with the fingers; 'japonica' which becomes a sticky mass once boiled; and 'javanica' which is between the other two in consistency. There are also three 'sizes': short grain, medium grain and long grain. The best varieties are grown in shallow, slow-moving water; this is accomplished in terraced paddy fields that are developed over large areas of what was once forested land.

Rice is regarded as a symbol of fertility and prosperity in much of South-East Asia. It is associated with Lakshmi, the goddess of wealth. She is represented in ceremonies and rituals by paddy stalks. Rice grains are showered over newly married couples as a sign of prosperity. Buddha was once offered a dish of milk and rice to strengthen him as he endured the rigours of his journey towards spiritual enlightenment; to this day sweetened rice is used in Buddhist ceremonies.

Mrs Grieve warns us of a truth we should heed nearly 80 years after she wrote, 'it should never be forgotten that the large and continued consumption of the white, polished rices of commerce is likely to be injurious to health.' She goes on to point out that 'the nations of which rice is the staple diet eat it unhusked as a rule when it is brownish and less attractive to the eye but more nutritious'. Despite the popularity of Basmati rice, it is refined white rice that is mostly cooked in Western kitchens and served in popular restaurants. While refined rice does not suffer from the growing reputation of genetically modified wheat as a trigger for multiple health problems, it nevertheless can slow down digestion and be a suspect in nutritional deficiencies if relied on too heavily as a staple. Rice bran contains a high percentage of fibre (up to 25 per cent) which is vital for the absorption of fats in the digestive tract. It also has a role to play in the reduction of so called 'bad' cholesterol in the bloodstream. White rice is not only of little nutritional value but it does not have these other properties either.

Mrs Grieve also tells us about the medicinal properties of natural rice: 'A decoction of rice, commonly called rice water, is recommended in the pharmacopoeia of India as an excellent demulcent, refrigerant drink in febrile and inflammatory diseases and in dysuria and similar affections. It may be acidulated with lime juice and sweetened with sugar. This may also be used as an enema in affections of the bowels.' She adds that 'a poultice . . . of finely powdered rice flour may be used for erysipelas, burns, scalds, etc.' Traditionally, not only brown rice and the flour from it, but also the oil made from rice bran feature in natural medicine prescriptions. This oil is made up of compounds that have antioxidant properties – which have led to rice being considered in the treatment of certain cancers (most especially of the stomach and bowel) – amongst which is found vitamin E. Because of this potential in the treatment of serious sickness there are controversial moves to produce genetically modified rice in vast quantities. The main purpose of this is to provide medicines for the specific treatment of patients suffering from dehydration due to a chronic susceptibility to diarrhoea. Recent studies by conventional medical scientists have begun to show results that not only suggest that rice has anti-cancer properties, but that it may also be useful in treating diabetes, heart disease and kidney stones.

Starch, oil and proteins from rice are used in cosmetics to soothe and improve skin quality and tone. A paste of honey and rice starch is recommended while the oil is used in a cream product to protect the skin from the harmful UV rays of the sun. Apart from this, rice also variously features in the tanning industry, as bedding for farm animals, in rope making, in the production of figures for ceremonies and, most famously, in paper making.

Keynote effects

Improves stamina in those who suffer from the inability to absorb nutrition through the gut wall; who are susceptible to food intolerance or other allergic reactions. It enlivens those who develop poorly, are weak and compliant or do not know any better (such as children of parents who insist that their children must be brought up as vegetarians when this does not suit their body type). Fosters a sense of self-confidence where there has been none to start with. The patient is given the opportunity to feel their individuality for the first time.

General symptoms

Poor nutrition. Debility from weakened digestive system. Emotional and spiritual disconnection as a result of a toxically compromised physical vehicle. Works on the whole of the alimentary canal. Calms the digestion and eases the passage of food through the gut. Calms the liver, spleen and pancreas. Useful where the solar plexus is affected in a strongly sycotic type. Hormonal imbalances in both men and women. Menopause. Asthmatic breathing due to fear. Diarrhoea from fear. Purifies the blood, the lymph, the major organs and the skin. Helps to integrate chemical and electrical activity within the brain.

Cleanses blood and lymph. Helps restore the water balances of the body. Useful after brain or head injuries. Autism. Asperger's syndrome. Anorexia and bulimia. Flexion and articulation problems; tendons and ligaments are painful or taut. Dislocation of joints; muscular dystrophy. Scoliosis and kyphosis.

Miasms

Psora, tuberculosis, leprosy and sycosis.

Mental and emotional symptoms

This is a remedy for the lonely child; loneliness in childhood and the memory of that. Anxiety and fear: fear of change; of lack of routine; of lack of discipline. Becomes very orderly, even fastidious. Has a need to do things in a proper fashion or in a correct order. Has faddish diet. Can become a fetishist. Gives great attention to detail. Works at very fine things such as a watchmaker or a miniaturist would. Works with great skill, delicacy and refinement. Meticulous. When thrown off balance from this activity they become nervous and anxious though they do not ask for any help and keep themselves to themselves. Can be thrown by interference in routine or by something coming up from the past that was thought to be finished with. Loss of bearings when change overtakes them. Lack of balance means that they feel unfocused, displaced, dislocated, ungrounded, even out of their bodies. Grief at the loss of children; sobbing. Fear of giving birth; fear causing difficulty in breathing. Fear with a sense of being squeezed; fear with nausea and diarrhoea. Can feel or look as if they have had a shock. 'I've lost my rudder.' A sense of being overburdened by anxieties but none so much that it could be specifically identified. Vulnerable to the point of being sensitive to the slightest cross word. Feeling of weakness and help-lessness with apathy and emptiness. Humble but not servile. Easily upset during the menopause, either physically or mentally. Slight mood swings that cause disturbance. Unaware of how they do not help themselves by staying in their set groove; this is especially true of their diet. Very helpful for those who are unable to control their eating habits; they suffer from their cravings but cannot stop. Tendency to comfort eat. Can clarify confused or blocked intuition. Sensitivity to beauty and creativity; can restore these attributes. Slow or difficult learning especially where there is defective nutrition. Poor memory or memory loss especially after head injury.

Physical symptoms

Head

Injuries when there is loss of memory or when other remedies do not complete their action. Headache with symptoms like **Belladonna**'s: throbbing and < bending forward. Tendency to faint. Light-headed.

Eyes

Cataract; blindness from cataract. (Exophthalmia)

Ears

Wax especially in children. Loss of hearing; 'selective hearing'.

Nose

Catarrh: thin and runny; watery. Snuffles in children. Loss of sense of smell.

Throat

Catarrh in the throat with coughing to clear the phlegm. Dryness with difficulty swallowing yet not markedly thirsty. Cannot swallow big mouthfuls; chews for a long time and may need water in order to swallow food. (Thyroid problems; helps to drain the thyroid gland.) Contraction in the throat at the same time as in the solar plexus.

Stomach

Sense of a heavy weight in the epigastric region. ++ comfort foods. ++ simple, bland food. Adults who prefer nursery food. Unadventurous appetite. (If given a diet, tends to neglect it.) Eating a little = full feeling. Ravenous appetite which disappears after a few mouthfuls. Thirstlessness: often uninterested in water though may like flavoured drinks.

Abdomen

Bloating and constipation. Water retention in the abdomen < before periods or at the menopause. Bloating feels < from eating only a little; < eating starchy foods. Restores appetite after a cold or after an acute bout of diarrhoea. Delicate digestion. Potatoes <. Worms. Candida. Intestinal parasites. Tenderness of abdominal walls. 'Tummy aches' before school; 'schoolitis'. Grumbling appendix. Sigmoid and splenic flexures feel tender or congested. Diarrhoea from fear. Contraction in the solar plexus at the same time as in the throat. Sense of terrible fear in the solar plexus.

Female
Shrivelled breasts at menopause. Dryness of the vaginal mucosa. Infertility.

Male
Underdevelopment; undescended testicles.

Urinary organs
Frequent urging with little result. Passes quantities of pale watery urine with no reduction of retention of water in abdominal cavity.

Skin
Useful in chronic skin eruptions such as eczema. Dry eruptions. Skin problems where nutrition is defective. Dryness of the surface with poor water balances internally.

Neck and back
Clicking and crunching of the vertebrae in the neck. Cervical spine is tense and cracks easily.

Sleep
Very drowsy especially after meals. Sleepy in the daytime but wakeful and restless at night. Hot in bed. Vivid dreams but of unconnected incidents; events in dreams make no sense. Dreams of losing things; of losing one's way. Dreams of being gripped at the wrist with someone saying, 'I am so frightened; help me! I'm going into care!'

Considerations for the use of the remedy

- Associated with **Okubaka** in the treatment of allergies and catarrhal states.
- Also works well with **Lumbricus** to which **Rice** is the vegetable remedy analogue though note that **Lumbricus** can be servile while **OBR** is more likely to be compliant from the greater need for security.

- **Silica**, as a constitutional remedy, is often associated with **OBR**; they share several fundamental constitutional and mental/emotional characteristics.
- **Thyroidinum** is also a remedy closely linked to issues of maturation and may precede or follow **OBR**.
- **Lycopodium** is a remedy that follows OBR very well; they share lack of self-confidence and some of the bowel symptoms. It is most likely to be needed when the newly found individuality of the **OBR** patient gives them a sense of adventurousness that is so unexpected that it causes them a moment of retreat, as if they were not sure if they can cope with change after all.
- **Baryta-carb** may well be the remedy to precede **OBR**; however, as it is compatible with this remedy, it may be considered as a support remedy in low potency (i.e. **Baryta-carb** 1M or 10M with **OBR** 6 daily). **Baryta-carb** has more struggle with mental acuity even if only from trauma rather than in the usual picture of dwarfism or lack of intellectual intelligence while **OBR**; is more in retreat.
- It has an affinity with the bowel nosodes, **Gaertner**, **Morgan Gaertner** and **Sycotic Co**.

Also related to **Medorrhinum** and **Nat-mur**. It is antidoted by alcohol. Patients do best on this remedy if they come off tea. The patient is likely to be dehydrated with the symptom of lack of thirst. A revision of the patient's diet is essential when considering this remedy; it is likely that the patient's metabolism is slow or sluggish even if there is a tendency at times to diarrhoea.

Esoteric therapeutics

Encourages the return of energy from the sacral plexus to the base centre in sycotic patients. Encourages the introduction of Eastern thought processes into Western minds. Willingness is engendered to continue on the path without pre-conceptions or preconditions. Having trust and faith in the shape of one's destiny. Encourages the return of the connection between spirit and physical body. It is also one of the remedies that ease the fear incarnated with the soul (like **Ayahuasca** and **Thymus Gland**).

Chakras

Crown
Leads the patient away from a potentially carcinogenic state. There is a greater awareness of a life path, of being an individual with a purpose. There is a shift away from nightmares to dreams of a more informative or even instructive nature. For the first time, perhaps, there is a spiritual choice in the patient's life.

Brow
The patient is better able to direct his or her own destiny; it helps him or her to find their way. Choice of pathway is more available. This chakra has been undeveloped in childhood; there is often a strong sense of not having been allowed or been in a position to make choices during this crucial time. The mind has been as starved of stimulus as the body may have been of nutrition. The eyes may have only a distant light within.

Throat
Poor self-expression. Things get stuck in the throat. Poor elimination from the mucous membranes. Lack of voice may lead to thyroid insufficiency or, more unusually, hyperthyroidism due to a determination to get everything done as a replacement activity for being able to express or demonstrate creativity.

Heart
There is grief in this centre that has most to do with sadness for what has never been accomplished or lack of opportunity not least due to lack of confidence and sense of being left untaught. In the extremity of this grief the patient may seem to be pining away (as in anorexia) or retreating from the harsh reality of the world.

Solar plexus
This centre is the main focus of this remedy's activity on the physical level. It restores integrity to the digestive tract when the patient has been starved of what is needed nutritionally. The liver pulse is likely to be hard and accentuated with a sense of a narrow edge; the spleen may have a weak pulse. It is another remedy to encourage the elimination of toxicity, not specifically from the liver but from the whole alimentary canal and even muscles (such as the psoas) that harbour toxicity readily. When prescribed because of indications highlighting this centre then a low potency such as 6x may prove of value over a long period.

Sacral

Lack of power in this chakra may lead to loss of libido or lack of any connection to the emotional aspect of the centre. Lack of physical development in young people may have much to do with a general lack of growth or poor nutrition. The patient may seem deliberately shut down in this area not least from lack of self-confidence.

Base

Rice is strongly featured in this chakra; the early learning of life is unfinished either because it was unavailable or withheld. The digestive system, the endocrine system, blood and the musculoskeletal system may all or individually show lack of development though it is the digestive tract that is the focus. When generally indicated **OBR** is not deficient in mental acuity but is into conserving what little strength or stamina there might be.

Case studies

1 'Girl of eight; Down's syndrome. Small and petite; friendly, confident and sympathetic. Suffers from persistent vomiting. Green watery vomit with froth. Mother had stopped Marmite, cheese, oranges and chocolate. Strong yellow urine. Poor eater. She was given **Medorrhinum Americana** 200 (single dose), followed by **Organic Brown Rice** 30 (one daily). The sickness stopped; she gained weight and her eating improved. She was then given **Silica** 200 (single dose) and the **OBR** was continued on a daily basis. All symptoms cleared completely.' **LR**

2 'Boy of four; had chickenpox followed by molluscum contagiosum. Poor eater with a bad diet. He was given **Variolinum** 200 (t.d.s. x 3) and **Thuja** 6 o.d. The skin improved but the eating habits did not change. He was then given **Variolinum** 200 (one three times a week for three weeks) and **Organic Brown Rice** 30 (o.d.). The skin cleared completely, he began to eat well and has continued to do so and an improvement at school has been reported.' **LR**

3 'This lovely little boy now aged five first came to see me nearly a year ago. His parents were already taking him through an American behavioural therapy system which involved intensive training and he was taking a variety of dietary supplements for a leaking gut and candida. His mother had had food poisoning when she was five-months pregnant and the baby was born three weeks late after an induction. His birth was very fast and he did not breathe until his feet were tickled. He then developed normally but had many ear infections and tonsillitis after his first year.

'According to his parents he was very bright and alert and his speech was advanced. His development was arrested by the MMR vaccination after which he was ill for a week with a high temperature, listlessness and loss of appetite; he ceased talking and started 'drifting off'. Six months later he developed meningitis and was diagnosed as autistic a month later. He was at his worst three months before and three months after the meningitis.

'His behaviour had improved enormously as a result of the behavioural therapy. His parents had brought him to see me to see if I could help primarily with his speech and secondly with his appetite. He talked a little gobbledygook to himself while playing but otherwise would not speak; he was much quieter than other autistic children I have treated but had enormous tantrums at home especially when he was pushed in his therapy. He had a very poor appetite; his parents had him on a completely organic diet that was dairy-, gluten- and sugar-free but he craved sugar.

'I started him off with **Nat-mur** 200 followed by **Sea Salt** 200, **MMR** 30 twice weekly alternating with **Syphilinum** + **Arsenicum** + **Thymus Gland** 12x twice weekly.

'His parents said he was lethargic after each dose of the [combination] remedy and "grumpy" after the **MMR**; he had yellow pus coming out of his eyes and all his autistic symptoms were worse initially. His speech had since improved dramatically; he was saying words and stringing them together and had far fewer tantrums. He had had a temperature at night for the first week and was restless and since then had slept better. The remedies were repeated.

'He had another aggravation with pus in the eyes, lethargy then aggression but since then he had made "fantastic" progress and his speech was improving daily. Autistic behaviour was less noticeable; he had become affectionate and cuddly with his toys and his parents. The only tantrums were over being forced to eat new food. After the last remedies he had had a temperature. Rx: **Medorrhinum Americana, Thuja** 1M, **MMR** 200 weekly.

'He again had an aggravation; lethargy followed by aggression with biting but was much better after the first and subsequent **MMRs**. His appetite was now excellent. He had had many sore throats with catarrh in the mornings; this was now better. His speech continued to improve. Rx: **Berlin Wall** 10M, **MMR** 200 weekly, **Syphilinum** + **Arsenicum** + **Thymus Gland** 12x weekly.

'There was another aggravation after the Berlin Wall and also after each dose of the **MMR**. His behaviour was quite wild and he liked spinning himself in circles. His parents were "staggered" at his progress with his speech and he was reading well for his age. He was trying hard to communicate, he had started blinking and screwing up his eyes. His play was not developing and his parents were trying to teach him how to play. He liked playing on his tummy with his bottom in the air and often slept like this. Rx: **Medorrhinum Americana** 200 weekly.

'He had now calmed down but was demonstrating more autistic behaviour than he had since he came to see me: shaking his head and limbs and banging his head now and then. He had had more sore throats but his speech and play continued to improve and his parents thought he was generally progressing well. He was going to school and holding his own but playing alongside children rather than with them. I gave him more doses of **Nat-mur** and **Sea Salt** along with **Rainbow** LM1 over the next weeks [and] then he had **Carcinosin** 1M.

'He was beginning to ask questions, wanting to play and wanting others to play with him although he preferred playing alone. There was more eye contact and he was looking from one person to another [while] following a conversation. He wanted to express himself more than he had the ability to and this made him frustrated. His parents said there was much more of his personality coming through and he was showing a sense of humour and saying "I" for the first time. The biggest problem was his sugar craving. Rx: **Saccharum Officinalis** 1M weekly and **Organic Brown Rice** 200 weekly.

'He said "Hello" and smiled when he came in and answered my

questions for the first time. His parents talked about him almost exclusively in terms of his personality for the first time. He was showing normal fears, emotions and character traits and was enjoying fantasy play. His listening skills were improving and his therapy was now taking the form of normal play and reading and talking games. He had too much energy at night and none in the morning. Rx: **Lumbricus** 10M< **Organic Brown Rice** 200 weekly.

'This boy's improvement has been staggering – greater than any other autistic child I have treated – and the therapy that he has been following has made an enormous difference to him. There is still some way to go and many remedies I can see he will benefit from. His parents have been very determined to "rescue" him and have put a phenomenal amount of effort into his behavioural therapy.' **AF** (First published in *Prometheus* No. 10 June 1999.)

24

PERIDOT

Olivine

The remedy was proved on 10 March 1995 by 11 members of the meditation circle, 6 women and 4 men with the medium. The crystal and an essence made from it were present in the circle and the remedy proved was of the potentized essence in the 30th potency. Each participant was given one dose before the meditation began.

The Background

Peridot has the chemical formula: $(Mg, Fe)_2 SiO_4$. It has the appearance of translucent pale green glass (though it can vary between a yellowish green and a bottle green), showing its high silica content. Its form is orthorhombic. It is of the hardness 6.5 – 7 on Mohs' scale. It is sourced from Brazil, Canada, the Canary Islands, Egypt, Ireland, Italy, Pakistan and Sri Lanka, and is found in areas where the igneous rocks are rich in iron and magnesium. One such is the island of Zebirget in the Red Sea where it was gathered in ancient times; another is in lava flows of the Hawaiian Islands.

Peridot is also known by other names: olivine (because of the colour association with the fruit of the olive tree); chrysolite (from the Greek *chrysos*, 'gold', and *lithos*, 'stone'); the 'evening emerald' and the 'gem of miracles'. Peridot was known as topaz by ancient people though there is no relationship with the stone we now know by this name.

The breastplate and ephod made for Aaron, written about in the book of Exodus, were sacred garments of the high priest of the tabernacle. The breastplate was studded with the twelve precious stones representing the tribes of Israel. A green stone, variously described as peridot, topaz or serpentine, was originally the second stone of the breastplate though it has now been superseded by emerald. In ancient times, when peridot was more highly valued than the diamond, it was a stone to 'drive away the spirits and influences of evil'. It 'protected against obsession and dissolved enchantments and phantoms of the night. It gladdened the heart with hope, strengthened the soul and inspired thought; it banished illusion, despair and madness and aided the faculties of inspiration and prophecy.' (Isadore Kozminsky quoting old manuscripts.) Others wrote of its ability 'to expel phantoms and rid people of folly' if one set it in gold and wore it. It was also recognized to be of service in healing the lungs and 'asthmatical complaints'.

Keynote effects

The remedy is most conspicuously useful in the healing of old patterns of hurt to the ego (see **Emerald**). It encourages the patient to soften and relax the protective emotional shield that has been reinforced following many hurtful incidents in the past. It helps to dissolve old patterns of negative expectation and reaction that prevent the patient from progressing. These patterns are otherwise virtually impossible to shift as they have afforded a degree of security till now. Another keynote is to do with vision: both ocular and spiritual. It clarifies what one sees and the way it is seen, allowing the person to progress with more confidence.

General symptoms

This is a remedy that is likely to be most obviously indicated on the emotional level. However, there are strong links into miasmatic territory and certain significant aspects of the physical body that are worth bearing in mind. **Peridot** is chiefly sycotic though beneath this layer will be the syphilitic state. It is as if the syphilitic miasm is using sycosis to hide behind. Mucous membranes become overactive causing congestion. Toxicity in the liver may have led to stiffness and pain in the muscles. The lungs become congested and susceptible to breathing difficulties and asthmatic troubles. Asthma in one with a history of a powerful mother figure. Shallow breathing or a sensation of holding one's breath; may be of value in cases where sleep apnoea is a main symptom.

Sleepiness from lack of movement. May be used as a drainage remedy for lung pathology; 3x or 6x potency can be used on a daily basis. There is a general state of fragility as can often be found in sycosis. The heart is affected by internal pressure either by sensation or actual hypertension or from pathology of the lungs. A state of lassitude with heaviness. The underlying syphilitic condition that may be manifest in the tissues of the heart and the bowel is the result of harbouring destructive emotions and allowing them to undermine the physical body over a long period. **Peridot** also has influence over the spine and the bones of the head: it can ease rigidity in the spinal structure and in the parietal and temporal bones. It effects positive changes in the pituitary fossa and internal auditory meatus. When indicated by rigidity of the pelvis and cervix it serves to open up the pelvic floor to facilitate the birthing process.

Miasms

Psora, syphilis, sycosis and tuberculosis.

Mental and emotional symptoms

Hurt and resentful though not necessarily expressive of either. A sense of pointlessness in those who feel unhappy. The patient finds it hard to shift from a negative state; they seem to be stuck in a condition of emotional inertia. They may feel boxed in and in need of more space. The patient feels 'blank' or 'nothing'; complains of 'emptiness'; may feel 'quite desperate' about the lack of emotional feeling. 'I don't know what the answers are; I don't know that I want to know the answers'. A sense of guilt from feeling of wasting time; feels lazy both in mind and body. 'There is a sense of space yet of being crowded.' Has a sense of not knowing what they can do for themselves to get things moving but also that it would be of no use to try. A feeling of being in no-man's-land. Emotional heaviness in the heart centre. Lack of self-worth. Weeping mood; tears lead to being more peaceful and calm. There is a reluctance to face challenges; to test one's own potential. Fear of doing what would cause them to be noticed as the result of old hurt to the ego (see **Emerald**). Emotional fragility; delicate and vulnerable (cf. **Thuja**). Easy embarrassment (cf. **Medorrhinum**). Envy and jealousy; herein may be the origin of the hurt to the ego. Envy especially of other people's achievements or good fortune. Tendency to be judgemental of others but from a position of weakness; easily intimidated by others' strengths. One of the blocks to progress can be the sense that others do things better. Fear of change; fear of breaking the habits of a lifetime. A darker aspect of the remedy brings up criminality: trauma in the past has led to warped morality in a fragile mind. There is unlikely to be any violence associated with this; more that the patient is habitually tempted through weakness and/or a sense of life's unfairness to carry out nefarious acts.

Physical symptoms

Head
Tension in the bones of the head < parietal and temporal areas. Headache: symptoms may be similar to either **Lycopodium** or **Spigelia**.

Eyes
Watery discharge. Dimness of vision. Floaters, cataracts. Glaucoma.

Ears
Blocked or feeling as if stopped. Wax builds up. Poor drainage from the ears due to lack of movement of the bones of the head. Hearing compromised; Eustachian tubes are full of catarrh. Tinnitus.

Nose
Watery discharge. Blocked nose with impeded breathing.

Mouth
Toothache: persistent and continuing after the tooth is removed.

Throat
A need to keep clearing the throat: hemming. Lots of phlegm in the throat; difficulty in clearing the throat. Watery mucus. Pain in the throat. A feeling in the throat 'as if something is held back'.

Respiration and chest
A sensation of a lump in the chest; a sensation of heaviness in the chest. Sharp pain in the chest that comes and goes. Shallow breathing; a sensation of holding one's breath or of not being able to breathe properly. Conscious of their breathing; a sense of not breathing deeply enough. A need to take a

deep breath in order to exhale. Asthmatic breathing. Heart feels constricted; wants to expand but cannot. Sensation of pressure on the heart.

Female
Twinges in the left ovary.

Neck, back and shoulders
Crick in the neck with tension of the upper body. Pain in the back and shoulders from tension held in the spinal column.

Considerations for the use of the remedy

It has been suggested that the remedy will be of use in certain situations, though only where there are clear indications for it.

- In pregnancy and childbirth; is said to facilitate delivery where there is stasis and tension. It has also been suggested that it promotes good bone growth and correct development of the central nervous system.
- Where there is misalignment of the spine; this is likely to become evident during or after cranial osteopathic treatment. (There is a likely connection with the problem having arisen during pregnancy and birth either in the mother or baby.) What is out of alignment in the spine may also affect the cranial base and the temporal and parietal bones. A comparison with **Sycamore Seed** (see *Volume I*) may lead to these remedies being used simultaneously to support cranial osteopathic work.
- In patients with hypertension due to emotional stasis.
- In AIDS when the emotional picture is marked.
- In those whose previous treatment has so far only had partial positive effects on the constitutional health but whose maintaining cause of buried emotional trauma has affected the energy of the thymus centre (see *Volume I*, **Thymus Gland**).

It was noted that the remedy is susceptible to frequent repetition in increasing potency. It is recommended in some cases[34] that the patient with a chronic

34 Knowing when to accept such a recommendation is largely a matter of intuition though, in this case, it may also be to do with knowing how anxious the patient is about change; the more cautious the patient, the slower and more deliberate the progress needs to be.

condition indicating **Peridot**, such as asthma or a heart problem, should begin by taking the remedy in a low water potency which would then be gradually superseded by a step-by-step rise through the higher potencies. An initial aggravation may appear to be that the patient shuts down even further in their emotional body but this would be a temporary habitual reaction and not an adverse one.

Peridot is chiefly a sycotic remedy; it shares aspects of this miasm with **Medorrhinum** and **Thuja**. However, as with these two remedies, **Peridot** is often indicated in those who have an underlying syphilitic tendency. The use of **Peridot** in a case may well begin to bring out this hidden state especially in lung and heart pathology. As **Carcinosin** is able to do, **Peridot** is capable of loosening the miasmatic 'knots' that in some cases threaten to confound even the most assiduous prescribing.

There are a number of remedies that bear comparison with **Peridot**:

- **Thuja** has the same frailty and vulnerability but where this remedy would be able to maintain a 'front' (at least for a while and particularly in professional circumstances), **Peridot** simply retreats beyond general view.
- **Lycopodium** is well known for shutting out what cannot be handled easily, just like **Peridot**, but it is far more forceful an energy. The usual time and digestive aggravations of this remedy are not likely to be present to anywhere near the same degree in **Peridot**. However, what can be confusing is that **Lycopodium** may well have been prescribed in the past, often quite successfully, for someone in need of **Peridot** at a deep, emotional level.
- **Carcinosin** has a similar degree of emotional suppression and weariness though it is much more likely to be passive-aggressive or passively victimized than **Peridot**. Nevertheless, this nosode can support, follow or precede **Peridot** very well.
- **Berlin Wall** may well be indicated around **Peridot** patients who have a history of criminal tendencies. The patient would have reached the state of needing these remedies through difficult past history involving trauma borne in on them from troubled family life during which the ego was severely damaged.
- **Sycamore Seed** is the main remedy of choice for influencing the bones of the head to move and realign. It has an affinity for the sphenoid bone and pituitary fossa as well as the parietal and temporal bones. It,

too, has influence on the pelvic bowl though it is more usually of use after a trauma (such as a difficult birth) has caused local tension and torsion. It is not unusual for this remedy and **Peridot** to be complementary in cases requiring cranial osteopathic treatment.

Esoteric therapeutics

In crystal healing it is said that Peridot 'emits a warm and friendly energy' (Melody) which is borne out by the general consensus of the provers who all felt the energy to be warm, light, calming and peaceful. It has affinities for the astrological signs of Virgo, Leo, Scorpio and Sagittarius. Its guiding planet is Venus (which associates the crystal with Taurus) which suggests that it is a stone for softening hardness, soothing agitation and fostering gentleness. The stone's influence on the chakras is said to be mostly on the heart, solar plexus and brow. It is recommended as a cleansing and protective crystal that is helpful in clearing the heart and solar plexus of negative emotions so that the mind is clear in matters of love and relationships. It encourages the ability to detach oneself from outside influences such as another person who maintains a negative hold. (This brings to mind one of the keynotes of **Olive**: subject to being in another's thrall.) 'Peridot teaches that holding onto people or the past is counterproductive.' (Hall) It affords auric protection in one whose energy field has been affected by feelings of jealousy, envy, anger, resentment and spite. It eases the burden of those who suffer from stress and it lifts lethargy in those who cannot cope especially when feeling frail and vulnerable; when suffering from lack of self-confidence. It can foster gentle assertiveness. It rebalances and realigns the structure of the physical body, the endocrine system, and strength-ens the connection with the subtle bodies. The crystal also influences the skin and tissue regeneration, the speed of the metabolic rate, the lungs, the heart and thymus gland, the gall bladder and the spleen. The activity of the intestines, especially in those who have a tendency to melancholia, is eased. More specif-ically, it is to be considered for those with eye conditions; it is seen as a crystal for improving vision both physical and spiritual. Another recommendation is that the gem essence should be given to pregnant women to ease the pains of contraction and open the birth canal.

In the proving various esoteric aspects were noted.

• The main purpose of **Peridot** is to open and lighten the closed and damaged heart centre while, at the same time, ensuring that there is

integrity in the energy that flows upward through the spine.
- The second principal purpose is to shift habitual patterns of suppressive or stagnant energy held in the heart centre that even the best-chosen remedies have not been able to influence.
- The energy of the remedy, like **Rainbow** (see *Volume I*), works downward through the body from the crown centre to the base. (This is opposite to remedies such as **Ayahuasca** and **Oak**. Remedies that work through the body in opposite directions are often complementary.) **Peridot** links the energy of the crown with the heart in order to foster openness and protection in the modern world while maintaining spiritual awareness. It is of great service in those who are negatively influenced by modern education, the effect of which is to curb or cripple such connections. This makes **Peridot** an ideal remedy for young people when indicated.
- The energy of **Peridot** is very gentle and pervasive. It softens hard tissue and relaxes tense energy. While this is effected and commensurate with it, a greater sense of connection is established.
- **Peridot** strengthens, reinforces and protects the heart chakra.
- **Peridot** is most likely to be indicated by those who are following a path of healing through transition, transformation and adaptation rather than simply seeking 'cure'. This is a remedy for healing journey-work.

Chakras

Crown
Peridot's journey into the body begins in the crown and works downward. Its purpose here is to keep the spiritual channel open while working on the heart centre to heal it from much past damage. The closing of the heart centre limits the capacity for receiving in the crown; the result of the remedy should manifest as greater understanding of life purpose and expansion of awareness.

Brow
Personal perception has been much reduced by damage to the ego; **Peridot** reverses this trend. Third-eye vision is enhanced. Fosters a more balanced view of one's place in the world and within one's life context so that, where change is necessary, it can be made with discretion and confidence.

Throat

Physically clearing the throat is part of the process of opening up this centre to greater awareness of one's voice; there is the sense that one can contribute meaningfully through this centre and be heard without being crushed or criticized.

Heart and thymus gland

The history of hurt in this centre needs to be cleared before major constitutional remedies can do all that they are capable of. **Peridot** can clear the path for remedies such as **Lycopodium, Nat-mur, Calc-carb, Sulphur** and **Thuja** to do their work thoroughly. The grief held in the heart is concerned with damage to the sense of self; unworthiness and lack of self-esteem are grief and sadness about one's inability to be effectual in the world. This is what most needs to be restored. When this is held at the deepest level of the heart and thymus then it is likely to be a familial trend which would need close scrutiny of past and family emotional history. Such cases may respond well to combining **Thymus Gland** with Peridot and, for example, **Medorrhinum Americana** or, perhaps, **Thuja** depending on the individual indications (that other remedies have been unable to shift).

Solar plexus

While there is little evidence from the proving of physical pathology in this centre, this centre is the physical core of the stomach meridian, the yang energy pathway that governs 'receiving' and causes 'ripening' both of which are compromised in a patient needing this remedy. In time, it is highly likely that symptoms in the digestive tract will have to be added to the general materia medica of **Peridot** and their absence to date should not deter the prescriber. Like the energy of the remedy, the energy that travels through the stomach meridian is downward in direction.

Sacral

Only one symptom in this chakra was noted in the proving: twingeing in the left ovary. However, as with the solar plexus, it is likely that further pathology in this area will be added to the materia medica in time. Being the centre most associated with the element of water and thus with creating elimination of stuck emotion, it is more than possible that a proportion of patients indicating the need for **Peridot** will have some symptomatology in this chakra.

Base

As a crystal remedy, **Peridot** is necessarily a base-centre remedy though its main focus is in the heart and crown. However, the net result of this remedy's work should be a gradual illumination of the need to be present in all senses, a foundation stone of the base chakra. As **Peridot**'s action is downward, the base centre is its destination.

Case studies

1   'A male with a very acute toothache. It felt like an abscess but an X-ray had proven negative. In fact there was nothing to indicate there was a problem with the tooth at all. On further discussion the patient explained that he was on a chakra course and was presently working on the brow chakra. I remember a colleague of mine having the same problem whilst also doing work on his brow chakra. His tooth flared up and regardless of what homoeopathic remedy he took, the pain would not go away. In the end he had the tooth removed but the pain still persisted. Another person I knew also began to have dental problems after working on their brow. Part of the process of working on the brow centre is that you are asking to clear dross from the head. This may happen on any level including that of toxicity. In the case of this patient presenting toothache, **Pyrogen**, **Gunpowder** and others failed to give any permanent relief. **Thuja** gave some relief but would not hold. My instinct finally took me to **Peridot** and after a couple of doses the patient's toothache was completely gone.' GM

2   'Female, 54, long history of ME. She practised a religion which involved special meditation on the heart chakra. She had been involved in this religion since the 1970s and the ME had started within two years of it. I felt that although the practice was helping her emotionally and spiritually it was somehow weakening her or disconnecting her from her physical body hence the ill health. The ME was very debilitating and as well as causing a lot of physical exhaustion, she also had severe digestive problems which were helped by her being on a very restricted diet. Anyway, she came to me in desperation as she had developed very

high blood pressure and no medical drugs had any positive effect on it at all and simply made her ME symptoms more severe. The next option was hospitalization. I initially prescribed **Aurum** 200c which made no effect and then decided on **Peridot** 30c. It worked within a few days and not only did the blood pressure improve but so did the ME symptoms. However, I only found this out five years later when the patient returned with the high blood pressure problems. She had not seen me since but told me that whatever I had prescribed five years earlier had cured the blood pressure and helped the ME considerably. I repeated the prescription: **Peridot** 30c daily and once again her blood pressure normalized and her ME improved. This time she followed up the visit and went on to tell me about the anger she harboured towards her husband, the father of her four children. And after years of trying to separate from him, as she felt he drained her, she did, and her energy levels have remained consistently better.' **HJ**

3   'Female, 46, patient in a state of emotional overload. **Phosphorus** constitutionally, originally presented with period problems and chronic chest problems which the **Phosphorus** cured but came with total emotional overload. A very spiritual person who overextends and likes to help everyone. Recently lost her father; had been nursing her sick mother; her husband was unemployed; her daughter having difficulties at school; her friend's daughter had died; her very close friend had been diagnosed with incurable cancer. She felt very angry with her dad for dying and with her husband for losing his job as well as for the fact that he had been totally unsupportive when her father died. She had become manic, was constantly busy, unable to sleep and felt utterly exhausted. As she said, anything to avoid the emotions. **Peridot** 30c daily restored her energy, released the anger and the tears.

   'I have found **Peridot** to be a wonderful remedy to reconnect the heart to the rest of the body, to raise the energy of a person to allow them to release emotions, particularly "difficult" emotions in people who are spiritual and don't find it easy to acknowledge anger, jealousy.' **HJ**

25

PLUTONIUM NITRICUM

The remedy was first proved by the meditation circle on 8 April 1994. There were 6 women and 3 men present each of whom was given a single dose of the 30th potency to take or not according to their individual preference. This departure from the usual protocol (in which every person in the circle invariably takes the remedy without being aware of the nature of the remedy) was because of the nature of the remedy of which everyone was aware. Some of the participants felt insecure about taking it but did so during the meditation. The remedy had been provided by John Morgan of the Helios Pharmacy.

The proving was undertaken before Ritzer and Eberle's proving was published in April 1995 in *Homoeopathic Links* 4/95. Their proving was completed by 11 people, all of whom were aware of the remedy's identity, and the homoeopathic picture was also based on 'the more than seventy cases where we prescribed Plutonium'. Their proving cannot be underestimated and an already invaluable description of it appears in Frans Vermeulen's *Synoptic Materia Medica II*. The quotations in italics that appear in the text below are taken from this excellent book in order to provide comparison and to establish what is missing from the meditative proving. Where the meditative proving differs is in expanding the nature of potential pathology, emphasizing the destructiveness of the energy of that pathology, broadening the mental/emotional picture and suggesting the implications of a spirit dimension. There is also the enormously detailed and invaluable Hahnemannian proving by Jeremy Sherr and his

Dynamis School. To have included quotations from this extraordinary publication would have expanded the consideration of this aspect of the remedy beyond the constraints of this book.

During the proving certain features that were not obviously symptoms to be cured became apparent. The majority of the provers experienced a shift in the perception of time: it was felt that time at first sped up (in some cases enormously) and then slowed down. Most also felt the sensation that they had grown in stature as if the remedy gave them greater height; in some cases immense height. Everyone also felt that the remedy they were taking was extremely and oppressively dark. Several of the provers had distinct visual awareness of certain colours. The most frequently witnessed colour was purple but there was also magenta and pink as well as green.

The Background

Plutonium (Pu) appears on the periodic table of elements at 94; it is the heaviest known naturally occurring element with an atomic weight of 244. It is an actinide metal with a silvery white appearance that quickly transforms into a dull grey or yellowish colour through oxidization. It has a number of unusual features unexpected in a metal: it has a low melting point (639.4°C) and a high boiling point (3,228°C); it does not conduct electricity or heat efficiently; as it melts its density increases and once liquid it becomes viscous. Plutonium reacts with the halogens: carbon, nitrogen and silicon. It is found naturally only in very tiny quantities within uranium ore which means that the plutonium used in the nuclear and weapons industries is synthesized. It was first synthesized in 1940 in the United States when uranium 238 was bombarded with deuterons. The discovery of this process was kept secret for six years because of the Second World War.

There are two different types of plutonium: reactor grade and weapons grade. They are achieved through different processes. Over one third of the energy produced in the majority of nuclear power stations derives from plutonium and is created as a by-product of burning uranium. One kilo of plutonium (Pu-239) can generate almost 10 million kilowatt hours of electricity. 60 tonnes or more of reactor grade plutonium is generated annually worldwide.

The half life of Pu-239 is 24,100 years. It is plutonium's habit of decaying due to the metal's instability that makes it hazardous through the emission of particles and gamma radiation. The risk of chemical toxicity from the metal is rather exaggerated due to its fearsome reputation as a weapon. However, the three forms of risk are through:

- Ingestion: it passes through the gut without being easily absorbed.
- Contamination of open wounds: this is rare as safety precautions are rigorous.
- Inhalation: the most serious threat as some particles can escape into the blood and lymph to affect the liver and most especially the bones for which plutonium seems to have an affinity.

However, the threat to life may be somewhat greater from unseen radioactive *energy*. There is still a vast amount of radioactivity in the earth's atmosphere from the numerous nuclear tests that have been carried out in various parts of the world, most particularly in the United States, Russia and the South Pacific.[35] If giving a name to something invests it with a powerful energy, as most people either believe or instinctively feel, then it is certainly worth looking at plutonium's etymological ancestry. *The Oxford English Dictionary* tells us that 'plutarchy' and 'plutocracy' are words to name 'the rule or sovereignty of wealth or of the wealthy (1643)' and that a 'plutocrat' is 'a person possessing power or influence over others in virtue of his wealth (1832)'. 'Plutolatry' is the worship of mere wealth (1889)'. These definitions lead us back to the Greek word from which they come, *ploutos*, meaning 'wealth'. The Greeks called the god of the underworld Pluto because it was believed that it was from this dark domain that wealth derived. Wealth in ancient days was often measured in produce that could be harvested. Pluto ruled over the energy that came from the depths of the earth to allow grain to grow. Then, on a different tack, the word 'plutonic' is descriptive in geology of what is 'pertaining to or involving the action of intense heat at great depths upon the rocks forming the earth's crust ... (1796)' or as in 'plutonic rocks (1856)'. This too is attributable to the Greek god; as lord of Hades, Pluto ruled over the heat of the

---

35 An especially telling comment that has been made by ground staff at various airports, when dealing with people carrying homoeopathic remedies that they do not want irradiated by the security X-ray machines is, 'There's more radiation up there in the sky than is ever in one of these machines!'

purgatorial fires that lay beneath. Plutonium was aptly named as it is a substance that creates a natural source of heat (if infernal) and, in replacing the vastly expensive production of fossil fuels, saves huge amounts of money.

Pluto, the Greek god of the underworld, was one of the sons of Kronos (Saturn) who, with his two brothers, Poseidon and Zeus, divided the world into three after Zeus had banished his father to earth. Zeus (Jupiter) became lord and father of mankind and god of the sky and thunderbolts and ruled from Mount Olympus while Poseidon (Neptune) descended into the depths of the sea to be ruler of the oceans. Pluto, loath to be alone in hell, ascended to earth in his chariot and abducted the lovely Persephone, daughter of the goddess of harvests, Demeter, and his own brother, Zeus. Persephone, blissfully unaware of her impending abduction, had been picking flowers with her nymph companions when Pluto erupted out of a cleft in the earth and swept her off to hell. Demeter was appalled and distraught; she had jealously guarded her daughter from the lubricious gaze and unsavoury attentions of the other gods and had refused their gifts and offers of matrimony. In her furious search for Persephone, Demeter allowed the earth to turn into a barren desert. Helios, the sun, eventually told her where she should look as he had seen all that had happened. When Demeter appealed to Zeus, and many of the other gods became aware of the starving plight of mankind below, Zeus obliged his brother to return Persephone to her mother. Pluto did so but not before he turned the situation to his advantage. One of the decrees of the Fates, to which even the gods were subject, was that anyone who ate or drank while in Hades should be condemned to remain there for eternity. Pluto tricked Persephone into eating four pomegranate seeds (a symbol of fecundity) before she rejoined her mother. This meant that she was forced to return to Pluto every year for four months, after the summer's harvest.[36] Thus the Greeks created a neat metaphor for marriage where there is a difficult mother-in-law and for the origin of the cycle of seasons.

Pluto is depicted throughout history as a chilling presence with an icy expression; his character is pitiless and implacable. The abduction of Persephone is one of only a very few legends about him. He is a shadowy figure and one invoked only with extreme caution or foolhardiness. He has little contact with the other gods though Hermes (see **Orange**) acts as guide to the underworld for the spirits of the recently departed. It was not Pluto himself but his judges who decided the ultimate fate of a soul: the good went to the

36 Persephone or Proserpina was also regarded as symbolic of the Renaissance.

Elysian Fields; the wicked were consigned to Tartarus, the place of eternal punishment; the indifferent were retired to the meadows of asphodel.

Pluto is also the furthest planet from the sun in our solar system. It was first discovered in 1930 though the search for it had been started by Percival Lowell as early as 1877. It had taken so long to see it because scientists, expecting to discover a planet of far larger dimensions, had not imagined a celestial body of such small dimensions having such great effects on the solar system. When it was discovered it was realized that it was a double planet due to the relatively large size of its moon, Charon (named after the ferryman who rowed departed souls over the River Styx, the border between earth and hell).

Pluto, lodged in the Kuiper belt, completes its orbit around the sun every 248.4 years. It has a highly eccentric elliptical orbit at a 17° tilt from the horizontal which means that it is unpredictable in its movements. This elliptical orbit, virtually a squashed circle, means that Pluto is sometimes closer to the sun than Neptune is. This happened last in February 1979 and finished 20 years later. At its furthest from the sun it is 5,906,308,000 kilometres away. It is likely to be composed of rock and ice which sets it apart from Jupiter, Saturn, Uranus and Neptune which are all gaseous giants. Pluto has recently suffered the indignity of losing its status as a planet. Luminaries of the astrophysical world have decided that it is no more than a dwarf planet. This remains a con-troversial decision even among scientists and so the debate rages on.

Whether it is a planet or not, there is no doubt that professional astrologers regard Pluto as vitally important as a natural influence on our lives. Pluto represents transformation in whatever guise it needs to take to effect necessary change. In this, like the god, it is utterly implacable. Pluto roots out and uncovers all that is worthless, parasitical, weakening and wasteful. It does this through degeneration, decay, putrefaction and death. It blocks the progress of what is unworthy and undermines anything that is avoidance of the inevitable. Pluto stands between what we may believe or desire to be our choice and the point where we have no choice to make. Though we may feel that Pluto is harsh and cruel, it is no more than what is required to purge and purify after corruption has set in. Humanity is not good at judging what to keep and what not to keep; human frailties and insecurity prevent us from being ruthless about all that is no longer valid. Pluto steps in as a correction. Though the mills of the god Pluto 'grind slow, they grind exceeding small'. It is, therefore, not just an influence of disaster as it at first appears. It is a force for renewal and rebirth. It is the planet most associated with the force of evolution. It is the closest thing astrologers have to describe the syphilitic miasm.

We experience Pluto's effects as obstructive; we fight with loss and illness, with handicap and pain, with all manner of imperfections and guilt and shame, thinking as we struggle, 'Why me?', 'When will this end?' and feeling overwhelmed, vulnerable and close to giving up. Yet where Pluto is concerned the end result is clarity, the free flow of energy, renewal of creativity and a chance to start afresh.

Pluto's chief areas of concern are in the eighth house, that section of a person's astrological chart that governs sex and sexual relationships, death and regeneration and resources brought within our reach by others (such as bequests, donations, benefits, etc.). The eighth house belongs to Scorpio which is ruled by Mars, Pluto's lower octave. There is a very strong link between the sign of Scorpio and Pluto. Scorpio's nature is to live with the prospect of loss and death though unlike Pluto it has great fear of these events. Like Pluto it is a sign of determination and obsession, invested with intense energy that may be loyal, passionate, exploratory, relentless and voracious or manipulative, devious, destructive and cruel. Pluto's purpose is focused on self-development, ultimately towards the expansion of spiritual awareness. It is also to be seen at work in the highest political circles. Scorpio is often found in places of high office or in positions where its energy serves to transform whatever comes within its orbit. Pluto stalks the same corridors of power when it comes time to clear out the debris and detritus of years of corruption.

The generation of children that was born between 1984 and 1996 is known as the Pluto-Scorpio generation as it was at this time that Pluto traversed the sign. People born within these twelve years are seen as strong willed, determinedly independent, intolerant of oppression and obsessive in their desires and interests. (Each of these attributes may just as easily be read in negative terms.) One of these interests is the sharing of resources such as wireless technology in order to maintain constant communication. It is also roughly during this period that there was an intensification of the awareness of problems that are associated with learning difficulties and when words that had been rare or non-existent became part of the vernacular: dyslexia, dyspraxia, dyscalculia, cross laterality, Asperger's, autism, etc. It also saw the dramatic intensification in the debate over controversial issues such as vaccination, pollution and other scientific endeavours that have had a questionable effect on the planet.

Pluto began to traverse Capricorn in November 2008 and will leave this sign in January 2024. The significance of this may be of interest in the understanding of **Plutonium**, the remedy. Capricorn is said to govern the British Isles. Capricorn is the star sign that has to do with organization in all the meanings of that word. People born in this sign tend to be in favour of tradition; they like what has been proved to work. They need to know that institutions that carry responsibility will not fail and they work hard within such enterprises to ensure the cogs of the machinery operate smoothly. Astrologers tell us that when Pluto is in conjunction with Capricorn we can expect massive upheavals in any institution, enterprise or government department that is not wholly accountable or that is not of unimpeachable integrity. Perhaps it is not surprising that in recent times banks have gone into receivership, the behaviour of some political figures has been exposed as discreditable and the obscure workings of the UK Parliament have been brought into question especially as far as its financial operations are concerned. Pluto has no truck with hidden energy. This is also true of the remedy.

Keynote effects

Like all radiation remedies, **Plutonium** reduces terrible fearfulness held in a patient's auric field. Exhaustion, lethargy, weakness, dullness and absence are all features that may follow on from violent and aggressive behaviour or may not. Either way they should be lifted leaving the patient more grounded and better able to cope with a daily existence that has become such a struggle.

General symptoms

At the core of this remedy is destructiveness and breakdown: this may be on the mental level or the physical. Physical restlessness yet exhaustion; cannot remain still for long yet too tired to be able to think. Blood, lymph, glands and skin are the chief areas of physical pathology. Eczema with burning pains and < water. Necrosis of the skin. Putrefaction of the flesh or from cancer. Black exudates especially of ulcerated flesh and of cancerous tissue. Warts, moles and naevi; dark excrescences on the skin. Glandular swellings. Hodgkin's disease and non-Hodgkin's lymphoma. Thyroid pathology; cancer of the thyroid. Central nervous system damaged by pollutants. Learning difficulties associated with neurological developmental problems; poor coordination and lack of balance. Pollution: electromagnetic and heavy metal toxicity. Nervous agitation with easy startling. Useful for the correcting of geopathic stress disorders.

A remedy for acute burns. Left-sided bias to symptoms.

Desire to lie down from feeling of extreme heaviness. Periodical or paralysing fatigue. Chilliness and shivering.

Miasms

Psora, syphilis, cancer and radiation.

Mental and emotional symptoms

Feelings of being slowed down or speeded up: disorientation in time due to losing the sense of one's usual pace. Restlessness. Sensations of being elongated and stretched. Extremely fearful; terrified; fear as if from an indefinite source; from the distant past. Fear of death and of dying. Feelings of being engaged in a constant struggle without end. Fear of not being able to cope or to come through the fight. A sense of having been tipped into circumstances that one has few resources to deal with. Indecisive; the decision process causes anxiety and tiredness. Jumbled thoughts with a feeling of the head not being connected. Sensations of being separate: body and mind are disconnected; body and soul are not in communication. Feels that the body is not connected to the earth. There is a feeling of being scattered. A feeling that the right side of the body does not fit with the left or sometimes that the top half does not feel congruent with the bottom. Sensation as if the interior of the body were an empty space. Confusion and feeling that one cannot access the truth. Thoughts are broken; one thought interrupts another. The mind goes blank, not with emptiness but full of things that do not make much sense. Poor memory; as if one is going senile. Senile dementia. A sense that one is the victim of lies; a victim of cruelty. Alienation between people in a family; children feel as if they have been born into the wrong family. Perverse need for pain and suffering, persecution and struggle. Apathetic and lethargic; lack of any motivation. Deep sadness with an inability to cry.

Obligation: a feeling of being 'externally forced to keep on going and do all kinds of things'; cannot live as she likes; a feeling of too much obligation. Fastidious: urge to put things in order. Feeling of decay, disintegration into different identities. Persistent feeling of existential threat: fears his own defeat if he dares to insist on his personal will and inclination; fear of ecological catastrophes. Claustrophobia. Aggressive, reckless impulses. Deep religious feelings or philosophical thoughts.

Physical symptoms

Head
Heaviness in the head. Pressure in the frontal area.

Pressing pain in the forehead. Pain in vertex comes up as if it would explode.

Eyes
Sensation of very cold draught of air passing over the eyes. Eyes feel 'incredibly cold'.

Face
Tremendous heat in the face. Strong tingling.

Chest
Fear felt in the heart or in the chest.

Sensation of heaviness and fullness in the mammae. Sensation of tension in the mammae, desire to wear a bra.

Abdomen
Pain in the spleen.

Cutting pain like knives > bending double.

Rectum
Sensation of insecurity in rectum when passing flatus.

Skin
Eczema < water; with burning sensation. Dermatitis. Allergenic eczema and skin eruptions. Warts; moles; naevi; dark-coloured excrescences.

Back
Paralysing pain in sacral region; pain extending to posterior part of thigh and popliteal region.

Extremities
Restlessness of the limbs especially the legs. Pain in the left wrist as if the hand had been severed from the arm (the prover had held the remedy in her left hand before eventually taking it).

Sensation of leaden heaviness. Pain in soles of feet on account of vesicles on toes. Sensation as if left leg were shorter.

Sleep

Desire to sleep from extreme tiredness. Difficulty in sleeping from feeling tired and restless at the same time.

Short sleep >. Sleeplessness and restlessness from pain in sacral region, tossing about to relieve the pain. Sleeplessness from feeling of heat.

Strange and peculiar sensations

- As if a mouse or rat was running up the left side of the body and reaching the throat with the feeling that it would throttle you
- A sensation of a bat hitting you in the face
- A sensation as if body and soul were separated
- A sensation of growing extremely tall
- A sensation that one is an alien; that one is being watched by aliens.

Considerations for the use of the remedy

Plutonium is an uncompromising remedy but not one that will inevitably cause difficult aggravations. It is more that, when well indicated, it will act on an energy system that is ready to adapt and move into a state of change. This is not to say that the patient who is manifesting those indications is *intellectually* ready. There may well be fear of change even after struggling so long with an untenable status quo. In all this it is like **Moldavite**.

Vermeulen makes a comparison between **Plutonium** and **Granite**, another 'heavy' remedy with aggressive tendencies and severe back pain. Other remedies to compare are:

- **Carcinosin** which shares the same sense of lost purpose; there is also the heaviness, weariness and weakness and it can also be passive-aggressive.
- **Buddleia** which is also 'never been well since' a devastating trauma.
- **Aconite** and **Ayahuasca** cover the same existential fear though they are different in most other aspects; **Ayahuasca** is complementary to Plutonium.
- **Opium** has the fear too, as well as all the heaviness and slowness and it

is also characterized by similar heat in the face, tiredness and sleepiness; however, it is a remedy of forgetfulness: there is none of **Plutonium**'s feeling that there is something more to life that should be lived.

- **Baryta-carb** and other non-iodide radiation remedies have the heaviness and apathy with slowness of thought and decision-making noted in the provings; however, **Plutonium** does not have the same degree of timidity or the lack of intellectual stamina or capacity.

Esoteric therapeutics

Where **Plutonium** is invaluable and without rival is in cases of 'heavy karma': where the patient is and has long been struggling with life lessons that are overwhelming and causing difficulties that threaten to consume all available energy. One primary indication is in a patient who has not only been unwell since some trauma but has lost all sense of either identity or purposeful pathway. There is also a possibility the patient feels that the life he or she is leading is not the one that they should be pursuing; that they are on the wrong road and can never seem to find the right one though they are not sure that they could recognize the way even if it was in front of them. They are so immersed in still dealing with difficult conditions thrown up since quite early on in life that they see no prospect of an end in view. The slow and ineluctable grind of their destiny seems stuck on a hamster-wheel. They know there is something more and this makes them very frustrated. **Plutonium**'s relationship with **Thymus Gland** becomes extremely important here. When these two remedies are employed as part of a strategy to unlock the deep past then the patient is able to assume his intended purpose. The following combination remedies may be used with discretion in cases of extreme difficulty where other familiar and well-indicated remedies fail to bring resolution:

- TG + Ayahuasca + Plutonium
- TG + Syphilinum + Plutonium
- TG + Carcinosin + Plutonium
- TG + Arsen-alb + Plutonium

Depending on the individual case and the homoeopathic intention behind the prescription, each of these combination remedies may be given in high or LM potencies. The first one on the list is particularly indicated in cases where the patient has otherwise been unable to access the familial and ancestral influences on his or her life history of accident, trauma or illness that have led to an intractable condition with a picture similar to that of **Plutonium** but with characteristics of **Ayahuasca** and **Thymus Gland**. If the patient is also born in the sign of Scorpio or its opposite and challenging sign of Taurus then this lends added urgency to the choice of this remedy. Combinations apart, if Scorpio and Mars are strongly present in a patient's chart then the likelihood of needing **Plutonium** is increased.

Chakras

Crown
Soul and body feel separate; there is little connection or communication between the spirit and the body. Even when the patient feels close affinity for spiritual matters there is poor ability to ground any spiritual experience.

Brow
Poor memory and confusion reign here. Intellect is fearful and intuition is asleep. Reason and knowing remain at arms' length. Restlessness of mind vies with desire for peace. The existential threat is most keenly felt in this centre.

Throat
This centre may be completely blocked and unable to function in any way except physically in the act of swallowing though even this may become difficult and a featured symptom of pathology. There is almost no real creative expression even in one who is full of creativity; it cannot be reached as too much occupies the time, energy and attention of the patient.

Heart
A deep sense of sadness lives in this centre; sadness that has no full expression. The grief most concerns what the patient is least sure or aware of: the causes of feeling so lost lie buried in history and family origins.

Solar plexus
Fear and anticipation are both felt here and can cause pathological changes to occur in the alimentary canal. Symptoms will mirror the sense of stuckness.

Sacral

Sex and sexuality and how they affect relationships or have hereditary connections may or may not be central to the patient's condition. If they are the focus, exemplified by any pathology of the generative organs, then it is likely that **Plutonium** will be supported by remedies such as **Lachesis, Thuja, Medam, Tiger's Eye, Senecio + Tyria** etc. There will also be a strong connection between or a parallel with the history of the throat condition and the problems in this chakra.

Base

There is precious little groundedness in **Plutonium**. The effect of past injury or stress on the spinal column may be crippling with severe pain in the sacral area (though this may also reflect the problems in the sacral centre). It is because the patient is so stuck in the severe Saturnian lessons of this centre that there is so little movement in his or her life. Saturn and Pluto, father and son, the influence of one generation on another, are at work mostly in this chakra hence the fearfulness that is at the root of so many conditions that this remedy is called for.

Provers' comments

1 'The remedy, when I took it out of the packet, felt as if it was burning a hole in my hand, not so much a flow of heat but piercing heat through the centre of my hand.'

2 'I thought I had to take the remedy because for the past six weeks my mind has just jangled as if my head and brain were not connected. I took the remedy and within one minute I felt an immediate calmness in my head [that] I have certainly not had for six weeks. I feel as if everything has come together. I have stopped being restless in the group. I could not sit still but as soon as I took the remedy I suddenly felt focused and back to my normal state.'

3 'I have this feeling of being very tall, of going up very high and not [being] connected to the earth. I have not got palpitations but I feel as if everything is racing.'

Case studies

1 'A woman in her 50s, a singer who had breast cancer in her early 30s and who had had homoeopathic treatment for 15 years, came for her appointment. She was in something of a crisis. She was highly sensitive emotionally and was much affected by her only son's swings of emotion and her husband's bipolar behaviour. There were also frequent ups and downs with her extended family which she felt keenly. Having been through a long period of trouble with her sister and mother and having had her hopes raised and dashed several times over auditions, she had discovered that her right breast was now "leaking".

'"The implant has lasted 17 years since they put it in when they stripped the glandy stuff away but then I was involved in a car crash and had to have another op. They removed some more tissue and warned me that water implants tend to rupture. So they haven't done so badly. My sister told me I should have had both breasts off." At this point she wept quietly and began to feel very shaky. "I feel rejected by my profession. I feel cut off at home. I'm all in bits; one bit here, another bit there. I went back to that place where the cancer happened. I've asked myself so many questions. I wept and wept. I blamed myself for the abortion. I have said 'goodbye'; that's at rest."

'She was given **Plutonium** 10M: single collective dose. She returned three months later and said that the remedy was "massive". She felt much clearer. "It made me really tackle all the problems. It made me look at the cancer and let it go!" She had had an operation to repair the breast and was now not at all concerned about it. "I've been looking after my body for the first time. My shoulders feel they have dropped. I'm giving myself time. I can be still inside. I feel wonderful! I don't know why I'm so optimistic; we've got no money." When asked what she felt she would most like to focus on with her treatment now she replied, "I need self-discipline. I need to work on my confidence and get some order into my life."' CG

2 'A woman born in Capricorn but with many Cancerian traits arrived to her appointment feeling very emotional. She was stressed at work with all the demands made on her at a time when she was trying to cope with a death in the family; her mother's step-son, a paranoid schizophrenic,

had hanged himself several months previously. She was very stiff all over and felt unable to straighten up; she was afraid that this was the first sign of arthritis. She complained that her brain was very slow.

'"It's as if my brain is getting arthritis. I get these headaches that come across my forehead over the eyebrow. They feel so heavy. I want to lie down and be quiet when I get them. I feel very withdrawn." She began weeping again and explained that she could not get over the thought that her 'cousin' (as she called him) had finished his life in such a way. "It was awful to think he wanted to harm himself like that. I can't bear the thought of him feeling so desperate; I can't grasp it. My mind goes blank. I blank it out."

'She had already had remedies for the acute grief and she did feel that they had helped. She was given **Plutonium** 100: single collective dose. When she came back four weeks later she was very pleased. "Those remedies were amazing! I feel so much more grounded; much more so than I've felt for years and years." What was even better about this remedy was that it seemed to release her energy to work better with other remedies. She had suffered from irritable bowel symptoms for years which had only slightly responded to indicated remedies. Now, having had the **Plutonium**, she did really well on remedies for the organs of the solar plexus and her lower bowel.' JM

3 'A young man of 24, son of a single mother, who had grown up unable to attend school due to his considerable learning difficulties and difficult behaviour had been coming for treatment for 10 years. His constitution was most similar to **Silica** though he had never seemed to respond to it particularly strongly. He had made considerable progress over the years with **Anacardium, Stramonium, Tuberculinum, Emerald, Lycopodium, Med-am, Arg-nit, Merc-sol** and others. He was now able to hold down a job and had learnt to drive: his passion. He spent any spare time he had working out in a makeshift gym he had at home in the garage. He was intense in everything he did but he was also extremely nervous and reticent. He suffered from sensitivity to the environment; hay fever was an annual problem. He also had food intolerance that restricted his diet. Usually when he came he was not particularly articulate and many points needed close questioning to clarify what he wanted to say. He would start sentences and then get tied up with the

search for words. On this occasion he came with his digestive problems that usually responded well to **Lycopodium** and **Morgan Gaertner**. He also complained that when he worked out he was pushing his body to the limit though afterwards he did not feel as good as usual: "I feel drained after a session." He also felt that he was missing out nutritionally: "I feel skinny. I don't feel quite me. I feel better when I'm bigger." He felt that his immune system was not doing well as he kept getting colds and sore throats. He also added that he now felt bothered by being single. When asked what he felt the focus of his present problems was he said, "I feel restricted." He was given **Plutonium** 1M with **Organic Brown Rice** 30, one three times per week for four weeks.

'When he returned he was quite different in attitude (and his gut did not feature at all in the session). His physical presence was more definite; he gave off a sense of greater determination and resolve; his verbal expression was not hesitant and needed no clarifying. "It's been quite an eventful period. I developed strong feelings for a woman at work which is not really me. I don't really feel much like that. She told me that there was nothing possible. I'm seeing someone else now."

'He then went on to say, "I don't know – when I get stressed I get a dark side. It's like a hatred – for humanity. I can feel strongly for good or bad. I can feel this hatred go through me; it's a contempt for the world. I wonder if I am denying who I truly am by not eating sugar. I find it stressful to be in a relationship and it makes this dark side come out more. When I drive I lose whatever it is that is holding me back all the time. I've always felt dead and monochrome. I've had this potential all the time but I've never let it out. When I have these dark thoughts I have this graphic image of a kneeling man who is being decapitated." After a pause he continued, "I am going to take up Thai boxing; I'm going to do cage fighting."

'In the months before he went to Thailand to study kick-boxing he began qi gong classes. He said that he became much more placid and patient with women he was attracted to. He found his job completely unfulfilling. When he got to Thailand he witnessed cage fighting and gradually realized that this was not what he wanted. He felt that it was all mindless violence. He also missed the girlfriend he had taken up with several months previously. He was slightly surprised to find that he missed having sex. He had suffered food poisoning while away and this had set him back in terms of his digestion. **Lycopodium** and **Morgan Gaertner** were able to settle this relatively quickly.

'This is not a case that is illustrative of cure. It is more notable for what the remedy brought out; the patient was at last able to express his darkest thoughts. He had always had latent aggression; his mother had pointed this out at his very first appointment. He had always been set apart from his peers by his difficulties; he led a very isolated existence for years only thrashing boxing-bags and lifting weights and reading magazines about cars and communicating with a computer. From the **Plutonium** this all gradually changed and he began to open out, to soften and to be able to look around at the world. He was able to sustain a relationship and live away from home. What is also worth noting is that he had no relationship to speak of with his father who by all accounts had been a feckless person. It seemed as if the **Plutonium** helped the patient to emerge from a chrysalis, to transform from boy into man.' **CG**

4 'I went to Cornwall on holiday with my husband and developed terrible blisters on the leg. When the blisters burst they behaved like necrotizing fasciitis. It was really scary. I went to the hospital just to see what they had to say and they thought it was very peculiar, had never seen anything like it and couldn't do anything for me except take tests. My legs were covered! Martin [Miles] gave me lots of remedies: **Arsenicum**, **Syphilinum** and lots more but nothing did anything. I went to my GP and all he did was to take pictures of it. Martin then suddenly thought of giving me **Plutonium** 10M. Within hours it was better and it completely cleared up within days just on the one dose.' **JM**

5 'A 28-year-old woman, a Taurus, came because she had developed a melanoma on her leg. She was a sun worshipper and used sunbeds all the time. She had **Carcinosin**, **Thuja**, **Thiosinaminum** and others. Nothing changed the melanoma till she had **Plutonium** 30: one three times a week. After a while on this prescription the melanoma disappeared and she has been well since.' **JM**

6 A child of seven came with asthma. He was a very sycotic kind of child with lots of mucus. He had **Thuja**, **Medorrhinum Americana**, **Nat-sulph**, **Spongia**, **Ant-tart** and others, all of which helped but none held for long.

The condition chuntered on for six months or so. Then it transpired that the father had worked in a nuclear power station for eight years. The boy was given **Plutonium** 1M, single collective dose. He had a severe aggravation. **Thuja** and **Nat-sulph** came up in this aggravation and he responded well to them in the acute. He had a repeat dose of the **Plutonium** when the aggravation had calmed down as his asthma started to build up again. After this second dose, followed a little while later by **Thuja** 10M, the asthma disappeared completely and has never returned.' JM

26

PUNICA GRANATUM

Pomegranate

Pomegranate was proved by the meditation circle on 23 February 2007. It was the inspiration of the late Michael Miles who supplied the fruit from which the remedy was prepared. The group consisted of 7 women and 3 men. The remedy is to be differentiated from **Granatum**, which is made from the pomegranate root bark that appears in Boericke's, Clarke's and Murphy's materia medicas. (The proving of this earlier remedy was not given any attribution by either Boericke or Clarke.)

The Background

The name Linnaeus gave to the plant was *Punica granatum*; the Latin name was *Punicum malum*, the Libyan or Carthaginian apple. The word *granatum* was applied on account of the seeds. Other folk names include grenadier and malicorio.

The plant's natural habitat is western Asia including Iran, Bengal and northern India (where it is dried to make the spice known as anardana). The pomegranate is a small, shrubby tree growing to no more than about 4.5 metres in height. Propagation is either by seed, from cuttings or by layering. It needs a sunny site in well-drained soil. The trunk is covered with a pale-brownish bark. The leaves are narrow and lanceolate and appear opposite each other; they are thick and glossy as well as being virtually evergreen. Buds and the young shoots are red while the large flowers are solitary and have crimson petals that alternate with the lobes of the calyx. The fruit is as large as an orange and has a thick, inedible reddish-yellow rind. The pulp inside is acidic and there are a large quantity of seeds each separated by a thin, bitter, cream-coloured membrane.

The roots are covered in a yellow-grey bark and have the appearance of quills. They have no odour and an astringent taste. The flowers are used to dye cloth a deep red and the bark is used in tanning leather a characteristic yellow. The bark is made up of 22 per cent punico-tannic acid as well as gallic acid, mannite and a variety of alkaloids. It is the admixture of tannin and the alkaloid, pelletierine, which acts so powerfully against worms and has given pomegranates a reputation for being a vermifuge. Pomegranates are also a source of vitamin C, folic acid, potassium, polyphenols and antioxidants.

Pliny prescribed pomegranate to expectant mothers suffering from morning sickness. The juice has natural antiseptic properties and recent research has shown that it may be a factor in inhibiting the development of prostate cancer while it has long been held useful in heart conditions. Boericke tells us that it is used 'as a vermifuge for the expulsion of tapeworm and homoeopathically for the following symptomatic indications. Salivation with nausea and vertigo.' He recommended the use of the first to the third potency. Meanwhile, Clarke tells us that 'Pomegranate is a well known vermifuge especially for the expulsion of taenia. For this a decoction of the rind is used or else *Pelletierine*[37] in the following manner. After a mild purge the previous night, in the morning 30 grams of Sulphate of Pelletierine is administered in a solution containing 50 grams of Tannic acid. This is followed by a glass of water in ten minutes and a brisk purge in half an hour.' He notes that 'the homoeopathic provings bring out many symptoms of helminthiasis as: pale blue rings round the eyes. Itching, crawling, tickling of nose. Ravenous hunger; craving for sour or juicy things; fruit; coffee. Loss of appetite. Nausea; fermenting in the abdomen; griping; dragging in the inguinal region as if hernia would protrude. Itching and tickling in anus frequently during the day. Emaciation. Convulsive movements.'

The fruit is used as a dessert while the juice is added to cooling drinks. The flowers, leaves and seeds were used in former times as an astringent (a contracting agent) and a vermifuge. The seeds are demulcent. The fruit is not only astringent, it is also a cooling agent in fevers, it assists in biliousness and, as noted, has been used to remove tapeworm. In India it is often combined with opium

37 Pelletierine is an alkaloid ($C_8 H_{13} NO$) discovered by Bertrand Pelletier, and obtained from the rind of the fruit.

and prescribed for diarrhoea or chronic dysentery. Dioscorides tells us that the pomegranate was good for the stomach. The juice was good when mixed with honey for mouth, anal and genital ulcers, including cancerous ulcers. It was thought to be useful in ear pain and for problems in the nasal passages. The flowers in decoction were good for loose teeth and weak gums. The rind was useful in helping to bind loose bowels while the roots were used as the vermifuge.

Traditionally, the pomegranate is associated with encouraging romance, longevity, fertility and sex appeal. The fruit was sufficiently prized by the ancient Egyptians for them to bury a stock of them in their tombs as food and medicine to accompany the dead on their journey in the afterlife. Around 300 BC, Theophrastus, viewed by many to be the father of modern botany, was one of the first authors to leave us a description of the pomegranate. It features in the Koran, being one of the fruits in the heavenly paradise of the four gardens. Mohammed ordered his followers to eat the fruit 'to purge the body of longing' as if the fruit were a desire suppressant, the very opposite of its reputation. In King Solomon's temple pomegranates were features on the supportive pillars. The robes of Jewish kings and priests were embroidered with the fruit and plant. For some, the pomegranate is the original of the tree of the knowledge of good and evil.

In ancient Greek mythology the pomegranate represented persistence of life, fertility and regeneration. In the story of Persephone, she it was who was captured by Hades and taken to the underworld. She was given four seeds of the pomegranate to eat without her knowing that they symbolized the indissolubility of marriage. By eating the seeds Persephone bound herself to Hades forever. Zeus recognized her distress and caused the seasons to occur so that she could return once each year to her mother Demeter, the goddess of abundance and harvests, at springtime.

For Buddhists the pomegranate is one of the three blessed fruits, along with peach and citrus; it represents 'the essence of favourable influences' and features as such in Buddhist art. In China a sliced pomegranate is a traditional wedding gift as it symbolizes fertility, abundance and a blessed future.

The script in italics interpolated into the following materia medica belongs to the comparatively substantial proving of the root bark and may be of value when studying the remedy made exclusively from the fruit.

Keynote effects

This is a remedy to foster calmness and stillness in those whose nervous system is overwrought with stress and hyperadrenalism. It encourages those who rush about too much to remember their need for rest. For those who speed about anxiously trying to cope due to a fear of change and the need to keep ahead, it is indicated as a balancing remedy. It encourages patience and stillness and not being afraid of facing what the past holds. Fosters a greater ability to create personal space so that others are less able to draw on one's own energies. Like many new remedies, it has been described as one to put oneself back in touch with soul purpose.

General symptoms

The nervous system is under strain from excessive adrenal output. The patient may not be fully aware of how far this is damaging to health. The other main systems that are affected by this constant demand for energy to keep going are the digestive system, the cardiovascular system and the urinary and reproductive systems. Chronic irritable bowel symptoms; excessive mucus in the bowel suggestive of hyperacidity; constipation; flatus and bloating. In low potency it can be used therapeutically to assist in the processes of assimilation, absorption and elimination from the bowels. It supports the liver, the stomach and the intestines.

The remedy affects the quality of blood and helps prevent excessive viscosity. Symptoms are also manifest in the reproductive organs, both male and female. It has been described as 'almost a specific for prostate cancer'. To be considered in a male patient who has had a high PSA (prostate specific antigen) count from a blood test. Can be used as a drainage remedy in low potency (3x or 6x) in prostate or uterine pathology. Also of value in conditions of the ovaries and testes especially in cases where there is a history of long-term emotional stress.

Of value in heart and circulation problems: reactions to emotional distress felt in the heart. Pulsation and palpitation felt in the chest often accompanied by feelings of fear or anxiety. Symptoms of indigestion and discomfort felt in the chest may call for this remedy.

Useful in allergic reactions. May prove to be of use in the treatment of histamine reactions even when these are serious enough to threaten anaphylaxis.

Pomegranate has been linked to the cancer miasm. It is said to be useful in any stage that potentially leads to the development of cancer particularly of any part of the reproductive system. It is most indicated when the cancer state has been fostered by unexpressed grief particularly when the emotional suffering has a connection with the bond between the patient and the maternal root.

It is said to be one of the few remedies that can cut through the drug layer of terminally ill patients who are distressed and confused and feel alone in their sickness and without help despite all the nursing. It is said to foster spiritual peace of mind.

Great weariness and exhaustion, scarcely able to keep upright. Trembling. Discomfort and nausea. Itching of the skin of various places, face and body, as if pimples would break out. Biting and itching in palms of hands. Yawning. Great sensitiveness. All symptoms < after dinner. Pain in abdomen is > after drinking cold water. (Clarke)

Miasms

Cancer, sycosis, syphilis and psora.

Mental and emotional symptoms

Grief: a sense that there is a well of grief that has yet to be expressed. Tearfulness helps to relieve the pressure of emotions but there is always more to come; the sense that if one began to cry about one thing then there would be a lot more that would have to be released in the same way. The patient may act out a lot of busy-ness as a way of avoiding dealing with a history of grief; layers of grief. Alternatively, the patient may complain of excessive tiredness and sleepiness for the same reason. The patient may say that they feel stuck or locked into their present circumstances and this is likely to be accompanied by anxiety especially about change. The core reason for this grief is the sense of separation from the mother, loss of the mother or never having had the benefit of the bond with a mother (see **Statice**). Sad mother syndrome: the child may have had a mother who suffered much but was unable to resolve her problems; witnessing the distress of a mother figure may be the underlying cause for the presenting pathology. A lasting misunderstanding of a mother's motives for her behaviour towards the child (now the patient) may also be an indicating factor. The role of a patient's imagination cannot be underestimated in considering

Pomegranate as it may be the cause of lifelong misapprehension of situations long past that were inexplicable at the time of their occurrence. The remedy is for those who feel profoundly in need of nurturing (see **Rhodochrosite**). The core mental symptoms include being busy to the point of not being able to cope with anything more, avoidance of emotional subjects to avoid opening up to grief and fears about change, about heart disease and cancer.

Great sensitiveness and impressibility (sic). Irritability and arrogance. Penurious and quarrelsome in humour. Hypochondriacal scruples. Melancholy, gloomy temper, dejection and discouragement. Stupefaction and intellectual embarrassment. (Clarke)

Physical symptoms

Head

Feels empty. Vertigo very persistent. (Boericke)

Vertigo especially during intellectual labour or in the morning on rising with obscuration of the eyes or with nausea and aching in the stomach. Sensation of emptiness in the head. Stupefying pain and painful heaviness in the head especially in the forehead. Pressure on the forehead and on the occiput. Acute drawing pains chiefly on the right side of the head. Shootings in forehead. Pustules on forehead and temples with pain as from excoriation, leaving small tubercles on drying. (Clarke)

Eyes

Has an affinity for the eyes and particularly the retina. Tired eyes < from overuse.

Sunken eyes; pupils dilated; weak sight. (Boericke)

Eyes hollow and surrounded by a livid circle. Itching and burning in the canthi. Dryness and smarting in the eyes. Yellowish tint of the sclerotica (sic). Inflammation of the eyes as in coryza. Convulsive movements of the eyelids. (Clarke)

Ears

Cramp-like squeezing, acute drawing pains and shootings in the ears. Tinkling and buzzing in the ears. (Clarke)

Nose

Burning heat and dryness of the nostrils or an accumulation of tenacious mucus. Crawling itching in the nose. Coryza alternately dry and fluent. (Clarke)

Face

Complexion sickly, yellowish and earth-coloured. Burning heat in the face, sometimes transient. Gnawing itching in the face and especially in the cheeks. Swelling of the cheek which is livid; burning heat, itching, tension and crawling as with chilblains. Squeezing and acute drawing pains in the face, in the cheek-bones and in the root of the nose often on one side only. Dryness of the lips and burning sensation in them. (Clarke)

Teeth

Acute drawing pain, tension and squeezing in the maxillary joints and cracking of the joints during mastication. Shooting pains in the teeth even at night in bed. The teeth seem to be elongated. Gums unfixed and easily bleeding. (Clarke)

Mouth

Excessive accumulation of saliva sometimes of a sweetish taste in the mouth. Tongue moist and white. Excessive spitting of mucus. (Clarke)

Throat

Sensation of astriction (sic) in different parts of the mouth and of the gullet. Contraction of the gullet. (Clarke)

Chest and heart

Has an affinity for the vagus nerve and for regulating the rhythm of the heart. Sensations of heavy heartbeat, uneven rhythm and fluttering heartbeat. Anxiety felt in the chest which affects the stomach. Sensation of tension in the sternum area.

Oppressed with sighing. Pain between shoulders; even clothing is oppressive. (Boericke)

Sensation of anxiety in the chest and groaning. Great oppression of the chest with lassitude in the legs. Pressure on the chest and across the sternum. Rheumatic pains shooting and drawing in the diaphragm. Shootings in the chest especially when walking. Tension and painful squeezing in the ribs. Palpitation of the heart sometimes on the least movement. Pains and cramp-like contractions in the muscles of the chest. (Clarke)

Appetite
Great variableness of taste; taste alternately acute and dull. Appetite alternately diminished and increased. Extraordinary hunger and voracity even after a meal. Desire for different things and especially for coffee, for fruits and for succulent and acid aliments. Great thirst for water. Liquid aliments and potatoes cause nausea and eructations. (Clarke)

Stomach
Frequent and noisy eructations. Frequent nausea, sometimes with lassitude, flow of water in the mouth, pain in the abdomen and in the stomach, frequent want to evacuate without any result, shivering, sickly looks and ill-humour. Vomiting even at night and sometimes with lassitude, trembling, perspiration or vertigo. Painful pressure, fullness, burning sensation and anxiety in the precordial region. Cramps in the stomach when fasting in the morning. (Clarke)

Abdomen
Irritability of the ileo-caecal valve. Both the small and the large intestine can be affected. Indigestion with a variety of pains. Grumbling and rumbling in the large bowel. Wind and bloating. Constipation with dry stools. Acid indigestion. Sensations as of hiatus hernia. Tendency to piles which may come and go depending on the amount of mental/emotional stress.

Pain in the stomach and abdomen; worse about umbilicus; ineffectual urging. Itching at anus. Dragging in vaginal region as if hernia would protrude. Swelling resembling umbilical hernia. (Boericke)

Copious evacuations of a deep colour. Diarrhoea with frequent evacuations and evacuation of fæcal matter and mucus. Before the loose evacuations, nausea and fermentation in abdomen; during the evacuations, burning heat in face and pressure in rectum. Tenesmus with movements and fermentation in abdomen. Prolapsus of rectum during the evacuations. Insupportable itching and titillation of the rectum. Burning itching in the anus, on the buttocks and perineum, on the scrotum and on the hair covered parts of the genital organs and especially on the thighs. Shootings in anus and rectum. (Clarke)

Female
Conditions of the ovaries, tubes and uterus. Symptoms < at the period. Thick and sticky menstrual flow. Cancer of the ovaries or uterus that stems back to unresolved grief.

Catamenia premature and too copious and accompanied by colic and pressure from the sacral region to the groins. Yellowish leucorrhoea. (Clarke)

Male

Prostate conditions are eased: hypertrophy, cancer. Difficulty urinating: long time to start the flow < night time; dribbling of urine. Little or no pain associated. Loss of sexual power. Prostate conditions stem from grief and loss.

Mucus oozing from the urethra as in gonorrhoea with burning traction in the cavernous parts as far as the glans. Excitement of sexual desire. (Clarke)

Urinary organs

Incisive shooting and gnawing pains in the urethra. Inflammation and swelling of the urethra. (Clarke)

Skin

Sudden acute histamine reactions: hives or urticaria. The remedy may be found most useful in supporting other remedies such as **Apis** and **Medusa**.

Gnawing and insupportable itching in the palms and the back of the hands. (Clarke)

Extremities

Traction, rheumatic pains, crawling and sensation of paralysis in the arms with difficulty raising them. Rheumatic pains in the joints of the hands and fingers as well as in the forearms. Painful and paralytic stiffness in the fingers. Swelling of the ball of the thumbs with livid colour, burning heat and marbled swelling of the veins. Sensation of stiffness in the hips as in sciatica. Acute drawing pain, paralytic pulling, heaviness and shootings in the knee. Pain as from a sprain in the instep. Painful corns on the feet. (Clarke)

Considerations for the use of the remedy

A number of remedies stand comparison with **Pomegranate**. They include **Nat-mur**, **Pulsatilla**, **Lycopodium**, **Rhodochrosite**, **Copper Beech**, **Statice** and **Chalice Well**. If we also take the information given us by Clarke and Boericke then we must add **Arsen-alb** as well.

- **Nat-mur** also covers such grief but in **Pomegranate** there is not the same degree of 'stiff upper lip'. Nor is there the same degree of 'greyness' that can manifest in a long-term **Nat-mur**. It is not as if the grief is calcified, more that it is deeply held and the patient does not know how to access it. **Pomegranate** has more in common with a recently formed **Nat-mur** than a truly chronic state of it.

- **Pulsatilla** will cry more readily than **Pomegranate** though once the latter has started to weep, the tears may flow for longer. **Pulsatilla** is usually distinguishable by its well-known general symptoms of dryness and thirstlessness as well as the variable nature of any pains or other symptoms.

- **Lycopodium** is most often mistaken for **Pomegranate** especially in the digestive system. The aggravation time of 4 – 8 may distinguish it from **Pomegranate**. **Lycopodium** can be just as tearful (and tends to be more so than the materia medica would suggest) but it is not so rushed and hurried. **Lycopodium** is less concerned with the grief at the loss or absence of the mother bond than **Nat-mur** or **Pomegranate**.

- **Rhodochrosite** is one of the first remedies to consider where 'nurture' or the lack of it is the focus of the case. This is not necessarily as rushed or hurried a remedy though it can be and there is not the same degree of avoidance in it as in **Pomegranate**. **Rhodochrosite** tends to be aware of how stressed they are and has the feeling that they just cannot cope with any more. **Pomegranate** does not have that same perception and is also more easily dragged down by the demands of other people while still trying to comply with them. This remedy is also more associated with the menopause than **Pomegranate**.

- **Chalice Well** covers the well of grief as much as **Pomegranate** but it is more general. There is not the same link to the mother figure as in **Pomegranate**. **Chalice Well** is also more a remedy of 'letting go' of interfering emotions while **Pomegranate** is more about bringing solace, equilibrium and more personal space to the patient. **Chalice Well** helps patients to see what they need to do; **Pomegranate** helps them to see how they need to be.

Pomegranate has been suggested as a remedy to consider in the treatment of men suffering from prostate cancer. It should be considered as a drainage remedy in such cases as it works on a body in which some cells have become cancerous due to unexpressed grief. This is to view the cancer as a layer of pathology in a patient who has much journeying to do in search of health.

Prostate cancer is for the most part a small cell condition that insidiously chunters away within, with little to be observed. What will be seen is a state of tiredness; of being a little fed up with being stressed and overwrought; of being easily drawn on by other people. This is a man who has little time for himself but has a history of hard work and responsibility. One would be able to see that he has had times of being typically 'Lycopodium'; that he might be easily described as 'Nat-murish'. He is sensitive, hard-working and inclined recently to getting muddled which bothers him greatly. He can be fearful and anxious especially about his condition but he is reluctant to deal with the changes that he really should be making: to his diet, to his routines, to his work schedule.

In prescribing **Pomegranate** for such a case, it is well worth considering the use of **Pomegranate** in combination with **Mag Poli Ambo** (the north and south poles of the magnet). This is said to be far more efficacious than **Pomegranate** on its own. The use of **Pomegranate** + **Mag Poli Ambo** + **Thuja** 6c as a layer case drainage remedy would support any indicated constitutional remedy. Others to consider would include **Pom** + **Mag-p-a** + **Carcinosin** and **Pom** + **Mag-p-a** + **Arsen-alb**.

Pomegranate is often of greatest use in a layers case as its use almost pre-supposes that there are deep-held patterns of negative energy to be brought to the surface and resolved. It is one to use in a genuine **Nat-mur** case where the patient simply does not have the resources to dig deep enough to deal with the long-held grief. Like many other new remedies it can be a remedy of preparation for the deepest possible work. Where it is especially indicated is in those cases where (like **Nat-mur**) there is a strong mother element, one that is run through with sadness and separation.

Pomegranate has also been suggested for use in acutes in the 200th potency particularly in allergic reactions.

Esoteric therapeutics

Pomegranate particularly works on the base, sacral, solar plexus and heart chakras. Its chief action on the base chakra is to ground a patient who has lost a sense of well-paced rhythm to life and to awaken or reawaken the energy of the other three chakras. Its energy flows upwards through the body. Whatever has occurred in the heart and sacral centres is responsible for the distress felt in the solar plexus. The most usual and often unspoken underlying causation is the broken link with the mother especially when that figure is one of sadness, ill health, confusion and distress. Pathology in the sacral centre may well have a hereditary basis that comes through the mother's line. The same is true of the disturbance to the heart centre though the patient's own grief may be enough to explain the distress felt in the heart and circulation.

Chakras

Crown
The overadrenalized state may lead to excessive sleepiness as a way of cutting off from an exhausting lifestyle. Alternatively, there may be poor sleep due to feeling 'wired'. Either way, the patient's crown centre is poorly connected with the brow, heart or base.

Brow
The brow centre is ruled by the adrenal glands: though the intellect may work fast, there is not much time to pay attention to the calming influence of the intuition which would counsel 'more haste, less speed' with more time for relaxation. The patient's mind is unbalanced by faulty judgements about past events that carry emotional significance. There is a tendency for the mind to gloss over what might be difficult emotional issues; it's as if the train is going too quickly to stop at the next station to alight.

Heart
Pomegranate is a 'key' remedy in that it unlocks that which lies buried especially in the heart centre. It should be considered in anyone who has had the usual range of grief remedies but who has not made the signal progress that might be expected. Think of this remedy when **Nat-mur** has been given more than once, even with good results, but needs to be repeated again as the patient has once more slipped into old patterns. The same is true of **Lycopodium**, **Pulsatilla** and **Lachesis** (though this latter often seems to be followed by **Nat-mur**). Too busy to realize that the heart needs a long period of recuperation.

Solar plexus
The remedy can appear to be like other irritable bowel remedies such as **Lycopodium**, **Chelidonium** and the **Natrum** remedies and may be arrived at

when these others do not achieve the expected relief from symptoms. However, much of the trouble that has brought on the **Pomegranate** picture is due to excessive adrenal output. It cools overheated blood energy which otherwise could lead to heart and circulation problems, histamine reactions and bowel symptoms.

Sacral

The remedy is as useful in male as in female patients. The chief reason for considering it in regard to this chakra is the stagnation of energy that leads to congestion of the tubes and organs of this centre and the consequent build-up of mucus and thickening of tissues. The eventual tendency for these to become malignant is part of the picture of **Pomegranate**. The origins of this condition lie in the cancer miasm and the lost or broken link with the mother figure.

Base

Pomegranate can engender patience and balance both of which can be invaluable in one who is in a state of not looking inward. It helps to quieten the fears of one who is unused to looking within for self-healing.

Case studies

1 'A 56-year-old Taurean woman artist, a melancholic with a history of grief, continued to come for treatment. She gave the impression of being very syphilitic; she was always grief-stricken and she seemed only to have very sad friends. Her choice of partners was also grim. She had done reasonably well on **Opium, Syphilinum** and **Tub-bov. Berlin Wall, Nat-mur** and **Rainbow** had also all made promising changes. In her pictures she painted her mother dying. This was a case of "never been well since" her mother's death 20 years before, yet she had never felt nurtured by her mother. She had two failed marriages; she smoked, she drank and was abusive when drunk. Though she was always weeping, tears never helped her. She liked coming for constitutional treatment but often forgot to take the remedies. She had had **Med-am, Thuja**, and **Carbo-veg** among others. She did well on **Statice** 30 o.d. for three

weeks. Two months after this she was given **Pomegranate** 30 – 200 – 1M over 24 hours. She immediately went into profound grief. She cried continuously for seven days. After this she went into anger and then resentment. She had dreams of being tortured by her mother which in turn led to a strong eruption of hives on her chest. She was only given **Nat-sulph** 6x (Taurus's tissue salt) to help her through this aggravation. When her reactions had all died down she became far less melancholic and much more positive. When she needs a remedy like **Nat-mur** now, she responds far more deeply and lastingly.' JM

2   'A 35-year-old Piscean lady came with fertility problems. She had never been able to conceive despite tests showing that she was physically well. She had been through IVF three times with no satisfactory result and was reluctant to try it again. Her own mother had died in childbirth though no explanation as to why was given. She was angry with her mother for dying and abandoning her. It was clear that her heart and sacral chakras were blocked. She was given all the salt remedies, **Carcinosin, Statice** and **Silica,** the last two of which did particularly well for her constitution. She was then given **Pomegranate** 10M, single collective dose. She phoned up two weeks later to say that she was much more philosophical and almost apologetically said, "Why all this fuss?" One week later she conceived.' JM

Janice Micallef writes: '**Pomegranate** supports the prostate well. In six cases **Thuja** in a high potency followed by **Pomegranate** in a low daily dose had proved decisive in resolving the symptoms. **Pomegranate** particularly helps patients with prostatic hyperplasia who have had antibiotics. Apart from this **Pomegranate** supports cranial osteopathic treatment given to patients with ileo-caecal dysfunction.'

27

PURPLE

The colour purple was proved by the meditation group on 7 February 1997. There were 7 women and 5 men present plus the medium who conducted the proving. The remedy was given to each participant in the 30th potency. A second proving was conducted with a mixed group 2 weeks later. The provers were aware of the name of the remedy they took before the meditation. **Purple** was the inspiration of Ruth Epps and was made by her.

The Background

Purple, the result of mixing the primary colours of red and blue in different proportions, varies according to the eye of the beholder as retinal sensitivity to red and blue varies from one person to another. Purple therefore must be defined by different shade names: magenta, mulberry, burgundy, lilac, mauve, lavender, claret, indigo, amethyst, violet, heliotrope, royal, Tyrian, imperial, aubergine, etc. The colour, as far as the remedy is concerned, is at the darker end of this range: Tyrian or imperial purple. Unlike indigo and violet, which are evoked by a single wavelength of light on the colour spectrum, purple is, according to colour theory, a non-spectral colour, being darker than either of the other two.

Tyrian purple was most famously produced as a dye and traded by the Phoenicians though archaeological finds suggest that before the Phoenicians and Romans, the Minoans of the 20th to 18th centuries BC already knew how to extract the dye from shellfish. *Murex brandaris* and *Hexaplex trunculus* are marine gastropods that produce a mucous secretion that provides the chemical base for the fast dye. The snails use the mucus both to surround their egg clusters as it is antimicrobial and as part of their arsenal in attacking other marine creatures they live on. It required huge numbers of snails to produce small quantities of the fabulously expensive colour.

Sumptuary laws in various cultures forbade the use of the colour by anyone other than royalty, the pope or the very high-born. The Romans took the use of purple as a social symbol to a very high degree. Silks particularly were dyed in Tyrian purple and as a result children of the later imperial court of Byzantium were said to be 'born into the purple' (*porphyrogenitos*). Closer to our own time, purple is much used in the church as a penitential colour; it is associated with Lent and Advent. It is also used in funerals. A purple stole is worn by the priest hearing confession. Inherent in all this is the concept of humility; the humility of Christ.

According to feng shui experts, purple is a colour of high vibration and should be used sparingly and with discretion. It is even said to trigger diseases of the blood if applied to living room walls. It is recommended as a suitable colour for spaces used for meditation as it raises the level of the awareness of spirit and of spiritual dimensions.

Keynote effects

Transformation on the deepest level of the spirit; fosters an inner awareness of spiritual reality. The remedy is seen most frequently indicated in those who, through fear, inertia and habit, have long been held back from making transformational changes in their lives that would help them to release from the grip of materialism and make a more spiritually orientated journey (often psoric or syphilitic patients). It is also seen in those who have made the break with materialism but who have become completely ungrounded so that their spiritual journey has little or no foundation (often sycotic patients). Blood/heart/circulation pathology in those who have ignored the spirit body in favour of more worldly concerns. Facilitates an easy sleep and access to dreams. **Purple** can bring to light much darkness held within especially in those with links into the syphilitic miasm. It is a remedy of illumination.

General symptoms

Physically there is weakness and lack of energy; enervation. Lack of stamina. Physical weakness in serious pathology. Blood disorders: anaemia and leukaemia; also in conditions where the blood is stagnant or sluggish with a tendency to clot. Alcoholism. Might be indicated in those who are on warfarin or heparin to prevent strokes. The remedy affects the return of venous blood towards the heart. Bruising and varicose veins when usual remedies fail to relieve the symptoms. Also may be indicated in those who have heart troubles that feature a tendency to mauve or purplish lips. Chilliness. Sleepiness from tiredness and weakness and as a means of avoiding responsibilities or wakefulness when troubled on a deep, unconscious level. Postviral syndrome; ME. Thyroid conditions. To be considered in the treatment of those with diabetic tendencies. **Purple** is one of the remedies to consider for those suffering from jet lag.

Miasms

Syphilis, cancer and psora.

Mental and emotional symptoms

Lack of self-confidence; a sense of having a weak personality that allows events or other people to sway them. Lack of self-knowledge. Humility and sadness. A sense of being small, insignificant or stupid. Very self-conscious; prefers to avoid the limelight and stay back in the shadows. Disappointment; a sense of having been led off course in life and that there is no going back to renew the journey. Grief. **Purple** encourages one to speak out about those things that have lain buried for ages; even those things that were never seen as blocks to healing – they are now revealed as the very thoughts and feelings that have been holding the patient back from moving on in life. Reluctance to change old patterns and routines; fear of change. **Purple** corresponds to the Tower card in the tarot: this is the vibration evoked by a sudden traumatic shock to the system that heralds inevitable change often first felt or thought of as a disaster or a destructive event;[38] 'death of an old life, heralding a spiritual unfoldment moving forward on the path'. Fear of death; fear of disease; fear of separation; fear of authority. Depression and hopelessness after periods of sacrifice or of feeling 'in the dark' and in those who lack faith in the spirit body or in those who have a religious faith that lacks the depth of inner strength. Lack of focus and inability to concentrate. Feelings of being held back. Is also indicated in

38 See **Buddleia** (*Volume I*) which is the plant most closely associated with **Purple**.

those who are held back by their antagonistic feelings and thought patterns towards others. Is useful in jet lag when there is lack of proper grounding, poor focus, enervation and little motivation. Miasmatically, **Purple** is a profoundly syphilitic remedy.

Physical symptoms

Head
Dizziness especially with headache. Headache: < on the left but later moving to the right. Headache < from crying for a long time; headache from grief. Sensations of drunkenness.

Eyes
Of possible value in retinal haemorrhage.

Throat
Sensations of a blocked throat; hard to swallow. Thyroid problems; will support other symptomatically indicated remedies, especially **Lachesis** and **Nat-mur**. Swollen glands on the left side with copious phlegm in the throat.

Chest
Deep aching in the chest: tenderness < taking a deep breath. Piercing sharp pains on deep breathing. Constriction around the heart area.

Skin
Dark moles; malignant changes to moles. Purple patches on the skin or bruising either spontaneous or traumatic.

Back
Vulnerable to back problems especially in the lower spine. Piercing pain in the right shoulder blade, deep within the chest cavity and < for taking an in-breath.

Sleep
Difficulty in going to sleep; hard to go back to sleep once woken in the small hours. Sleepiness especially in the daytime. Unable to remember dreams or to understand their significance.

Considerations for the use of the remedy

The effects of the remedy can be enhanced and amplified with the use of **Clear Quartz**. If **Clear Quartz** is used in a case marked by structural anomalies (such as scoliosis) then a period of physical adjustment may be part of the overall effect of the prescription (see **Clear Quartz**) in which case a course of treatment with a cranial osteopath would be complementary. **Purple** also complements **Blackberry** especially in blood disorders and can work on the patient's higher vibration while the fruit works on the physical level.

The common remedies most likely to be compared with Purple include **Lachesis, Arsenicum, Syphilinum, Carcinosin, Platina, Phosphorus** and **Carbo-veg**. New remedies that should be thought of include **Amethyst, Buddleia, Holly Berry, Sequoia** and **Plutonium**.

- **Lachesis** can be one of those remedies that are best given after some preparation as an aggravation from it can be distressing. While it is indicated by incipient or actual heart pathology with all its characteristic symptoms, when it fails to relieve or make much impression, **Purple** might be considered as a support remedy in low potency. This is also true of other viper poisons or of the less often used **Latrodectus Mactans**.
- **Aurum**, too, is followed or preceded well by **Purple**. Gold and purple, in metal and coloured cloth, have much history in common; both were the preserve of royalty. However, in terms of homoeopathy, **Purple** is able to amplify the beneficial effects of a remedy that so often, these days, does not always appear to fulfil reasonable expectations; the **Purple** seems to be able to 'shine a light' on a higher purpose than simply to recover self-worth.
- **Arsen-alb** is much more anxious and restless though **Purple** has both these characteristics. The facial expression and complexion are pinched and pale in **Arsenicum** but in **Purple** they are more likely to be depressed and dusky.
- **Syphilinum** is just as likely to be used as an intercurrent in serious heart pathology. What might differentiate it best are the typical < at night and night sweats. **Purple** is an excellent support remedy for **Syphilinum**.
- **Carcinosin** is something of a skeleton key remedy; it covers so many different aspects of a constitution that is only able to throw up a

confused picture. Where it is successful in serious pathology is in putting a case back on track; in clearing up the confused signals put out by a body unable to illustrate its distress with a discernible likeness. **Purple**, too, has the ability to put a case back on track but the variety of symptoms for consideration would not be nearly so wide. With **Carcinosin** there is more a sense of muddle; with **Purple** there is more a sense of darkness.

- **Phosphorus** might look like **Purple** but only when seriously unwell; when all the sparkle and sensitivity have been damped down or expunged.
- **Carbo-veg** has breathlessness, cyanosis and chest symptoms like **Purple** but it is far more likely to have its typical digestive symptoms that **Purple** has not been noted for to date.
- **Amethyst** is more noted for its effects on the central nervous system than **Purple** despite the fact that the two remedies share a similar vibrational force. There is more of a tendency towards addiction in **Amethyst** and it is more likely to be useful before serious pathology sets in or in phases of relative symptomatic calm in those who suffer chronic illness and depression.
- **Buddleia** not only shares the attribute of colour with purple but also the aspect of 'disaster'. While **Buddleia** is known rather dramatically as 'the bombsite remedy' and is prescribed after a terrible, destructive and devastating trauma,[39] **Purple** is more likely to be of service in one who has suffered from self-sacrifice but without recognition or who has some inner, potentially spiritual crisis either of faith, conscience or self-worth from serious news (see 'Case studies' below) or deep personal realization.
- **Holly Berry** is a remedy of extraordinary protective influence on the chakras and on the aura in general. It combines extremely well with **Purple** and **Syphilinum** in supporting those whose constitution is deeply compromised by the syphilitic miasm. Often best given in the 10M.
- **Plutonium** is, like **Holly Berry**, suitable for combining with **Syphilinum** and **Purple**. In this case the combination is a deep and subtle healer of a constitution devastated by much trauma, surgery, drugging and environmental pollution.

39 For example, **Buddleia** was useful to relieve those who were traumatized by images of the Twin Towers disaster that appeared on TV screens.

- **Sequoia** is equally known for humility and gentleness but it is a remedy that has more to do with growth and development at a lower vibration than **Purple**.
- It is also worth noting that **Purple** has a place in the healing of skin symptoms that may appear in cases involving **Thuja** and **Medorrhinum Americana**[40] (as well as **Carcinosin**): moles and naevi. **Purple** will follow well or even supersede the use of **Thuja** in moles that are purple and turning black and/or cracking.

Esoteric therapeutics

Purple is a subtle healing vibration that does not necessarily present itself for consideration all that readily. It has a great affinity for all things hidden, unspoken or buried. It is deeply syphilitic in this aspect as in other things. It is often, therefore, a remedy that is thought of after other, more conventional remedies have been given with more or less success without removing the blocks to healing. Astrologically it is associated with Scorpio, the most sensitive, anxious and easily threatened of the 12 signs. It is also associated with the 12th house: that which governs seclusion, secrecy, spirituality, self-sabotage, death and karma. It is also related to Pluto, the celestial body that governs the unearthing of all that is hidden, all that requires transformation as a natural process of maturation, all that is essentially corrupt; it governs that which must be transformed from the basic elements of earth, water, fire, and air into the ether of spirit energy.[41] It is associated with the conception vessel and governor vessel meridians. **Purple** is also a remedy of silence; although it is indicated for the release of held, stuck emotions and trauma or karmic familial patterns, it is also a remedy to engender the peace, tranquillity and silence after the struggle. In this it is associated with the moon which is, in some aspects, the planet of detachment, cool reasoning and instinctual reaction.

---

40 **Medorrhinum Americana**, being more syphilitic and carcinogenic than regular **Medorrhinum**, is sometimes called for in the treatment of people who have moles or naevi that threaten changes.

41 See references to Pluto in **Plutonium**.

Chakras

Crown

This chakra is the one that is most affected by the remedy. It can respond by becoming open and receptive, affording the patient more spiritual insight, peace and harmony than has been known. It lifts depression and eases troubled sleep. It fosters calm reflection on even the most problematic worldly issues. Achieving this also heals the heart and base centres that have been so stressed by material concerns.

Brow

The struggle in this centre is about the quality of light that has hampered the ability to find one's way in difficult circumstances. This chakra has been trammelled by the sense of working in the dark; it is as if one has been forced to live in a dimly lit room into which the light of day seldom penetrates.

Throat

This centre is blocked from chronic inability to find the right expression. Energy cannot flow easily in either direction as there is so much in the heart centre and in the brow that is held back. This chakra may be a focus of pressure that is manifested in the ears, Eustachian tubes, thyroid or the cervical spine or in the poor quality of breathing in the upper respiratory tract at the level of the thoracic inlet.

Heart

Heaviness and weakness of this chakra concomitant with depression and lack of expression may call for this remedy either as the main similimum or as a support to one of its relations (see above). Too much worldly trouble has darkened or dimmed this centre in one who once had a brighter prospect in view that has never been fully realized.

Solar plexus

The liver is congested and return blood through the portal system is slow. This leads to the threat of varicosity; either varicose veins in the limbs or haemorrhoids. The challenge in this chakra is the memory of past conflict; the habit of struggling continues with few resources to cope leaving the chakra in a chronic state of tension. The fire element is dimmed and there is the threat of stagnation.

Sacral
The lack of movement in the throat chakra is mirrored by the stagnation in this centre.

Base
With so much to preoccupy the patient in the upper chakras, there is little sense of solid grounding; personal development and growth are stagnant.

Case studies

1 'Purple for acute depression. A female patient (73) was facing her third major abdominal surgery for cancer. She had been quite clear when opting for the surgery that it was the only option for her and while she was naturally feeling apprehensive her attitude was very positive and determined. However, a few days before the surgery she was gripped with a deep, black depression. She said it was as if part of her just wanted to leave her physical body. The acute and sudden nature of the depression frightened her and she wanted to regain her previous positive attitude before the surgery.

'This patient had a history of clinical depression, obsessive and self-destructive behaviours and in "homoeopathic speak" was deeply syphilitic. The first thought for a remedy was, of course, **Aurum**. However, she spoke of how she had been recently drawn to the colour purple instead of her usual preference for red and had purchased cushions and candles in this colour. She was even uncharacteristically wearing purple. I prescribed **Purple** 30c (being the only potency I had in stock) three times a day. Within two days she had completely returned to her normal positive outlook and went ahead with the surgery.' **CAB**

2 'Having treated lots of drug addiction and alcoholism, I have realized that a great number of addicts fit the **Lachesis** picture. What I have also discovered is that combining **Lachesis** + **Purple** + **Syphilinum** works fabulously for healing the **Lachesis** addictive personality type.

'Current case, male 42, started drinking heavily at 13 then went on to try every drug to the point of almost death with each one. Eventually couldn't tolerate any drugs so has only had alcohol since the age of 37. Since then he has drunk about a bottle of spirit a day and mainly avoided drugs. During this time he has also got married and had two children; recently his wife has become pregnant again. The fact that he has disgraced himself in front of his children with drunken behaviour, as well as his wife telling him to leave unless he stops drinking has brought him to me. The drinking began as he grew up in a very wealthy but regimented family. He is a very gentle, spiritual, artistic but rebellious person. He has been taking the **Purple + Lachesis + Syphilinum** mix daily for three months. Has not touched a drink at all and feels calmer than he has ever felt in his life. He has realized he used to drink and take drugs to avoid a terribly depressed feeling that he was a failure to his family as he was never interested in wealth or the trappings of it. He has three older brothers who are all hugely financially successful but he works as a landscape gardener and tree surgeon, is very creative and inventive, specializing in building tree houses from the wood he cuts doing his tree surgery. He is a really special, gentle, kind soul with a huge affinity for nature. He is really coming to terms with his own beauty since being on the remedies. I feel the **Purple** is a very important part in that.' HJ

3 'Purple** is often useful for those who have the sun in the 12th house on their chart. This usually indicates that the person finds it very hard to "find themselves" till they are in their 50s; they cannot "get into" their life fully. It is also a remedy that helps to clarify which miasm is uppermost in cases where there is an obvious miasmatic block to cure but it is difficult to tell which; when **Carcinosin** has been unable to do this job.

'A woman whose son had developed a tumour on the tibia came for treatment. She had gone through the trauma of her son's various treatments and was in need of constitutional support. Nothing was of any help until she was given **Purple** 30. On her return she 'confessed' to the four abortions she had undergone before her son's birth. She was able to talk of these traumas and to say that she felt as if the guilt that had weighed her down for so long was lifting. Within two days of having taken the **Purple** the specialist in charge of her son's treatment gave her a far more positive prognosis than he had done before and he has since made a full recovery.' JM

4 'An 81-year-old Libran woman who had been coming for constitutional treatment for a long time, characteristically never said much about herself; she "didn't give anything away". She would appear to be most similar to the picture of **Kali-carb**. After a long list of remedies over the years she was given **Syphilinum** 30 and, eight weeks later, **Purple** 200. At her next appointment she was clearly different; she proceeded to relate all the terrible things that she had suffered through her long life. Most obviously she was far less rigid.' **JM**

28

RED

....

The remedy was proved on 20 September 1996. Five women and four men and the medium participated. Each was given the remedy in the 30th potency before the meditation started. Everyone was instructed to take the remedy again at the end of the meditation and to record other symptoms of the proving over the following week.

The Background

Red is the colour evoked by the longest wavelengths of light discernible by the human eye. (Anything longer is known as 'infrared'.) It shares with blue and yellow the status of being a primary colour. Blue and red are complementary. When red is removed from white light, the result is a greeny-blue light known as 'cyan'; a term that gives us 'cyanosis'. Turquoise and aquamarine are both in this range and are capable of absorbing red.

One of the reasons for primates to have developed sensitivity to red is for them to be able to distinguish between edible and poisonous foods, red being one of the most typical colours of toxicity in nature. (Blue is often the colour of the result of poisoning: cyanosis.) Rod cells in the human eye are not sensitive to red. This means that red light can be used to enhance night vision.

Red is strong in symbolism. It denotes danger, sin, guilt, anger and sex. While yellow and black are arranged by nature to give warning, red signals actual or imminent danger. Guilt is illustrated by the story of Mary Magdalene, the original 'scarlet woman', who was outcast in the stories of the New Testament for having been tainted with the sin of prostitution. Red is associated with passion, either negative or positive, and courage, sacrifice and blood brotherhood. Of all the colours it causes the most reaction in people. It stimulates and quickens the action of the heart; it stimulates activity by provoking the production of adrenalin; it stirs emotional responses. The greatest number of road accidents involves red vehicles. Thieves target red cars more than other colours.

The positive attributes of red include courage, leadership, will power, confidence, energy, determination and spontaneity. The negative attributes include fear, ruthlessness, aggression, domination, resentment, obstinacy and self-pity. In crystal therapy red stones have gained a reputation for healing haemorrhages and inflammatory conditions as well as stimulating libido and creativity. Stones used to enhance the vibration of red in the body include carnelian, jasper, garnet, ruby and red tiger's eye.

Keynote effects

The remedy transmutes the fiery energy of anger, resentment and malicious negativity that is centred on the solar plexus, particularly the liver and gall bladder, into a creative harmony; the patient finds it possible to relax from a state of inhibiting angry tension into a more general feeling of acceptance of the status quo. It is also noted for the contrary: those who are incapable of showing opposition where they might be expected to are able to rise to the occasion and focus their inhibited self-assertiveness in a reasoned and non-aggressive manner; they are able to feel their own power but without causing any emotional havoc in others. Red heals the heart centre through its effect on the solar plexus.

General symptoms

Blood purifier. Improves circulation through working on the organs of the solar plexus: liver, spleen and, to a lesser extent, on the stomach and pancreas. Also works on the small intestine where much of the fire element of digestion takes place. For those with digestive problems that are the result of inflammatory processes; where there is continually stoked anger, resentment and hurt held in the liver and gall bladder. Heat, redness and swelling but most particularly in the internal organs. Heals burns especially those from the sun. Hot flushes; useful in the menopause when other symptoms agree. Unwell while on or from having taken HRT. Heat in the face and in the head with a sense of congestion. Sense of the blood boiling. High blood pressure. The tendency to prolapse from pressure built up in the solar plexus generally and in the liver particularly. Also the opposite: anaemia, a sense of blood draining away; faintness from lack of blood to the head. Loss of blood;

haemorrhage. Chilliness and pallor from poor circulation. Coldness of lower extremities with heat in upper half of the body. Useful in most pathologies of the heart and circulation especially where there is a clear psychosomatic link. Blood disorders including leukaemia. Nervous system function is compromised from constriction of the diaphragm with digestive and nerve symptoms in lower half. Restores rhythm to the tides of the body including heartbeat, the intercommunication of liver and spleen and the digestive processes. Restores elasticity to arteries that have borne ebullition of blood especially in the brain; damage to the brain from high fevers in children. **Red** is a syphilitic and tubercular remedy mainly but also sycotic especially in menopausal states. Useful in dealing with patients who have cancer where tumours have a plentiful blood supply. Very important in treating patients with AIDS.

Miasms

Psora, syphilis, tuberculosis and cancer.

Mental and emotional symptoms

The division between the yin and yang aspects of this remedy is obvious in this area. Separation is a strong theme: not in the sense of sycosis but more to do with physical and emotional separation. There is the expression of anger, fury, rage; resentment and contempt. Tantrums in children who have had high fevers that have dehydrated the tissues of the brain causing the patient to be quick to react, irritable and sensitive. Anger, petulance and resentment in teenagers who have not received love and attention. There is also the lack of expression of these negative forces through the proper channels so that the fire of the negative emotions is not allowed to be burnt off thus causing the patient to suffer physical symptoms and to struggle on with a lack of balancing power. **Red** is useful, therefore, in those whom one would expect to feel anger but, in the absence of genuine and convincing forgiveness, claim not to. Anger that is born on a rising tide of resentment from the will being frustrated. For situations where anger has been useless; the patient was in a position where their anger proved to be impotent so that there is a loss of personal power. Road rage. Restlessness and irritability. Irritability causes flushes of heat. Useful for those who are in a constantly competitive environment in which adrenalin is being pumped all the time. This stimulates the body to produce too much heat for an excessive amount of time; it also encourages the consumption of foods high in proteins such as red meat. Mood swings between indifferent passivity and fury. Moods subject to sudden switches of hormones especially in those who suffer hot flushes and anaemia. A strong sense of guilt and/or shame which may be from a historical root or they may be inexplicable with the patient being unable to express where they may stem from – in which case they may be due to karma or ancestral problems. Strong sense of dignity, loyalty, friendship and brotherhood. Ailments from shame and dishonour. The patient is very affected by honour and dishonour and takes such things seriously. Companionship and comradeship are social priorities. Suffering from not being able to feel connections with others; suffering from separation. Where communications have broken down especially between family members. Frustration at not being able to say what one feels or being unable to say what one feels to the person who needs to receive it. The more negative the state of the patient, the nearer to the syphilitic miasm and the further from the truth. Distortion of truth. Egotism. Arrogance. Miasmatically the remedy is syphilitic and tubercular mainly but also sycotic especially in menopausal states. Useful for patients dealing with cancer where tumours have a plentiful blood supply. May prove to be very important in treating patients with AIDS.

Physical symptoms

Head
Heat and congestion. Headaches from excessive blood in the vessels of the brain. Pounding head. Vertigo and fainting from lack of blood to the head.

Eyes
Redness of the conjunctiva. Heat in the eyes and the sockets. Glaucoma. May be of help in those who suffer from poor night vision.

Face
Redness and flushing. Heat. Acne rosacea. Thread veins on the cheeks.

Mouth and throat
Red or pale lips; red or pale gums; red or pale tongue. Chronically swollen and red tonsils. History of fiery, red, sore throats. Numb sensation of the tongue.

Chest
Tightness and constriction in the thoracic cavity. Diaphragm feels constricted.

Heart
Irregular heartbeat; arrhythmia. Constriction or fullness of the heart. Might be considered in aortic aneurysm. 'Wind round the heart' sensation: due to a tightened diaphragm.

Stomach
++ Chocolate; ++ red meat; + carbohydrates. < salt; should be taken off salt. Hiatus hernia and acidity.

Abdomen
Liver feels compressed; liver capsule is constricted and in torsion. Pain in the gall bladder region. Duodenal ulceration; works well as a support remedy for other well-known ulcer remedies. Ulcerative colitis. Crohn's disease. Heat and soreness in the abdominal viscera. Bloating from allergic reactions to certain foods: < excessive proteins; < dairy products and red meat. Slow digestion with constipation or diarrhoea. Cannot finish sensation after passing a stool. Bleeding after or with stool. Piles: tend to bleed more than itch. Sensation of heat and pressure in the anus. Spleen enlarged or displaced with discomfort. Poor immune function due to compromised spleen energy or its absence.

Female
When anger and resentment have built up in and from this area. Supports **Staphysagria** and **Tuberculinum** when they are given for healing sexual abuse. Prolapse. After history of excessive uterine bleeding either from operations or fibroids. Useful after patient has come off HRT and is suffering from hot flushes. Prolapse of the uterus.

Urinary organs
Useful as a kidney drainage remedy where the patient has a history of urinary infections which might feature in a 'return of old symptoms' situation after other indicated remedies are given. Useful also where the patient might be expected to process a lot of anger about family disunity. Support remedy for the kidneys

in those who have no 'fire'. Encourages enfeebled constitutions to use the eliminative processes to support the emotional body in expressing excessive negative energy. Prolapse of the bladder.

Skin

Sunburn. Psoriasis when the skin is hot, dry and flaky and is < sunshine or heat. Not suitable for eczema as **Red** has a reputation for aggravating it without cure – though this caveat is based on the effects of using Red cream (6x) rather than the higher potencies.

Considerations for the use of the remedy

This remedy is clearly defined by its two extremes: the yin and the yang, positive and negative aspects. There is a duality that needs to be identified in the patient; a duality that is not necessarily to do with the sycotic miasm but is more to do with paradox. The theme of separation is inherent in the divide between the top and bottom halves of the body, separated by the tension held in the diaphragm; by the divide between the organs of the solar plexus and the emotional heart; by the divide between the mind and the heart. There is the aspect of ascending energy which seeks to fulfil aspiration and there is the aspect of consuming energy which seeks to purify and burn away that which belongs to the past and is of either no further use or is a hindrance to the further development of the patient's healing. Negative karma or emotions, held in the solar plexus and particularly evident in the tension of the thoracic diaphragm, prevent the rising, aspirant energy from carrying positive energy towards and through the heart and up into the higher centres and also from consuming (burning away) the negative energy harboured in the solar plexus and lower centres. The remedy's specific affinity for the diaphragm dividing the lower chakras from the higher ones, gives us means to establish greater flow between the upper and lower body. The heart centre is healed through the healing of the solar plexus and the lower chakras. Like **Emerald, Ruby** and **Green,**[42] **Red** is indicated in those who have the tendency to relegate negative emotional experience to the liver and the gall bladder leaving these organs to produce symptomatic evidence of distress. In **Red's** case, it is the tension and torsion

42 Also **Berberis Vulgaris, Chelidonium, Hepar-sulph, Kali-carb, Lachesis, Lycopodium, Mag-mur, Nat-sulph** and **Nux Vomica** all have the same negative tendency.

in the thoracic diaphragm that is particularly evident as this causes the liver and gall bladder to be squeezed and even twisted within its capsule and provokes distortion of the viscera as a result; all of which may lead to pain in the acute or irritability of the gut in the chronic phase.

Should be considered as a useful addition to the treatment of those who suffer from AIDS. It can be used in a triangle of remedies: **Red, AIDS nosode** and **Arsen-alb; Red, Syphilinum** and **Ayahuasca; Red, Tuberculinum** and **Lycopodium; Red, Medorrhinum Americana** and **Thuja.**

Red and **Green** are complementary; **Green** follows the successful use of **Red** and encourages and establishes equilibrium after the upsets treated by **Red.** The three fire signs of the zodiac are Aries, Leo and Sagittarius. The tissue salts associated with these three are, respectively, **Kali phos, Mag phos** and **Silica.** Each of these remedies is associated with some degree of exhaustion and weakness. **Red,** as a main prescription, is supported by any of them in cases where the yin aspect of the remedy is the indication for its use.

Esoteric therapeutics

Of all the new remedies, **Red** is most associated with the element of fire.[43] This may be the raging fire of temper or the embers of exhaustion and loss of identity; the fullness of hot flushes or the weakness of anaemia. Paradoxically, **Red** may be a remedy to help heal the very absence of fire. A study of the patient's circumstances will betray reasons for either passion or passivity. If the latter, there will be found ample reason in the case history to *expect* the former if **Red** is going to be effective. Though the focus of action of the remedy seems to be so strongly in the solar plexus, the purpose of the remedy is to open up the heart centre to feelings of unconditional positivity and to affect blood, the vehicle of life force and all that it carries of ancestral karma.

Chakras

Crown
Lack of fire in the system may lead to vertigo, light-headedness and poor memory. Allowing the energy of creativity to rise enables the crown to receive. Sleep may be affected by dreams with a theme of lacking courage. Loss of

43 **Sodium Bicarbonate, Cardamom, Med-am, Pomegranate, Senecio + Tyria** and **Tiger's Eye** all have aspects of fire in their make-up.

creative drive has lessened the ability to reflect coolly and has dulled the receptivity of this centre.

Brow

Hot-headedness has led to erring on the side of being destructive in relationships and in making life choices. Emotions that have long resided in and been stoked by the energy of the liver divert one away from rational thought and sensible reaction. Otherwise this centre may be enervated by the habit of compliance which happens readily in those who have lost will power through suppression by one means or another.

Throat

There is a deep block in this centre which prevents the clear and mature expression of thoughts and feelings. Instead, thoughts and feelings are either not expressed at all or they are delivered with negativity: anger, frustration and resentment. This lays the chakra open to physical symptoms of inflammation, swelling and pain or to suffering from a relaxed throat where the voice is without energy or its pitch is difficult to control.

Heart

Either too much or too little fire in this centre disturbs its balance. It might be hard to find unconditional compassion due to the complexity of emotional history or it might be difficult to discover any strong emotional reaction because of the history of keeping emotional expression to the minimum for fear of reaction or reprisal. In either case the net result may well be conditions of the tissues of the heart and the arteries leading into and away from it.

Solar plexus

Anger and resentment that may have arisen during childhood or in the teens have stayed so long burning away in this centre that pathology inevitably results. Acidity of the system as a whole or particularly felt in the stomach and oesophagus might be a primary result. Liver fire has invaded the stomach and prevents the qi required for the disposal of waste (descending qi) from clearing the system; toxicity builds up. Spleen and kidney qi is expressed too soon in negative emotions to have matured enough to rise up into the heart centre and beyond for purely creative purposes. The net effect of this turmoil is that the diaphragm becomes a wall of tension.

Sacral

Symptoms deriving from hormonal imbalances may arise in this centre especially if they manifest as a result of hormone replacement therapy or from other interference with the natural rhythm of the body clock. Is useful in helping to drain the kidneys when there has been a history of anger and frustration that has damaged liver function.

Base

With the profound disturbance in the solar plexus and the heart chakras, the base is unstable. There is so much to challenge the Mars centre that the constant swing between defence and attack undermines the centred calm of groundedness. This embattled state may not be evident visibly on first acquaintance due to taciturnity, wariness or the patient's need to remain in control and dictate, at least initially, what they feel they need treatment for. In one who is suppressed and quiescent, there is a lack of self-confidence and volition that does not immediately call to mind the colour of this remedy. In either type of patient, there is a likely tension in the diaphragms of the body which would be responsible for pulling the musculoskeletal structure of the body out of alignment which, in itself, would be capable of destabilizing this centre.

Case studies

1   'Young man (18): he came for treatment for pains in the abdomen which were intermittent. There were flatus and grumbling in the gut as well as more pain when expecting to pass a stool. The symptoms had begun while he was in France to work in a law firm as part of his work experience. He was given very menial tasks to do and made to feel "like a spare wheel" in the office. He found that he had little chance to improve his French and that he was ignored by the rest of the staff. He became angry but had no one to whom he could let off steam. When he returned from France he felt deflated by the whole experience, the abdominal symptoms continued and the psoriasis he had always suffered from got temporarily worse; he had patches all over his torso. On examination it was clear that he was unable to stand with his feet together in a balanced posture: there was an internal rotation of his right

shoulder and his right hip rotated in the opposite direction causing a torsion and twist on his liver and a tendency, on closing his eyes, to fall to the left. He could only shallow breathe due to the tightness of his diaphragm. He was given **Lycopodium** 1M (single dose) and **Morgan Gaertner** 30: one three times per week for two weeks. The result was unsatisfactory. He was then given **Red** 30: one three times per week for four weeks. Within ten days the abdominal and digestive symptoms were completely removed. There was also a temporary aggravation of the psoriasis which then abated leaving the skin much as it had been before he went to France.' **CG**

2   'A young man of 25, who is engaged to another of my patients and getting married this summer, came to see me. He is of slight build, with dark hair and presents as a very shy, nervous, sensitive soul but has almost a sulky demeanour. He will barely have any eye contact. He has come to see me for stomach problems with loose bowels, bloating and explosive wind.

'He also has anger problems. At times he loses control and isn't aware of what he does. He has been known to hit walls; he says he bottles things up and then hits out. He often feels people, especially bosses, pick on him. His first job was driving a bus but had one incident where someone ran out in front of him and he ran the person over. Later he had another accident in which he dislocated his right shoulder and tore all the ligaments and also had whiplash. He was unable to work for several months. He then trained as a driving instructor as he felt this would help him to learn to control his temper when he is in a car. At home he can be quite volatile but says he becomes angry over trifles, for example if his fiancée hasn't cleared the washing from the washing machine. But he says he tries to hold his anger.

'His history shows that he was a very happy child until the age of six when he was playing a game of kiss chase with older children. They caught him and pinned him down and stripped him naked. This affected him greatly and any relationships thereafter. He put on a lot of weight and then started being bullied at school and this continued throughout his school life. He learned to control his emotions; he felt that fighting back was useless. His relationship with his dad deteriorated as he says his dad was always telling him what to do. He started lashing out and when he was 16 years old he started fighting back but this only got him put into isolation. A PE teacher helped him by getting him to play rugby and gradually, as he became good at sports, the bullying stopped.

'At 18 years old the bullying started again by his friends over his weight. All his friendships broke down and he found himself being nasty to all his friends. He was nasty to all the people he worked with in the bus garage and after the accident he didn't want to drive the same route. He became very depressed and suicidal and felt he could not talk to anyone except his mum. He had antidepressants and counselling which helped but when he went back to work he had another accident which shocked him even more deeply. His blood pressure went very high and he was constantly on painkillers. During the time he was a bus driver he was continually bullied by other drivers. But at home or with friends anything could trigger his rage and especially when he was driving.

'Not long after he retrained as a driving instructor he had a disagreement with the driving school over money they owed him. He left and went back to bus driving. When he started he was very wary and expecting trouble. He can also become very anxious and panicked very easily.

'In the first three months he was given **Lycopodium** and **Ruby** both of which helped a lot. He also had **Staphysagria** and **Buddleia**. Then he came in one day and said he had something he wanted to share with me: that although he loved his fiancée he also was gay; he had not had a relationship with any men although he had kissed a few. He said his fiancée was aware of this and didn't mind. He felt shame and guilt about this and couldn't talk to his family as he knew his dad would probably disown him. He felt his mum would understand and support him no matter what but was worried about causing her grief. Following this he had **Red Chestnut Flower**.

'Then he was given **Red** 30c twice weekly and reported back that this had helped him to feel more comfortable with himself and his work colleagues. He has started making friends at work and is finding he can talk to people a little more easily. His demeanour is more open now. He has been calmer and as the **Red** was increased in potency the road rage began to calm down. Recently his father died very suddenly and so he has had grief and shock remedies but at the last consultation he reported that his road rage has been better and he is trying to act more maturely when he is in a vehicle and to realize that there are all sorts of drivers on the road and this awareness has made him more tolerant and patient.

'This is a case in progress but I feel **Red** has most definitely played a very big role in helping to balance this young man.' JL

3   'A 65-year-old man, an outspoken, outgoing Aries with a history of liver stasis, came feeling shocked after a falling out with his best friend. His liver function was upset and the liver pulse was dysfunctional. He was given **Nux Vomica** 200 – 1M – 10M after which the liver pulse was restored to normal. However, he was still extremely angry. Neither **Staphysagria** nor **Nat-mur** nor **Anacardium** made any difference. He was unable to see why the incident had happened. He was then given **Red** 200. After this he was much better. His heart chakra was more open and his solar plexus calmed right down.' JM

29

RUBUS FRUTICOSUS

Blackberry

Blackberry was proved by the circle on 9 October 2009. The remedy was taken in the 30th potency at the start of the circle. The provers, 8 women and 3 men, were then instructed to take further doses of the remedy: one, three times a week for three weeks afterwards. The remedy was made from berries picked in autumn 2008 and potentized after a three-month period of maceration in ethanol. The bottle containing the fruit and ethanol was of amber glass and left on a windowsill throughout the time of steeping. (All the berries used for the remedy are likely to be of the same subspecies as they were all gathered from a small area of woodland on the same occasion.)

The Background

There are 400 different types of *Rubus* in Britain of which there are a number of subgenera including cloudberry, raspberry and the black raspberry (distinguishable from the ordinary blackberry by the silvery backing of the leaves). The full, proper nomenclature for the blackberry itself is *Rubus fruticosus* (or *fructicosus*) agg. This is because it is an aggregate plant: the species is made up of many different subspecies. This has come about as the result of its varied methods of reproduction.

The plant has a perennial underground rootstock which throws up biennial shoots. In the first year of its growth, which can be up to 4.5 metres, these produce only leaves that are compound and palmate of which there are five to seven on each leaf stock. In the second year lateral shoots extend from the first year's growth and these bear the flowers and fruit. These secondary leaves are smaller and three to five in number. Flowers form in late May and are either white, pink or mauve depending on the species. The berries, green and red at first, form through the summer and are ripe by late August and September.

The first method of reproduction is for the tips of the first year's shoots to bend and reach the ground. Where the shoot touches the soil fresh roots develop and form the stock of a new plant. It is the profusion of these rooted shoots that then creates the hectic, tumbling bramble bushes so familiar to us in woodlands and unkempt hedgerows. *Rubus* also reproduces by the more usual method of pollination of flowers, bearing of fruit and propagation by birds or by apomixis which is virtually asexual propagation. Some bramble plants are polyploid which means that the chromosome numbers in their genetic make-up have doubled. This variety of means of reproduction has meant that many different subspecies of blackberry have developed and has led to the different sizes and flavours of the fruit and the differing degrees of prickliness.

The blackberry is not, strictly speaking, a berry in the botanical sense; it is more a mass of tiny berries clustered together, each bulb (or drupelet) of black juice holding a seed within it. The fruit, like the plant itself, is an aggregate.

Bramble plants have an important role to play in the ecosystem. They provide food, shelter and protection. Bees and other insects raid the flowers for pollen; flies and wasps congregate to savour the juice of the fruit; various species of moth deposit their eggs on the underside of the leaves; most common small birds eat the fruit as do dormice, mice and foxes; small birds (especially robins and wrens) nest under its protective cover; deer browse on the leaves.

Blackberry has always been known to medical herbalists. The leaves contain tannins. This chemistry makes the plant useful as an astringent and a diuretic; it also has the effect of constricting blood vessels which means that it has anti-haemorrhagic properties. Gallic acid, citric acid, pectin, niacin, flavonoids and anthocyanins are all constituents of the leaves. The leaves can be chewed to heal sores in the mouth and for indigestion; when either dry or green they can be made into poultices (to ease the lesions of shingles, boils and acne) or infused to make a tea (to relieve the symptoms of cough, cold or influenza). The root bark is also antitussive (useful in whooping cough) and can help to counter diarrhoea. The berries can be made into jam, jelly or wine.

Culpeper is enthusiastic about the bramble. He tells us that the green buds, leaves and branches are good for 'ulcers and putrid sores in the mouth and throat and of the quinsy and likewise to heal other fresh wounds and sores; but the flowers and fruit are very binding and so profitable for the bloody flux [dysentery], lasks [diarrhoea] and are a fit remedy for spitting of blood [consumption].' He goes on to say that the root 'is good to break or drive forth gravel and the stone in the reins and kidneys'. Next he tells us that whether green or dry, the leaves and brambles 'are exceeding good lotions for sores in the mouth or secret parts' and 'for too much flowing of women's courses [menstruation]'. He recommended blackberry as a 'powerful remedy against the poison of the most venomous serpents'; whether drunk internally or applied topically to 'help the sores of the fundament [anal fissures] and the piles'; the distilled water of the leaves, branches and flowers or fruit as 'very effectual in fevers and hot distempers of the body, head, eyes and other parts'. His cure for an itching scalp with sores was 'the leaves boiled in lye [a cleansing wash] and the head washed therewith . . . and makes the hair black'.

Culpeper introduces the bramble by telling us that 'it is a plant of Venus in Aries. If any ask the reason why Venus is so prickly? Tell them it is because she is in the house of Mars.' Venus rules the sign of Taurus and **Blackberry** is often of great use to Taurean patients especially if they have Mars strongly in their astrological chart.

One curiosity about the blackberry is worth noting: it has been reported that the bramble shows signs of a significantly higher uptake of pollutant-heavy metals than other plants. In a paper read to the proceedings of an international symposium on trace elements in the food chain in Budapest in May 2006,[44] it was stated that higher than usual traces of aluminium, copper, iron, lead, zinc and cadmium were found in brambles tested on a waste-disposal site in comparison with other plants. Perhaps this might one day prove to be of significance to our materia medica if it is discovered that the potentized remedy has an influence over the elimination of heavy-metal toxicity from the body.

There is a superstition that blackberries should not be picked after 10 October (Old Michaelmas Day), the day Satan was defeated by the archangel Michael. Tradition says that on being cast out of heaven, Satan fell into a bramble bush and stamped on, spat at and cursed the plant for the pain and ignominy he suffered.

44 Published by the Working Committee on Trace Elements of the Complex Committee, Hungarian Academy of Sciences.

Keynote effects

This is a remedy rich in physical symptoms stemming from negative energy in the blood, the heart, the spleen, kidneys and pancreas. It restores integrity to the blood, to the immune system and to the digestion. It calms the nervous system and the emotions of those who live in a state of anxiety. It is also a remedy that can help to restore a person's sense of direction and foster their ability to take the first steps to change.

General symptoms

Toxicity of the system is manifest on the skin: boils, abscesses, carbuncles, sores and ulcers. Black excrescences and skin cancers that do not respond to treatment; rodent ulcers (cf. **Rad-brom**). Discharges from lesions that are dark red, purple or black; also with pus or blood and pus mixed. Burns that do not heal with indicated remedies may well respond to **Rubus**. Mucous membranes that show no sign of healing where there are sores, ulcers or other lesions. There is venous stasis leading to congestion and poor drainage of the lower extremities and liver toxicity; varicose veins; haemorrhoids. Pockets of pus may be held in any part but are likely to be found in lung tissue; bronchiectasis. Heart tissue is damaged; weak from a history of myocarditis. Weak kidneys after a history of kidney infections; **Rubus** is a kidney drainage remedy and will also serve to clear the ureters and the urethra of toxic waste such as pus. Encourages the sphincters to act more efficiently. Like other drainage remedies it can be prescribed in the 3x or 6x potency. The spleen is directly affected: the formation of new blood cells is fostered in the bone marrow and the quality of fresh blood is greatly improved in the spleen; the immune system's response to infection is enhanced. The digestive system is similarly affected. **Rubus** is a remedy for dysentery, diarrhoea and stasis of the bowel. It improves the quality of nutritional absorption and assimilation; the distribution of blood to the vital organs ensures that essential biochemistry is maintained. Parasite activity in the gut is reduced. Heat which floods the system with nausea. Fevers where there is heat in the head and a sensation of tightness of the scalp; a sensation that the skin would burst. It may be of service in patients whose fever has only partially responded to other indicated remedies. **Rubus** also encourages the pancreas to secrete both insulin and digestive enzymes. It is useful in those who have a strong craving for chocolate and sugary foods. It is a supportive remedy in diabetes (see **White Chestnut Flower**, *Volume I*); it can be given in low 'x' potency to support other indicated remedies such as **Phosphorus** or **Phosphoric Acid**. **Rubus** is calming to the central nervous system. It affects the workings of the brain; it covers weak memory and poor concentration. The secretions of the pineal gland are improved which may well mean that **Rubus** is a remedy to consider in depressive states especially in those who suffer considerably from anxiety. Cancer comes into the sphere of this remedy: cancer of the brain, of the kidney, of hollow organs, of the skin (basal cell carcinoma). Cancer metastasis.

Miasms

Psora, cancer, syphilis and sycosis.

Mental and emotional symptoms

Anxiety that is often well concealed; fear that may have no obvious root but that arises in patients whose inheritance includes fearfulness. Fear that underlies lack of self-confidence; fear of participating in life. Anxious about having to speak out; anticipation of saying something wrong; failure to speak up for oneself. Also pleasant feelings of anticipation. Poor motivation. Lack of joyfulness. Defensive attitude with prickly lack of humour. Pent up anger. Panicky feelings; sense of something dreadful going to happen. Panic with palpitations or racing heartbeat. Mood swings between feeling that one must be defended and guarded and feeling indifferent and needing comfort and solace. There is a tendency to eat comfort foods. Poor concentration, poor memory and poor focus on a given task. Feelings of being rushed and hurried; feels under too much pressure. It is a remedy for those who fail to listen to their own intuitive thoughts; for those who get things wrong yet blame themselves for having known they should not have acted in the way they did. For those who refuse to listen to sensible advice and put themselves at risk in some way for their obtuseness. Sensitive people who have difficulty with the pace and noise of modern living; this is especially true of children who need this remedy. Hoarding of stuff that has no further use; the remedy can encourage the desire to spring clean. Has a feeling of wanting more space; room to move or to stretch. Nostalgia.

Physical symptoms

Head

Head suddenly feels full of blood, affecting the ears. Transient ischaemic attack (TIA) especially in those who have a tendency to high blood pressure. Headache < temples or sides of the head; usually on one side only. Poor drainage of blood from the head with feeling of thickness, dullness and fullness in the cranium. Heaviness and oppression in the head with a sense of nausea. Faintness.

Eyes

Glaucoma; sensations of pressure in one eye.

Ears

Feel full of cotton wool. Sensation of fuzziness in both ears with sensation of fullness in the head.

Nose

Peculiarities of the sense of smell; aware of 'a smell that gets into my nose and I cannot get rid of it'. Watery nostril < left.

Face

Acne: pustular. Black mark on the lips. Sallow complexion or greyness.

Chest and heart

Sharp pain in the centre of the chest and slightly to the left; in the heart region. High blood pressure; < stress and irritability. Sensation of tension in the heart area that is associated with emotion. Weeping eases the tension held in chest. Constriction of the chest on the left side with sensation of tension in the head. Contraction in the heart. Breathlessness with palpitations. Unable to take a deep, full breath. A feeling that the chest has caved in. Strong need to take a deep breath with the sensation of constriction; air hunger. Wants to expand the whole chest; to stretch against the intercostal muscles. Left lung is subject to infection: pus-filled mucus from the left lung in pneumonia or chronic airways disease. Bronchiectasis.

Stomach
Sugar craving.

Abdomen
Diverticulosis and diverticulitis. Nagging, sore pain in the descending colon. Bleeding from the rectum on passing a stool; bleeding from diverticula. Dark blood-streaked mucus on stools. A remedy for the spleen: strengthens the spleen's ability to supply the immune system with lymphocytes. Piles: purple, full, external and with a tendency to bleed. May ooze dark blood.

Female
Infertility in those who feel at odds with their environment; in those who fear that pregnancy would be detrimental to their health or because of a fundamental lack of 'likeness' with the partner. Fibroids that cause slow, dark bleeding which may be part of the menstrual flow or not. Malignancy of the generative organs especially within the uterus or Fallopian tubes.

Back
Sudden stabbing pain in the right side of the back just above the kidney area. Wanting to stretch.

Skin
Acne; facial or on the torso. Pustular spots that may bleed < on scratching.

Extremities
Varicose veins < on the left leg: dark blue veins ('almost black') showing through very pale, even white skin in a network.

Considerations for the use of the remedy

Blackberry is a remedy for the fear of change when the necessary change for the sake of well-being requires the patient to alter their way of life; to undergo a revolution of purpose within. The situation will probably be of long standing and therefore the physical body's eliminative system is likely to have become overburdened due to the delay in making such changes. So there is likely to be toxicity either in the physical body that is manifest in the blood, skin or in the behaviour of the liver and spleen or in the emotional field where there is a state of constant mental aggravation. Physical and mental toxicity are often present together though in an otherwise healthy constitution, emotional toxicity may be all that is apparent.

In cases of longer-standing stagnation this is a remedy that may be needed on a drainage level first; frequent doses of low potency will encourage the physical system to eliminate from the blood and the liver. The spleen can be helped to improve both the immune system and its activity of replenishing the body's supply of fresh blood cells. Once the cleansing of toxicity is well under way, higher potencies of the remedy may be needed to do a similar job on the emotional level. The fear factor will probably be well rooted in the kidney energy; thus it will be partly the result of ancestral fear inherited from family.

The patient who needs this remedy is one who is likely to require patience and persistence on the practitioner's part. The use of **Blackberry** may well follow after using **Lachesis** or, indeed, any of the snake remedies. However, it will also be called for in those who have a history of drinking excessive quantities of alcohol or eating too much blood-intoxicating food. **Blackberry** is complementary to **Morgan Pure**. A patient likely to do well on an indicated prescription of **Blackberry** will need blood cleansing and plenty of emotional support. Referral to complementary practices such as acupuncture, craniosacral therapy or shiatsu is often invaluable.

Esoteric therapeutics

Blackberry is a remedy that has an effect on all the chakras but particularly on the base, sacral, solar plexus and the heart. Its chief action is in the heart, spleen and kidneys. It strengthens a heart that is weakened by fear and anxiety that emanate from the kidneys: kidney fear is usually ancestral and karmic in origin and can affect every aspect of the energy centres. Blackberry can be used as a kidney support remedy just on this indication alone: the 3x or 6x can be given daily to ease hidden anxiety especially about health in one who is anxious about making changes that would mean departing from all that he or she has been in the habit of doing.

Chakras

Crown
A remedy for the pineal gland and its secretions; balances the relationship and fosters communication between the pineal and the pituitary (and thus the rest of the endocrine system). Helps to discourage those who are susceptible to becoming ungrounded from getting into difficulties with losing their bearings either geographically, emotionally or spiritually. For those who are disturbed by magnetic fields or whose body clock is upset (possibly due to night shift work). Draws light into the being so that the tendency to prefer darkness is eased away.

Brow
Blood cleansing and easy drainage from the head. Cerebrospinal fluid is kept flowing through the ventricles especially after the use of **Rainbow** (see *Volume I*). Memory and concentration are both helped in those who have confusion of busy thoughts that is fed by anxiety.

Heart
Can bring the life force back into the heart centre when it has been weakened by fears: fear of life; of speaking one's mind; of being here and of what is expected of one. When the energy relationship between the kidneys and the heart is affected it leads to an imbalance between yin and yang and stagnation of heart energy. Lung energy is improved when the remedy is prescribed for drainage.

Solar plexus
Greatly supports the activity of the spleen in the maturation of fresh blood cells. Improves the function of the pancreas and the output of its secretions. Pancreatic trouble is often emotionally manifest as a lack of joy; here joy has been ousted by anticipation, anxiety and fear. **Blackberry** is well indicated when both spleen and pancreas give rise to concern especially in one whose stress levels have long been high; adrenalin is antagonistic to insulin. Continued use of a low potency can help to minimize craving for sugar and sweet things such as chocolate (see **Sodium Bicarbonate**). Supports the action of remedies indicated in diabetes. The remedy helps the body distribute blood to the digestive system correctly so that stagnation can be prevented.

Sacral

Stagnant energy in this centre leads to lack of expression (verbally in the throat centre or physically as difficulty in menstruation or infertility). Drains the tubes associated with this centre. Weak kidney energy following earlier infections.

Base

Its action on the elimination system makes this a remedy for the base centre. Improves the central nervous system's conductivity, cleanses the blood and has an effect on fearfulness that disturbs the mind.

Provers' experiences

1 'For three weeks following the proving I experienced huge waves of extremely powerful energy and emotions. I have been engaged all week in throwing out binfuls of old papers; desire to spring clean every single item in my house – the expression "spring clean" doesn't come anywhere near what I have been feeling. I am completely consumed with the many tasks that absolutely must be completed. One strong thought is that I cannot possibly leave all of this for anyone to sort out after I pass on. Feelings of responsibility for those who will be left behind. There is a huge satisfaction while engaged in this long-overdue activity. There are very deep emotions stirred up by coming across old photographs. Someone came to the door selling poppies in remembrance of those who died in the two World Wars. I bought one . . . and was overcome with such compassion for all those who fought to save their country . . . I have no memory of ever feeling like this before . . . such depth of feeling! Impossible to fathom it. It was passionate, compelling, voracious (and) all-consuming while it lasted. Surprisingly I was not left with uncomfortable feelings of nostalgia while clearing things out – but I did ponder over my marriage, wishing that my ex-husband was still alive so that I could be with him. (Feelings that soon passed . . . still have a few more pills to take.)'

2 'Dream: (My husband) was making a wetland centre. There was a lot of marshy water about. We were showing people around but it had a

strange feel. Then I was looking around some stalls which had a Moroccan feel; I felt that the goods were not "fit for purpose" and what was being sold related in some way to what we had been learning in the circle but I can't remember what. There was a link with the wetlands and these leaves and skeletal gourd-like things that were to be used to build things. Evening came on; it was damp and misty. There was a driveway with roses like espaliered fruit trees. I looked closer and they were all blackberry bushes covered in mildew.'

Diary of continued physical effects
10/10/09 Pain above the heart during the proving.
11/10/09 Heart pain, out-of-body sensations; the body became concerned about its survival.
12/10/09 Pain at times above the heart.
13/10/09 No heart pains. Out-of-body sensations.
16/10/09 9pm slight pain above heart like a dull toothache.
21/10/09 Notice that it is much easier to formulate words and respond more clearly to questions.
25/10/09 Heart pain again.

'Overall comments: the dull pain above the heart continues to appear from time to time for short periods. Brain function is more clear and concise. (On 11 November had an ECG and was diagnosed with "thickening of the heart": hypertrophic cardiomyopathy. Had gone to the surgery to enquire about a recurrent spot of solar keratosis expecting to be referred to a clinic to have it frozen off.)'

9/10/09 (day of proving) had to stop car twice on the way home due to exhaustion. >> after taking the dog out: felt re-energized. Was awake between 1.30am and 5am with mind churning over all the things needed to be done.
10/10/09 Dream: needed to catch a flight but there were lots of obstacles that made it impossible.
12/10/09 Dream: carried a large unconscious dog to the vet.
16/10/09 Awake 11pm to 4am feeling very cheerful.
21/10/09 Couldn't get warm with occipital headache.

22/10/09	Unwell; something brewing: hot and cold, lethargy, headache.
24/10/09	Awake between 11.30pm and 2.30am.
25/10/09	Woke every hour; feel a failure.
29/10/09	Woke 2am with intense itching, right upper arm; scratching = no >. Burning shoulder and armpit, down arm. Lasted for days and spread across left breast and posterior left ribs – the site of shingles 2½ years ago (that came on after the proving of **Rosebay Willowherb**).
5/11/09	Red, raised, itchy spot left upper arm (on the site of the BCG vaccination); still there on 19/11/09. Redness around the vaccination site (lasted a few days). Moods: either very good or very low. Generally for the first two to three weeks: intense anal itching waking me between 12.30am and 2.30am.
19/11/09	Coughing all last night; throat and upper chest very dry. Tickly cough. Woke with no voice. Hoarse all day and kept feeling hot/cold. (Felt that fearfulness stemming from a professional problem that called her credibility into question – and that brought up "a huge fear of authority" – had affected the throat.)

'(There has been a general sense of) being pressured and rushed – no time to get everything done. The sense of time has been distorted in the last three weeks (whilst taking the remedy).

'The same prover also reported developing small, dry eczematous patches of skin on the outside of the left breast, at the base of the spine on the left and on the right thigh; they were not visible but felt.'

Case studies

1   'Though it is difficult to separate out the effects of **Blackberry** alongside the other remedies, this lady is very sensitive to remedies and she did say that the Monday and Friday remedy had a big effect on her emotions.

   'Female: 50 years old and a Capricorn; one of six children: four girls, two boys. She does very well on **Lachesis**. This is an overweight woman who has been coming for many years. She and her mother both used to come regularly for treatment. She and a younger sister lived with the mother; the sister moved out; the mother developed an ulcerated leg which was intensively nursed by the patient with homoeopathic treatment only. When the mother died a few years ago the family fell apart as the colours came flying out in enormous clouds of jealousy over the mother's will. It's never been the same since!

'The patient has never left home: the house which the mother left to her and her sister. She used to work in her parents' greengrocers shop and has never had any other outside job of work. She made some attempt to buy another house so that she could pass on her sister's share of the inheritance but her heart was not in it and she was full of fears about change and moving on. The buying of the house did not materialize. And there was much blame, judgement, anger and a deep sense of injustice in her. "She [the younger sister] has done nothing [for her money]. She doesn't deserve it. I've earned my money ten times over [looking after the sick mother]."

'She has frequently talked of ending her life because she finds it too hard to be here. She has had many minor accidents; often falls and damages her legs or head.

'August 2009: diagnosed with blood clots in left leg. Prescribed warfarin for three months. She came to see me in November 2009 when she said, "I can't forgive her [younger sister]. Don't want her near me." (Because sister had asked her to sell the family house so that she could have her share.)

'Rx: **Nat-mur** 10M: one dose; **Blackberry** 30 Mondays and Fridays x six weeks.

'Visit December 11 2009. Arrived in a very cheerful mood. Said she was in a much better emotional state after the Monday and Friday remedies. The younger sister came to see her (this, after a long time) – but the patient couldn't bring herself to kiss her. Passed an enormous stool, about 36 centimetres long. Things "out of perspective, not logical". (At long last the beginning of movement away from her stuck state.) Rx: **Blackberry** 1m.

'Visit January 22 2010. She said a massive amount going on. More very long stools. Has begun walking in the local park (previously unheard of!) three or four times a week. Rx: **Lachesis** 1M; **Blackberry** 30, M & F for six weeks.

'Visit March 19 2010. Bumped into her sister. (Universe wants them to settle their differences!) Let her friend take her for lunch. Friend couldn't believe it – so her receiving hand is beginning to open!' **ST**

2 'Not long after having done the proving I gave this remedy to a woman I had been treating for a long time. She was a Virgo who was remaining in her marriage for the sake of the children. (This was causing her distress.) She had fallen out of love with her husband and despite counselling and both being honest about their feelings, there was no physical attraction between them and she wanted to live together as just friends.

'[I remember that] there was a lot in the proving of **Blackberry** that was about facing changes that are coming by dealing with them truthfully; by not letting anything become obscured by old attitudes or patterns of reaction. It was stressed that this remedy can help people to not live their lives as a lie any more. It resonated with what I thought this woman needed. I gave her **Blackberry** 30 once a week for six weeks.

'She returned saying that she was "ready to move on" though she knew she didn't want to be impulsive and she wanted to bide her time. She said that it was now about being "disciplined without having emotional enjoyment". **GM**

3 'A woman, born in Aries, was at a desperate crossroads in knowing whether to push her music or her yoga career or have a child. She was wrapped up in the allure of fame and fortune from being in a band when the music press and exposure had dried up. First of all I gave her **Blackberry** 30 once a week for six weeks and then twice a week for six weeks. The result was a tremendous change of focus, decision-making, realizations and optimism. She is now six months pregnant.' **GM**

4 'A woman of 35, a Pisces, whom I describe as "an anxious mouth". She has been thwarted all her life. She was repressed as a child. She was never able to stick up for herself. There is a lot of grief in her life. She admits to having a fear of life. She always reacts in a prickly manner to any challenges. She suffers from piles and varicose veins. She has a sallow

skin with outbreaks of pustular spots on her face. She has a weak heart. There is considerable venous stasis. She needs a lot of support in her heart and the solar plexus. She has been a patient of homoeopathy for a considerable time and has taken, with varying degrees of success, **Sepia**, **Nat-mur**, **Carcinosin**, **Calc-carb**, **Hamamelis**, **Aesculus**, **Ignatia**, **Ceanothus**, **Berberis Vulgaris**, **Triple Salt** and **Silica**. However, her general condition, though eased, has never fundamentally changed.

She was given **Blackberry** 30: one each day for a week and then three times a week for eight weeks. When she returned she said her piles were completely better within a week of taking the remedy. The veins on her legs were now a lot less blue. She said, "I don't feel anxious any more. I've got more confidence and I've been sticking up for myself." She agreed to the plan of staying on the **Blackberry** for a while longer.' JM

5 'A 54-year-old man, a Pisces, had been coming for constitutional treatment for years. He had diabetes (late onset) and suffered from loose motions. He had a strong craving for sugar. Suddenly, seven years ago, he developed a black mark on his lower lip which he felt was disfiguring. He had various remedies that might have covered this symptom (though there were often other matters to consider as well): **Thuja**, **Nit-ac**, **Hydrastis** and **Carcinosin**. The **Carcinosin** appeared to cause the mark to be more pronounced. The patient became increasingly concerned and wondered if he should try conventional medicine. He was then given **Blackberry** 30: one daily for seven days followed by one three times a week for four weeks. The black mark disappeared within days and his sugar craving was reduced to nothing.' JM

6 'A young man of 17, a Taurean, came for severe acne. He had spots with pus all over his face and neck. He had a very grey complexion and looked unfit and unhealthy. On reading his pulses it was evident that his spleen and lungs were all deficient. He had constitutional treatment for a while which included the use of **Syphilinum**, **Clay**, **Pulsatilla** and **Silica** among others. He also had SSC (**Silica** + **Sulphur** + **Carbo-veg**) and **Gunpowder**, neither of which made a great deal of difference. He was given **Blackberry** 30 one a day for three weeks. His skin completely cleared of acne and his lung and spleen pulses improved by about 50 per cent.' JM

30

RUTILATED SMOKY QUARTZ

The remedy was proved in circle on 1 December 2006 by 8 women and 6 men with the medium. The 30th potency was used. All participants had been asked to take the remedy for a month on a daily basis before coming to the circle. Each one was given a further dose at the start of the meditation. It was recommended that each should take **Black Obsidian** 200 (one daily for 3 days) after the meditation in order to antidote the effects of the proving. This was the first time such an instruction had ever been given to the circle.

The Background

Rutilated Smoky Quartz has been known variously as angel's hair, the net of Thetis or love's arrows. It was also known as Venus' hair or sagenite, a word derived from the Greek for 'net'. These descriptive names illustrate the qualities of this translucent crystal (often clear quartz) with its fine golden fibres that appear to be like a tangle of hair. It does not give any idea of the smoky form of crystal that can appear to be shadowy, dark and with sharp spikes of needle-like metal fibres that seem to be strewn haphazardly into a frozen state of pik-a-stiks. It was a large stone of this kind that provided the remedy.

The word 'rutile' is derived from the Latin for 'red'; it was first applied to minerals in 1803. It refers to filaments of fine fibrous rutile crystals that are enclosed within and by rock crystals (such as clear quartz or kunzite) and smoky quartz. Such crystals are formed magmatically in pegamites or hydrothermally in clefts. The rutiles are a form of titanium oxide (TiO_2) which is at 6 to 6.5 on Mohs' scale of hardness. Smoky quartz (which can appear without any rutiles) is a form of silicon dioxide (SiO_2) and this is set on Mohs' scale at 7.

There is little in history to tell us how this crystal was used in earlier times. However, its use is suggested by the fact that ancient people wore rutilated clear quartz as a charm to foster the growth of hair. It was also considered to be under the influence of Sagittarius. It was believed that the rutiles were captured sunlight; the effects of wearing such a stone were believed to lift dark moods and ease coughs.

It may be worthwhile considering the remedy, **Titanium**, even though this is made from copper-red crystals obtained from the slag at the bottom of a blast furnace; not exactly the needles of naturally occurring titanium oxide contained by smoky quartz. **Titanium**, the remedy, is a composite of titanium cyanide and titanium nitride. According to Dr Clarke the remedy 'stands between silicon and tin in some of its relations and in other respects it is closely related to iron, chromium and aluminium.' He noted that 'one symptom was remarkable: "Imperfect vision, the peculiarity being that half an object only could be seen". Another symptom, which Burnett has turned to good account in cases of sexual weakness is "Too early ejaculation of semen in coitus". Clarke goes on to list other symptoms that may have relevance to **RSQ**: giddiness, loss of appetite, nausea and discomfort in the stomach as well as feeling generally 'greatly disordered'.

Keynote effects

Creates the conditions for personal understanding of the origins and process of one's disease state. It helps people to discriminate between those things they need to focus on for healing and those things that are not relevant. It affords a patient answers when they are stuck in asking 'Why me?' It can release the patient from the sense that they are the victim or the prisoner of their body's sickness.

General symptoms

The remedy has affinities for all the miasms but most particularly for the syphilitic and carcinogenic miasms. It has strong influence on the psyche but is also of use in pathology of the central nervous system, the blood, the heart and the endocrine system. It is especially noted as a thyroid remedy when it is afflicted by deep pathology. There is also an affinity for the organs of the solar plexus, particularly the stomach. Nervous disorders come within its sphere of action: nervous tics, sensations on the skin and within connective tissue; burning sensations; problems of spatial awareness, dizziness; visual disturbances; Bell's palsy; multiple sclerosis. Nervous disorders that can be traced back to periods of severe stress. Nervous exhaustion; adrenal insufficiency. Lack of libido. Early signs of ageing. Gout and other disorders of the liver due to a lifestyle that is no longer viable for the constitution. Cancer: of the thyroid; the stomach.

Miasms

Psora, syphilis, sycosis, tuberculosis and cancer.

Mental and emotional symptoms

Strong feelings of being unworthy; unworthy to be counted among their peers. Asks 'Why am I here? What am I doing here?' Says: 'I don't want to be here' and 'I don't want to be doing this!' Uncomfortable feelings of being out of place. Anguish; aware of one's mortality. Unable to see the point of existing as they do. Loss of motivation; lethargy; disconnection from (rather than separation from) reality. Depression stemming from lack of motivation even with suicidal thoughts or tendencies; feels lost in the murk of their own negativity with feelings of wanting to die. Feels lonely and alone; desolation. Confusion and anxiety with nervous anticipation. Confusion about sexual orientation. Irritability especially with other people who show lack of respect, lack of seriousness or other superficial behaviour. Introverted and given to negative speculation. Feels withdrawn and wants to run away or to avoid difficulties that seem to have no solution. Ambivalent towards opportunities; uncertain what they can get out of a situation and therefore reluctant to show commitment. Feel they have been sabotaged by events or by others. Ruminates about the past and goes over and over how things might have been if they had done things differently. Would like to go back and do things again to put things right. Tends to be agnostic; easily put off by formal worship. Prefers not to be in large groups of people; finds it easier to be in smaller gatherings or amongst family. Communication skills are weak. There is too ready an acceptance of the status quo in which the truth does not necessarily feature strongly. There is no strong personality to this remedy. The patient who needs it has been through experiences or associated with people that have caused the true personality to be subsumed in a plethora of worldly attitudes and assumptions. Though they can be sceptical, especially of an individual with independent views, they are susceptible to taking on the common delusions of our time; they find it hard to accept that there is any other opinion than the commonly held one. Poor discrimination; content to go along with what they have always thought rather than employ critical or intuitive thinking. They are victims of their own brain chunter; it is hard for them to switch off the negative thought patterns they are so used to rehearsing all the time. Very little self-reflection. Waves of panic especially when there is depression and a sense of being thwarted.

Physical symptoms

Head
'Splitting' headaches. Dizziness. Pounding in the heart from the strength of the heartbeat.

Eyes
Watering of the left eye. Rings of light on the periphery of the visual field in the left eye.

Face
Paralysis of the facial muscles: Bell's palsy < left side.

Mouth
Sensation of the teeth falling out.

Throat
Feels aware of the thyroid as if there is something in the throat around it or pressing on it. Thyroid pathology; cancer of the thyroid.

Heart
Awareness of the heart; of the heart's action. Palpitations: continuous or coming in waves. Fearful of the heart beginning not to function properly.

Stomach
Dreadful nausea especially when it comes on with vertigo. Acid indigestion; heartburn. Cancer of the stomach with nausea and sharp needle-like pains.

Abdomen

Aware of the spleen: pain in the spleen area with a feeling of a big ball pressing into the heart from below and under the ribs. Feel uncomfortable in the liver. Sensation of spinning in the solar plexus like a washing machine.

Skin

Tingling on skin exposed to air: face, neck, hands and legs; sensation of breath of air being blown on the skin but coming from within. Sensations of tremor just under the skin associated with hair follicles. Sensation as if the skin would slough off.

Extremities

Buzzing that goes down through the legs and also into the hands which leads to a feeling of weakness and then general lassitude. Tremendous weakness in the legs with a 'humming' running through them from the hips downwards. A creeping weakness from the hips and thighs which causes restlessness of the limbs with aching in the bone. Limbs feel as heavy as lead. Multiple sclerosis. Gout in the left big toe; in the left knee and little finger of the left hand.

Sleep

All symptoms are > for sleep. Prefers to sleep than to remain awake especially when stressed. Dreams: of people; of someone dancing very fast and continuing to go faster and faster.

Considerations for the use of the remedy

Rutilated Smoky Quartz is often of use in those who have more than one focus of pathology. In most cases the central nervous system and the endocrine system will be part of the picture. There is also very likely to be an aspect of depression which may not be apparent at first; the depressiveness is usually concealed and seems to be motiveless or to do with things lost to the past. There is also a slight (or not so slight) air of irritation or impatience with the process of talking about their symptom state as it conforms with the feeling of not wanting to be where they are; this may be added to by a degree of scepticism.

It is very usual for the patient needing this remedy to present as some other remedy personality such as **Thuja, Lycopodium, Arsen-alb, Aurum, Phos, Calc-carb, Nat-mur** or **Sulphur**, for example. It is as if they accept the status quo of their constitutional state as one or other of these remedies and cannot see how there is a bigger picture to their lives. **RSQ** is something of a joker in the pack of cards. It does not have a particular personality picture such as we find in other polychrests with their well-known 'essences'; it has a 'skeleton key' aspect that is its peculiarity. It seems that this attribute is necessary for its place in the homoeopathic canon as a remedy that in its action sheds light on the reasons for the pathology; and thus on the deeper meaning of their lives. The patient is not in connection with the full process of their disease; this is most obvious in those who are unaware of the emotional and psychic causes of pathology or even of any idea that there might be hereditary, miasmatic or ancestral links (and perhaps do not want to know). Part of the value of **RSQ** is as a key that opens the door of understanding about the full implications of healing, implications that are so often left unexplored through fear and the need to maintain the status quo of superficial knowledge offered by an official diagnosis. In essence, **RSQ** prevents us from hiding from the underlying truth about our condition. This can also be true about one who is not suffering particularly from physical illness but is disturbed on the level of the heart and the psyche.

In much of this, it is clear that **RSQ** is close to **Thuja**. Both remedies are multi-miasmatic but have a strong affinity for the cancer and syphilitic miasms. However, **RSQ** is more obviously represented by problems in the nervous system than **Thuja** and is more likely to be closer to a diagnosis of depression even if it is difficult to see. Furthermore, **Thuja** is more separate from reality while **RSQ** is disconnected. In other words, there is a degree of unawareness in the consciousness of **Thuja** while **RSQ** is aware and observant but unable to put thoughts and feelings together for not accepting or understanding the truth of the past. They follow each other well and are compatible when **RSQ** is required to support **Thuja** in a high potency.

RSQ is susceptible to repetition especially in potencies up to the 30th. The 200th is of particularly penetrative vitality[45] and quick in its action. If there are aggravations that cause the practitioner to be concerned, **Black Obsidian** is the antidote to be used.

45 During the proving it was received that the potencies to be used are the 30, 200, 10M and LM3. It was not explained why this should be and the information is added here for the sake of completeness.

Esoteric therapeutics

There is a consensus about the efficacy of RSQ among crystal healers that is congruent with the homoeopathic remedy. Melody[46] tells us that 'it assists one in getting to the root of a problem and, hence, provides access to the reason for a dis-ease or discomfort so that one can remedy the situations.' She goes on to say 'rutilated quartz provides for insight into the reasons for visiting the locations and viewing the scenes; it stimulates an awareness of connections between this physical life and the situations viewed.' It fosters new hope and independence. Judy Hall[47] writes that 'it opens the aura, allowing healing in, and filters negative energy from a patient, supporting emotional release and confrontation with the darker aspects of the psyche . . . soothes dark moods and acts as an antidepressant.' Hall adds that it 'promotes insights into events in past lives affecting the present life.' It is said to be a crystal that 'dissolves hidden, unacknowledged fear and liberates us from feelings of anxiety and constriction'.[48] On the physical plane it is used for the healing of respiratory diseases including chronic bronchitis; for strengthening the immune system; for loss of libido, impotence and premature ejaculation; for cell regeneration and energy depletion; for establishing greater core strength so that an upright posture is maintained. Hall further recommends its use in cases of mercury poisoning when that has affected blood, nerves, muscle and intestinal tract.

Chakras

RSQ is associated with the base centre primarily but also the solar plexus (through the physical symptoms), the heart and the thymus centre. However, it is also a remedy that balances and harmonizes the energies of all the chakras.

Crown

It is chiefly of value in this centre through its ability to facilitate meditation. It encourages awareness of the link between the base and the crown and brow and fosters self-reflection. It also manifests in dreams that can be interpreted for positive understanding. Dreams are likely to be about or with people, known or unknown, usually from the past.

46 *Love is in the Earth*
47 *The Encyclopaedia of Crystals*
48 *Crystal Power, Crystal Healing*, Gienger

Brow

Much of the disconnection of this remedy lies in this chakra: the intellect has been conditioned to accept what appears to be the truth or seems to be the majority opinion. RSQ encourages people to be more independent-minded and more confident in their individuality. Understanding that the unwilling-ness to face the truth has been due to the fear of having to face their darker side lies at the heart of **RSQ**'s effect on this centre.

Throat

Thyroid trouble is a manifestation of a person's inability to express him- or herself in a manner that commands attention or, at least, is noticed. **RSQ** helps with self-expression.

Heart and thymus

There is much disharmony within this chakra and it is chiefly to do with the darkness that casts a shadow over the person's emotional conditioning and family (ancestral) history. The depression that is a feature of the remedy may well be a reflection of what was running as a theme in past generations or in past lives. For this reason **RSQ** is a remedy that can be usefully combined with **Thymus Gland** and **Syphilinum** to form a remedy for the unearthing of past unresolved troubles that are consistent with (i.e. homoeopathic to) emotional difficulties lying unearthed in personal or family history.

Solar plexus

RSQ is a remedy for the stomach meridian. This meridian is primarily concerned with receiving the energy of food and discriminating between what becomes fuel (qi) and what goes for waste. This power of discrimination is difficult for the patient who prefers to persist with what has always been accepted. It is worth suggesting dietary changes that would not be too onerous to put into practice as this would bring in an early shift in consciousness. **RSQ** patients often 'can't stomach' this or that.

Sacral

Impotence, premature ejaculation, frigidity, infertility all suggest that this centre is strongly influenced by the remedy, particularly in men. However, the underlying causative factors are less within this centre than in the base, brow and heart; the lack of free spirit, independence, creative thinking and the suppression of the intuition all point to the patient being somebody whose strings are pulled by assumed attitudes and preconditioning.

Base

The foundations of this patient's life are laid on prejudice and insecurity that may be just a thread running through the weave or most of the tapestry. The central nervous system, the endocrine system and the musculoskeletal system are all potentially affected. The patient is seeking to become independent, self-confident, well established and no longer affected by commonly held belief structures. They are seeking to be more upright physically and emotionally. They may well be unaware of the origins of their troubles if these lie deep in the family past or in a past life of the patient himself. Here is a patient who is seeking a life correction.

Case studies

1 'A 37-year-old man with a history of being sexually abused had been having regular treatment for some months. He was a Sagittarian with his moon in Scorpio. He lived on edge suffering fear and anxiety with low self-worth. He had done well on **Syphilinum** and **Thuja** as well as other sycotic remedies. The anxiety affected his digestion. He felt much worse when his relationship ended. He reacted negatively to **Nat-mur** 10M with no amelioration. He did better on **Winchelsea Sea Salt** 10M when it was supported by **Ignatia** 10M. Nevertheless he became suicidal. **Aurum** 10M and then 50M made some improvements but then failed and he felt even worse. He took **Syphilinum** 10M and felt much better for ten days but then became worse again. It was apparent that his thymus, base, crown and brow centres were all closed down; there was no energy movement in or between them. He was then given **Rutilated Smoky Quartz** 30 b.d. for ten days. The improvement was immediate. Though he developed palpitations he became much calmer and said that he felt far more philosophical about life. He lightened up in his mood and demeanour and his self-esteem was strengthened. He continued with the remedy for another ten days, taking one a day. He continued the general improvement when he was subsequently given **RSQ** 30 – 200

– 1M in 24 hours. His heart chakra became lighter and then all the others went into alignment. He continues well.' JM

2 'A girl of five, born a Pisces with the influence of Pluto[49] strongly in her chart, was brought for treatment suffering from fearfulness. From her pulses it was evident that her spleen and blood were troubled by sluggish energy. After the vaccines were 'dealt with' by constitutional remedies and nosodes along with **Ceanothus** Ø, she still continued to be sad, lonely and friendless. She found it impossible to play with other children. Despite **Sulphur, Calc-carb, Tub-bov, Phosphorus** and other well-indicated remedies her aura remained very heavy and dark; she was not a happy child. She then had **Rutilated Smoky Quartz** 30 o.d. for seven days followed by three times a week for four weeks. For the first time she began to smile; she was then able to integrate with other children and to make friends. When she next needed constitutional treatment, **Phosphorus** worked really well and deeply.' JM

---

49 Pluto's influence is transformational. It is associated with elimination, destruction, regeneration and renewal. It rules Scorpio, and astrologers see its influence at work in processes marked by purification, purging and renewal. It dredges up to the surface for illumination all that has lain hidden and corrupt. Negative sentiments and emotions are often manifest as a result.

31

SENECIO JACOBAEA + TYRIA JACOBAEA

Common Ragwort and Cinnabar Moth

The remedy was first proved during a week's postgraduate course run by the Guild of Homoeopaths on the island of Paros in Greece in May 2005. It was chosen as one of two remedies to prove through meditation by two groups of 12 students who were attending the course.

The Background

This remedy is unique in that it is derived from two sources, one vegetable and the other animal. The common ragwort is here united with the caterpillar of the cinnabar moth which feeds on the golden-yellow flowers and glabrous leaves of the plant. They were chosen together as the moth's life cycle is so intimately connected with the plant. The caterpillar was feeding on the chosen plant at the time of collection; they came from an area of mixed woodland far from the likelihood of any pollution from pesticides or other chemicals.

The cinnabar moth lays its eggs on the leaves of the plant so that the hatching caterpillars have an instant source of both food and protection. The caterpillar is approximately three centimetres long, it is bright orange-yellow with almost black bands around each segment. This coloration acts as a deterrent to any predators and the toxicity of the moth's foodstuff makes it unpalatable. The ragwort is its most favoured food though it will also eat groundsel and other related plants. Its habitat is waste land, meadows, pastures, heathland and dunes in the south of England though it can be found in coastal areas in the north. It is widespread in Europe.

All parts of the plant are poisonous being full of pyrrolizidine alkaloids which, when ingested, have an accumulative effect in the system and block the liver's ability to regenerate itself. Thus the liver suffers permanent and potentially fatal damage. The caterpillar is able to store the poisons harmlessly in its body so that it provides a natural protection against predators such as birds. This toxicity is passed on through the pupa stage and into the adult moth. Both the adult and the caterpillar make use of red pigmentation to add a visual warning to predators. The caterpillar is striped yellow and brown while the moth has a brilliant vermilion underwing that is visible during flight.

The *Senecio* is a member of the Compositae family. The species of *Senecio* is possibly the largest of the plant kingdom having some 2000 members which range from tiny weeds to large tree-shaped plants; some are climbers and others are decorative garden varieties. Common ragwort is a native of Europe, Scandinavia and western Asia as well as northern Africa. It grows on waste ground, meadows and pastures, even shorelines. It grows in heavy soil, clay or light sand. It prefers acid or neutral soil. It tends to colonize an area; neglected meadows may sometimes be covered with the characteristic metre-high, bright yellow-blooming plants. It is a hardy plant and can withstand frosts. It flowers from June to October and produces seed heads from July to the end of October. The flowers are hermaphrodite; the plant is self-pollinating. It is visited by many varieties of insect including bees, flies and moths all of which help in the pollination process. It is regarded by farmers and livestock keepers as a considerable nuisance as it is poisonous to cattle, sheep and horses. Though livestock tend to avoid the growing plant because of its unpleasant, acrid smell, once it is dead and dry the odour and any bitter taste disappear. The plant remains poisonous and when it is inadvertently fed to animals the characteristic effects of the toxins become evident. The poison causes weight loss, jaundice, photosensitivity, dermatitis, depression, sleepiness, aimlessness, excessive yawning, staggering gait, abdominal cramps, convulsions, constipation and frenzy.

Senecio has been used medicinally despite the toxic nature of the plant. It is astringent, diaphoretic, emmanagogue and expectorant. The plant is dried before use. An emollient poultice can be made from the leaves; it is used to soothe burns, sores and cancerous ulcers as well as inflammation of the eyes. It has even been used as a gargle. It has been used to soothe bee stings. A decoction of the root can be used to treat internal bruising. However, warnings are always given in the use of the plant; even touch can cause an irritating rash.

Senecio + Tyria shares several aspects with **Senecio Aureus** which is already a proved remedy. This latter remedy has been called the **Coffea** for women's complaints. It is indicated by conditions of the female urogenital tract, the bladder, mucous membranes of the nose and lungs and the lumbar spine. It is comparable with **Pulsatilla**, **Kali-carb**, **Calc-carb**, **Sepia**, **Ferrum-phos**, **Helonias** and **Ferrum-ars**.

Keynote effects

It has a calming, revivifying and protective effect on those who have suffered abuse and/or suppression in the sacral centre. This is so especially in those whose childhoods bear the history of damaged innocence and suppression. It is useful in restoring confidence to those who feel that their true voices have never been heard. There is a strong aspect of duality in the remedy; it helps to create a greater sense of balance in the hormone system as well as in the psyche; between yin and yang. It encourages the return of 'flow' to the system that has tended towards stagnation.

General symptoms

A remedy for any or all forms of abuse to the generative centre. This is true for both women and men though it will probably be more often seen indicated in women. Physical trauma or chemical abuse to the sex organs: < HRT, the Pill, frequent use of the morning-after pill, surgical intervention that has left scarring, prolapse contributed to by frequent pregnancies and psychological trauma. It is indicated in menstrual disorders especially when characterized by haemorrhages with dark, stagnant blood, dysmenorrhoea and putrid discharges. It is particularly indicated in women whose personalities have altered due to suppression of the generative sphere and usual expressions of femininity: they have become intense, driven, distressed and they may be depressed or appear manic, overstimulated, gabbling and subject to mood swings. In men it helps to protect the male organs from developing pathology particularly the prostate. Useful in sensitive men with low libido. Rheumatic conditions; muscles become stiff and even rigid with wandering pains. Osteoporosis. Frequent colds with no proper resolution.

The remedy has a strong influence on the bladder, especially when there is a history of cystitis or damage to the urinary tract. There is a possible history of nocturnal enuresis. In the generative organs, the urinary organs or the mucous membranes of the lungs and sinuses there is the tendency for discharges to become putrid and malodorous. Mucus in the nasal passages can cause foul taste in the mouth. Vaginal discharges may be excoriating. Oedema may result from the general state of stagnation: of the extremities.

It is a remedy for children who have never had breast milk; who have been brought up in one-parent families and thus been without the balance of male and female role models. It is useful in children who have had their natural confidence suppressed by parental expectations or even abusive attention. It is also for parents cowed by domineering, manipulative children. It is likely to be indicated in those going through some transformative phase in life such as puberty, childbearing or menopause.

It might be called for by patients who have had several or many blood transfusions and have subsequently had personality changes. This is most likely to be indicated in those whose sweat and other excretions have become foul and whose skin has become unhealthy.

The remedy is deeply sycotic and carcinogenic though it is also tubercular and syphilitic. A patient in constitutional need of **Senecio + Tyria** is likely to be heading towards the carcinogenic state. The remedy is supported well by an appropriate nosode. The remedy should be considered when two or more of the following remedies are indicated or have already been prescribed with indifferent or no result: **Pulsatilla, Sepia, Secale, Folliculinum, Oopherinum, Cimicifuga** or **Lachesis**.

Miasms

Sycosis, cancer, psora, leprosy and tuberculosis.

Mental and emotional symptoms

Confusion with a feeling of not being oneself. A sense of being nobody and nothing. Either sitting and looking into nothingness or dashing about being busy and fast becoming exhausted. Restlessness and fidgetiness as if in search of something; a longing for a sense of purpose. May express themselves by saying that they have never really found out what it is they want to do in life. Feelings of desolation. A strong desire to go home. A feeling of having been damaged during childhood that may feel similar to being lost. A deep sense of shame but unable to identify the origins of the emotion; shame that bursts on her in waves. A deep sense of mistrust in the opposite sex. Distrust in men since experiences of abuse; a history of suffering since being seduced; feelings of emptiness and waste since realizing husband has had several affairs. Grief expressed in tears while alone. Feelings of darkness and loneliness with a strong desire to escape. Fear and anxiety with a need to run away and hide. Terror. A feeling that one's head would split in two. Schizoid feelings. Schizophrenic tendencies; feels as if possessed by some dark, sticky, heavy energy. Feeling of being dirty, unclean. (The remedy may be found to be·of value in those who have difficulty in coming to terms with being of mixed parentage or of mixed cultural background.) Loquacity; gabbling. Find themselves talking to fill the void; talking about inconsequential things, knowing that they want to talk about deeper, more meaningful things. Fear that they don't fit in; that they may not be able to take advantage of all that Nature and life have to offer. A feeling of having been put down all their life. A need for clarity; to be able to see things in black and white. A desire to sleep as it is so difficult to cope with one's problems. May want to be alone but never finds the opportunity. Feels very old.

Physical symptoms

Head
A sensation of tight binding around the head. Headache from dehydration. Stabbing pains into the head directly from above through the vertex.

Eyes
Tickling in the eyes; < right. Weepy right eye.

Ears
Acutely sensitive to sounds. Bubbling sensation.

Mouth
Foul, putrid taste in the mouth. Slimy mucus; mouth feels full of sticky saliva. Nausea from foulness of mucus and saliva. Pricking in the lips as if herpes would break out. Taste of blood. Acidic taste with nausea.

Throat

Congestion in the area of the thyroid. Constriction of the throat with mucus and salivation. Wants to retch from the saliva and mucus.

Chest

Burning in the area of the sternum. Encourages the return of breast milk when it has been suppressed. Tightness and pain around chest especially on the right side. Cough < from mucus in the throat. Back of the heart area feels tight.

Stomach

Nausea, vomiting and belching. Borbyrigmi: lots of rumbling and grumbling in the stomach and the intestines. Wants to vomit especially after traumatic emotions. Cramp high in the stomach area.

Abdomen

Dragging down as if an abortion or miscarriage were about to happen.

Female

Dysmenorrhoea: pains in the abdomen but particularly felt in the back. Menstrual blood may be black, foul, putrid. Ovarian pains especially when associated with emotional anguish. Excoriating discharge from the vagina with putrid smell. NBWS the Pill, HRT, the morning-after pill, etc. Late or absent periods. Dark, sluggish menstrual flow. Awareness of womb and ovaries. A feeling of being congested in the pelvic area. A sensation that the period is about to start.

Male

Low libido. Prostate symptoms; **Senecio** may well prove itself to be useful in preventing the patient who is headed towards prostate cancer.

Skin

Perspiration: clammy or running with sweat especially accompanied by nausea or faintness. Hot and sweaty generally. Small eruptions that are weepy on the right hand. Burning welt on hand.

Back and shoulders

Heaviness and aching in shoulders with weakness. A sensation of the spine cracking in two. Aching in the right shoulder. Pain from right shoulder that extends down arm to elbow.

Extremities

Hands are hot, sweaty, clammy. Hands or feet feel oedematous. Puffiness of the right hand. Pins and needles in the right arm from shoulder to elbow. Pain extends down the legs from the lower spine. Painful feet. Rheumatic pains in the limbs especially wandering pains.

Sleep

Sleepy in the daytime. Sleepless at night from worry and churning mind. Gets hot in bed. Dream-filled sleep with exhaustion on waking. Dreams of never being allowed to rest. Insomnia from frightful dreams.

Considerations for the use of the remedy

Senecio + Tyria should be compared with **Senecio Aureus** as they are so closely related. S/T is richer in the mental and emotional sphere. **Senecio** is related to **Folliculinum** and **Oopherinum** and follows both well. **Sepia** and **Lachesis** also have an affinity with the remedy as do **Carcinosin, Syphilinum, Medorrhinum Americana** and **Tuberculinum**. Patients may be in need of **Senecio** if they have a general tendency to show indications for **Pulsatilla**.

- **Folliculinum** shares the NBWS hormone changes brought about by drug therapy. Both remedies have symptoms in common with **Lachesis, Sepia** and **Pulsatilla** and can be confused with these. There is just as much exhaustion, instability and sensitivity in both but **Folliculinum** is likely to be less inclined to garrulousness and fidgety nervousness and more interested in sexual activity. There is more of a tendency to chronic headaches.
- **Sepia** has more indifference and resentment while **Senecio** is closer to feeling mad or confused at least.
- **Pulsatilla** is more dependent and tearful; more inclined to want company while **Senecio** wants to be left alone but cannot find space to be alone. **Senecio** feels less abandoned than downtrodden and ill-used.
- **Lachesis** has more viciousness of temper and is more likely to use

vitriol in attacking others. Both remedies have trouble with making clear sense in talking but **Lachesis** is more likely to jump from subject to subject in swift succession. **Senecio** rambles on about superficialities.

- **Helonias** has a strong sense of the womb and has problems with the urinary and pelvic organs.
- **Gratiola** is said to be the **Nux Vomica** for women. It shares the hysteria, irritability and apprehension but it is for women who are peevish, out of sorts and worried about their health. There is more likely to be a strong sexual appetite which **Senecio** does not have.

The remedy is very successful when combined in triad remedies in cases with multiple foci where no similimum presents itself unequivocally:

S/T + Thuja + Carcinosin
S/T + Tiger's Eye + Moonstone
S/T + Syc Seed + Syph
S/T + Thuja + Med-am
S/T + Ayahuasca + Rhodochrosite

Esoteric therapeutics

This is particularly a remedy to heal damaged yin energy, the feminine principle. It positively influences both men and women in this aspect. When yin is out of balance in the body, it does not necessarily mean that yang is predominant (as it can be with a remedy such as **Oak**) but it can result in 'dark' and heavy energy given off by and holding back the patient. There is a lack of flow in the whole system; there is stagnation in the lower three chakras and almost certainly consequent frustration held in the heart centre. This is a major remedy for those who have never felt complete autonomy of their own energy; they have existed but in thrall to a tradition, another person or a traumatic situation or from the suppression of part of their energy field (as might happen after drugs or surgery to treat the sacral centre). The characteristic emotions locked into the chakra system are distrust and shame; feelings that may not be overtly present in a consultation as they have been buried away from the heart centre.

Chakras

Crown

Tendency to cancer. Brain tumours. Deep sense of worthlessness rooted in the base => deep suppression of the psyche and the stirring of the cancer miasm. Sleeplessness. Dreams of anxiety and fear. Mental instability << for any suppression especially of menstruation; delusions and illusions; peculiar behaviour; feelings of unreality; madness. Multiple personality disorders. Possession: the aura can be blown open due to severe suppression which leads to the attachment of entities; the remedy can help to release entities engrafted on.

Brow

Misunderstands and misinterprets what others say and do. Contraction of pituitary; the body clock is deregulated. < the function of the hypothalamus. > the flow of cerebrospinal fluid.

Pituitary < since the Pill, HRT, etc. Remedy awakens pituitary function after it has become chronically blocked. 'Moral fixity'.

Throat

Blocked expression; negative expression. Emotional expression is blocked due to blockage in the sacral centre from artificial hormone interference: the Pill, HRT, sterilization, etc. Thyroid gland is destabilized. 'Though she speaks it is hard to understand what she says or to make sense of the thread of what she wants to say.' Thwarted femininity. Always in a hurry. Remedy encourages expression of aggravations through the throat centre: colds with thick catarrh.

Heart

Grief from suppressed feminine energy and expression. Feels downtrodden; << from abuse. < from dictatorial fathers; < absent fathers. Remedy is helpful to women who suffer from their partners having had affairs. Deep sense of sadness. Weeping, sad mood. <<persistent criticism; << lack of parental (paternal) support and love. Feels worthless. << mental and physical abuse. Aversion to children. Hard and harsh emotionally in those whose femininity is suppressed through the need to be self-protective. Strongly self-protective and combative. Remedy can foster or recreate the mother-child link when that is damaged by antibiotics or other treatment during breastfeeding. (Spiritual ether is carried by mother's milk and is thus important in integrating the energy between the chakras.) NBWS traumatic birth. Useful remedy in breast cancer cases especially with blocked glands. Congested lungs. Circulation tends to stagnate. Asthmatic.

Solar plexus

Blood flow is suppressed which has a knock-on effect on the psyche. Blocked liver. Pancreas, liver and spleen are all unbalanced. Blood sugar problems: hypoglycaemia. Digestive disorders. Gall bladder problems. Sticky blood: clots. Ascites. Sepsis in the lower centres.

Sacral

Heals the feminine energy in both women and men; sensitive men with low libido. Tendency to haemorrhage; spotting and irregular periods. Foul-smelling menstrual and vaginal discharges. Infertility. Does not want to have children. Symptoms or suffering (physical or emotional) from IVF. Hysteria from suppressed menses. Amenorrhoea. Dysmenorrhoea. Menopause that threatens to come on too soon. Hot flushes, suppressed by drugs or shock are restored by the remedy. NBWS the Pill, HRT, the morning-after pill and other drug therapy. Excoriating vaginal discharge. Bladder and kidneys stagnate. Offensive urine. Cystitis. Remedy can help in the prevention of prostate cancer. Restores the flow of energy in the pelvic organs. (In the treatment of suppressed menses the remedy may have to be repeated over several months and in conjunction with other remedies such as **Folliculinum** and the nosodes.)

Base

Lack of self-confidence; severely restricting, self-imposed limitations which keep the patient from moving forward. Sepsis. Stagnant lymphatics. Chronic degenerative diseases; osteoporosis. Hereditary genetic destabilizing of the reproductive system. Lack of fluid energy. Tendency to become stuck. Rheumatism; stiffening of muscles. The remedy encourages eliminative reactions. Sweating is restored. Useful in children who are fearful due to the lack of connection between them and their mothers; useful in one-parent children. Children who suffer from adverse criticism and punishment; they easily feel too overexposed to criticism. The remedy is multi-miasmatic; has an affinity for the nosodes.

Case studies

1 'Woman aged 70 who had had cervical cancer at 34 (treated with radio-therapy) and then suspected though incorrectly diagnosed with Crohn's disease at 44 that led to surgery, came for treatment for intermittent diarrhoea (during which she passed blood), incontinence of bowel and recurrent anal fistula. She had undergone a colonoscopy which had found scar tissue causing intestinal stricture, and then the reversal of an ileostomy which was carried out successfully. Scar tissue was also responsible for bladder incontinence. It was admitted in a histology report that the radiotherapy had caused damage to the bowel. She was distressed by the incontinence and admitted to considerable anger at the treatment she had been given and "state I've been left in". She felt that her health was more fragile as a result of the surgery and the medication that she had felt obliged to take over several years. Also over several years of homoeopathic treatment she was variously given **Carcinosin**, **Radium Bromide**, **Arsenicum**, **Pulsatilla**, **Thuja**, **Phosphorus, Sulphur, Alumina, Lycopodium, Baryta-carb** and **Aurum**. She reported improvements with all these in one aspect or another and her bowel problems ceased to be problematical.

'What remained to trouble her was the onset of peripheral neuropathy (the result, according to osteopaths, of a spinal fusion in her lumbar spine) and her continued sense of outrage not only at the doctors who had treated her but at her body's inability to function well enough for her to continue with her work; she saw herself as an invalid. She felt that the radiotherapy had blighted her life and been partly to blame for her inability to have children. She also deeply resented anyone patronizing her, something she felt acutely sensitive to; she even felt her husband was guilty of this. She admitted to feeling unable to let go of these emotions; it was as if they were frustrating her sense of creativity. **Staphysagria** was unable to effect any change whatever so she was given **Senecio + Tyria** 30: one three times per week for six weeks. She reported that she felt much better and "more on an even keel". She no longer suffered from any cramp in her legs, her energy had improved despite the continued weakness in her legs. A routine blood test at her GP's surgery had shown that her kidney function was considerably improved. "I feel emotionally so much stronger. I'm more myself and

I'm enjoying going out again. And I surprised myself by being able to take the tube and then walk ever such a long way the other day. I thought I'd be fatigued but I managed really well!"' CG

2 'A woman of 30 came with continued uterine and breast pains that had started in the same month as she had had a termination the previous year. She had thought that she was pregnant again and became almost distraught with the thought of it. She felt worse when her partner not only became unsupportive but had an emotional crisis over the prospect of fatherhood. Physically "I feel like I did when I took those tablets for the termination." She was exhausted, enervated, hot, sweaty, thirsty and felt that she couldn't be bothered any more. She had **Sulphur** 1M which brought on the missing period and relieved all the symptoms except the uterine pains which she felt were phantom as she had had a scan and two more pregnancy tests, both of which were negative. Her breasts were still engorged and sore and she had pains in the area of the pubis: a sharp line of pain from the low abdomen to the pubic bone. She had become very tearful and lonely as her partner had made her feel that "it was all my fault". She had also gone back on the Pill as she felt she could not risk any further pregnancy scares. She was given **Pulsatilla** 50M which completely changed her mood for the better but did nothing for her pains. The pains were either continuous for a while or they became intermittent while she was occupied at work. Her breasts remained swollen and sore but less so. She still felt that she needed more energy. She was also due to go for a further scan on the following day. She was given **Senecio + Tyria** 30: three times a week for three weeks. When she returned she said that she had had no further uterine pains, that her breasts were back to normal and that her periods were now back to 28 days exactly and without any pain. For the first time ever the period started suddenly and stopped within four days. She had no menstrual acne or sore gums and she had not been on any emotional roller coaster as she was used to. Her energy was now back to full strength. The only problem she had had was looser bowels. 'CG

3 'A Gemini woman who had had **Staphysagria** 10M for acute problems in a relationship came for her appointment and explained how she had been. She had had several bouts of cystitis while seeing her present

partner, an older man who was looking after his dying mother. She felt that the relationship was not going well and that she was, in some way she could not understand, being manipulated. "This chap has a lot of issues with anger. I'm in a constant battle thinking 'Why am I letting this man get to me?' Last weekend I saw a side of him which made me feel very uncomfortable. I see him as quite selfish on the sexual side. I'm disappointed with myself that I can't cope with that; with the anger. I can't deal with confronting anger from someone else." She had become violently sick on two occasions. "When I was sick the first time I was bringing up my ex-husband. This time was connected with the hurt he had caused me physically during sex." She was now worried about going on holiday with the new boyfriend. "I don't feel that I can walk away from the relationship altogether." She was given **Senecio + Tyria** 200: one each day for three days. When she returned she had had no further sickness, no further bouts of cystitis and at first never mentioned anything to do with the boyfriend or the holiday. She was more concerned to relate all she was doing about her diet as she had discovered that she was dairy intolerant. When prompted she mentioned that she had thrown out the boyfriend, felt much better "in my bladder and 'gynae' area and I no longer feel confused. I'm more attuned to what I want." CG

32

SEQUOIADENDRON GIGANTEUM

Sierra Redwood

The remedy was proved by the meditation circle on 17 November 1995 by six women and five men with the medium. Each was given a single dose of the 30ᵗʰ potency at the start of the meditation.

The Background

The remedy was made from wellingtonia; giant sequoia; big tree; mammoth tree; Sierra redwood or, in its Linnaean name, *Sequoiadendron giganteum* (*Sequoia gigantea*). The *Sequoiadendron* tree is a single species that was formerly associated with the *Sequoia sempervirens* (coast redwood). The *giganteum* differs in that its foliage is entirely of branchlets with cords of scale leaves while the *sempervirens* has branches with fern-shaped shoots with serried rows of hard, sharply pointed scale leaves with further side shoots. Other differences are that the *sempervirens* has a less compact 'crown' while the 'crown' of the giant sequoia is conical at the top, more dense and with a tendency to be more 'upswept' than its cousin. The giant is slower to grow in its early stages. While the coast redwood boasts the tallest tree in the world ('Howard Libbey') at 112.4 metres, the giant sequoia is the longest lived at up to 3,400 years old. It can grow up to 100 metres and more and its girth is anything up to 27 metres. It is capable of growing outwards at the rate of 8 centimetres each year and upwards by 45 centimetres or more. The natural habitat of both trees is the western seaboard of Canada and the United States at 1,500 to 2,500 metres above sea level. The environment is particularly foggy and this has contributed to the tree's longevity and its ability to continue growing and reproducing even into extreme old age. The moisture carried by the fog keeps the ground wet and reduces the loss of water from the leaves. In spite of its great size the tree blows down far less frequently than might be supposed. The bark is extremely tough and thick yet it is fibrous and can be torn off in shreds. Being up to 30 centimetres thick, the bark protects the tree from forest fire damage and the depredation of wild animals. The tree is also very acid which prevents the growth of fungi though these have been known to be the cause of death. Giant sequoia trees are particularly susceptible to being struck by lightning (like oak). Unlike other conifers they have a marked ability to grow fresh trees from their stumps and have been known to produce several trees from the one stump. In 1853 the first examples were introduced into Europe. Though redwoods and giant sequoia have colonized well, they do not fare so well in big cities. The cones take two years to ripen but they can remain on the tree for up to 20 years before they drop; in European examples the cones only stay on the branches for a few years.

Keynote effects

Worries and fears are placed into a proper perspective so that any inhibition about growth and development is eased; it helps patients to limit their negative reactions to external circumstances or incidents and to let go of negative attitudes that are held within and that have had little chance of being aired. Revitalizes flagging energy in one who needs to pace their life better. Has an affinity for the pituitary gland and is noted for correcting dysfunction of this organ.

General symptoms

Sycotic: affects the water balances of the body. Excessive mucus production especially in the lungs. Rheumatic complaints. Voracious appetite. Sycotic/psoric: exhaustion, heaviness and enervation with sense of inadequacy; oedema with sinking sensation. Also has marked effect on the five senses; especially vision. Has opposite effects: can feel lightness of being; ethereal, delicate or heavy, earthbound, solid. Can switch from one extreme to the other in these effects though in the mental/emotional sphere this is less obvious. Fleeting or wandering pains which are often constrictive or cramping. Parts can feel pressure: heart or lungs. Right-sided. Periodicity: two-year cycles or nine-year cycles; also seasonal changes with physical pathology. Detoxifies the system by helping to control the water balances. Acidosis without reflux. Also reduces radiation poisoning. Is useful in those who seldom become ill or in those whose illness does not curtail their creative energy and activity; who are very strong and gentle: 'the gentle giant' type. A very important remedy for those who are growing fast; encourages strength of all tissues. Pituitary function is faulty though this may only become obvious or be diagnosed during cranial osteopathic treatment. Can be given safely to babies still in the womb who are suffering from foetal distress especially if this is of emotional origin; parental difficulties that are registered by the foetus. It is a remedy of growth and development, helping to slow down the rate where it is too fast and to balance it when it is uneven (growing upward without any broadening). Can also be used for mental and spiritual development when new pathways are being explored but are leading to confusion. There is a curious quality that can be perceived in the patient that what is not yet revealed is more important than what is obvious or on the surface; can be used when superficial symptom pictures do not add up to much or to a variety of remedies and when no miasm is obviously a block to healing. The remedy tends to 'illuminate' what has not yet been treated because it was hidden but which is nevertheless vital to the progress of treatment. Can be used when other remedies seem to fail to complete their action. This is particularly true in those who have taken **Sulphur** and/or **Oak** but have not derived as much benefit as they might. Useful in cases of high blood pressure as it tends to encourage the general metabolism to slow down. Can be given in high potencies alongside other remedies that are more specific to reducing blood pressure levels such as **Spartium.**

Miasms

Psora, sycosis and tuberculosis.

Mental and emotional symptoms

The main keynote to the remedy is naivety. With the general strength of the remedy goes a state of childlike innocence and gentleness. For those who suffer but who do not know why they suffer; the heart is open and vulnerable and there is no comprehension as to why this should be abused by others. Grief from past occurrences which have not been resolved due to misapprehension of other peoples' intentions. Sadness, loneliness and emptiness. Sadness felt in the solar plexus. Heaviness and solidity which make the patient feel as if 'cast in stone' (affinity with **Granite**). The remedy encourages the patient to see events in a different light while still maintaining an open heart centre. Where lack of comprehension leads to a desire to 'give up the struggle'. A sense of futility. Strong desire to go to sleep. Sense of confusion; difficult to finish sentences or the task in hand. 'Can't be bothered' attitude. Vague and absent-minded. Feels things strongly but is unable to describe them or to understand them. Trusts in the beauty of the world in a childlike way but is aware of a sense of insecurity. Unable to detect sarcasm. Can be impish and mischievous but in a teasing manner rather than from a negative motive. Some of these feelings are exaggerated in those who would prefer to live at a slower pace than modern life allows but who feel chased and harried by worries; the speed of the vibrations of anxiety do not match with the rhythm of the constitution. Often such fears as they have come from within and may have little to provoke them in external circumstances. Has great compassion for others in spite of own suffering. Empathizes strongly with others even inappropriately. Strongly attached to children or has a childish attitude. Can feel a sense of separation and as if 'cut off' (**Thuja**). Seldom angered even when this would be expected. Mute even in rage (see **Red**). Tends to grow away from those who cause emotional hurt but without expressing anything. Becomes averse to certain company. Develops a complex about people: feels that he or she is not cared for any more by someone close but cannot think of any reason why this should be. Prefers not to think of emotional things too deeply; distrustful of their ability to handle emotional issues. (Can be confused with **Puls.**) Can be aloof and even apparently haughty as they are shy of approach. Great patience; has the ability to wait for enormous lengths of time (**Oak**). Has a great determination to succeed though not in any material sense; is more concerned with other values. Forever wants to improve on existing achievements. Indecisive. Has a sense that everything is slowed down, even that things are going along in slow motion; this can be the result of the remedy as well as a symptom. A sense of being old; expresses this with a feeling as if the oldness contributed to their sense of separation from others. Senility.

Physical symptoms

Head
Vertigo: a sense of turning in a circular motion especially while standing. Has a need to stand or sit with something to support the back. Splitting pain in the middle of brain which seems to separate the occipital area from the frontal. One of the main remedies for poor pituitary function. (Has been known to work well with **Anterior Pituitary** in asthma.) Acromegaly. Developmental learning difficulties.

Eyes
Misty vision; blurred. Light sparks before eyes. Dimmed vision with emotional blockage of years' standing. Pains (fleeting) in the right eye. Perfect sight; long-sightedness.

Ears
Buzzing. Hollow or full sensations (with pain). H/o ear infections.

Nose
Catarrh. < wet weather.

Face
Wears an innocent expression. Can also be weather-beaten.

Mouth
Dryness with a sour taste of lemons. (When the leaves of the tree are crushed or rubbed there is a strong smell of aniseed.)

Throat
History of septic throats. Nausea in the throat pit with anxiety felt in the solar plexus.

Respiration and chest
Asthma: sycotic in origin. Oppressed breathing with desire to take deep breaths. In-breaths are more difficult than out-breaths. Also feels as if there is an enormous capacity to take air into the lungs but this causes 'headiness'.

Hyperventilation. The more air they take in the more air they want. > steam inhalations or breathing into a paper bag for a short time. Very affected by Ventolin and steroids.

Coughs up thick mucus. Tightness in diaphragm that causes the patient to want to expand chest and take deep breaths as this is an exercise in stretching. Draws shoulders back (rather than up) in taking deep breaths. Palpitations. Oppressed heart from grief. Bradycardia and tachycardia. Useful after strokes especially when the patient's nervous system is left affected.

Stomach
Anxiety. Feels waterlogged. Heaviness especially after heavy meal. Thirstless. Thyroid insufficiency due to pituitary dysfunction.

Abdomen
Unexpressed emotions tend to cause liver and gall bladder problems. Bitter risings in the throat. Acid digestion. Sinking in abdomen < after a meal. Digestion < oily food.

Dried and crumbly stools with constipation or shredded, fibrous stools with burning sensations.

Urinary organs
Retention of urine or desire to go almost straight after having been. Split stream especially with prostate problems.

Female
Period pains: sudden onset; felt in rectum and down the back of the thighs to knees. Heavy flow. Fibroids. Poor lactation; improves the flow of milk – this is often the remedy for this problem when there is difficulty in bonding between mother and child.

Male
Lack of libido. Improves erectile dysfunction in impotent men (see **Clear Quartz**).

Neck and back
Inability to sit up straight. Needs spinal support. Pains felt in the cervical, dorsal and lumbar regions that shift about. Drilling pain in the right trapezius muscle

where it leads into the cervical area. Desire to stretch upwards especially on waking in the morning or after sitting for any length of time.

Sleep

Insomnia or its opposite, sleepiness. Dreams of: astral travel; of ancient civilizations; of transmutation where the dreamer becomes something other than they really are; of enlightenment. Also has dreams that seem real on waking and that remind one that something that should have been done has not yet been done. Wakeful from difficult breathing.

Considerations for the use of the remedy

In spinal trouble it can be compared with the following:

- **Ayahuasca** which is more known for twists and torsions in the musculoskeletal system and which carries implications of deeper emotional trauma than **Sequoia** which is more inclined to suffer from weakness and pain in the spine due to rapid growth or from lack of growth.
- **Salix Fragilis** holds more of a sense of burden than **Sequoia** even though both may have pains in the spine; **Salix**'s troubles are likely to stem from distressing events that pile one problem up on another while **Sequoia** struggles more with what prevents development.
- **Silver Fish** is known for being indicated in whiplash or, less superficially, for growth and development in children who suffer from excessive hyperadrenalism.

Sequoia can also be more generally compared with the following:

- **Thuja** is easily confused with **Sequoia** due to their similar spheres of action: sycosis, confusion, fear and worries that threaten security, mucus production, asthmatic breathing, etc. What differentiates them is **Sequoia**'s slowness and lack of drive. It does not suffer from **Thuja**'s feeling of being separate from reality; they are simply 'far off' like the lonely child on the playground.
- **Clay** is far slower, more stuck and heavy than **Sequoia** and the 'can't be bothered' attitude is tinged with truculence, a sentiment that **Sequoia** does not share.

- **Medorrhinum Americana** is far more volatile than **Sequoia** though it may be called for in supporting or underpinning a prescription of the tree.
- **Nat-sulph** is far more orientated towards the liver than **Sequoia** and holds a lot of dark energy that borders on depression in that organ. Nevertheless, **Nat-sulph** (in low potency or as a tissue salt) may be useful as a supporting liver remedy for someone who needs a constitutional dose of **Sequoia**.
- **Pulsatilla** is differentiated from **Sequoia** by its characteristic clinginess, dependency and tearfulness, all of which it has more strongly than the tree. Nevertheless, they are both known for the production of mucus though **Puls** is more likely to fill up in the throat and sinuses while Sequoia tends to have mucus in the upper respiratory tract of the chest and lower throat.
- **Rose Quartz** is just as quiet a remedy but its action centres mostly on the heart; there is more likely to be a feeling of wanting to be near home or of homesickness.
- **Granite** suffers from extreme exhaustion and weakness and the patient tends to be introverted and detached in a dark manner. **Sequoia** is not nearly such a dark remedy, not as spaced out and not nearly so miserable.

Sequoia is preceded or followed well by **Green, Emerald, Clear** and **Smoky Quartz** and **Sodium Bicarbonate. Baryta-carb** is said to be inimical though this is not qualified by any negative experience to date.

Esoteric therapeutics

Heals all the chakras and every level of the aura. Particularly heals the heart and sacral centres. The energy of the remedy can stretch up beyond the crown chakra in order to draw down into the subject that which needs to be known for spiritual development (see **Purple**). Can help wishful thinking to become practical reality in the mental and spiritual sphere. Can restore faith in spiritual values and engender more overt expressions of compassion and love.

Chakras

Crown

The remedy works to open this centre in those who would stretch their enquiring awareness beyond their normal fixed boundaries of routine and familiar territory. It allows for exploring the loftiness of spiritual philosophy without becoming ungrounded as most sycotic patients would. It awakens or reawakens awareness of spiritual values in one who has lost them or never had them particularly when the sycotic miasm is a strong influence on the patient's life.

Brow

The yin nature of the patient's naive state of acceptance of anything or everything they have been told is transformed to allow for discrimination without harsh judgement; the faculty of being able to reject that which prevents growth and development is allowed to flourish. The memory of negative experiences is given a filter of understanding, the absence of which up to now prevented being able to move on with independence and self-confidence.

Throat

There is a deep well of self-expression to tap into in this centre that has not been allowed light up till now. Expansion through opening this chakra results in rapid changes in all other aspects of the being without necessarily speeding up the system generally.

Heart

Peace and harmony are established in this centre to replace any fear that has contributed to its being so vulnerable. The positivity of this chakra is then at the disposal of others as the patient has a preternatural abundance of generosity of spirit and compassion. The purpose of the remedy is expansion in this chakra which, once established, begins to ease any difficult breathing. There may well be much ancestral grief in this centre confirmed by the history of previous generations of the family.

Solar plexus

Sadness felt in this chakra. The challenge faced in this centre is to be able to cope with the difference in speed between the inner person and the outer world which seems to go so much faster. This dichotomy gives rise to symptoms such as acidity and discomfort in the intestines.

Sacral
This centre can be slow to awaken. Sexual naivety.

Base
Awareness and understanding are geared to a slower rate of reaction than the speed at which the world goes now. There is a naivety which is not to do with slowness or stunting of development but to do with the inherent slower rhythm of the constitution that is left feeling puzzled and bereft by outside circumstances.

Case studies

1 'A woman of 45 who had come for treatment following severe emotional trauma and whose demeanour was rather wary and mildly cynical, was given **Sequoia** 1M when she complained of back trouble. She could not describe any specific injury or cause for the general weakness and aching she endured and she was inclined to be dismissive of her back's significance in her general condition. There was a suspicion of **Arnica** about her state. Her tendency was to veer either towards the tubercular or sycotic. When she returned in five weeks for a follow-up appointment she said that her children had thought that she had grown overnight; on measuring herself she found that she was standing an inch taller than before. The pains in her back had gone.' **CG**

2 'Female, politician, 58, chairs debates on alternative medicine, vitamins and minerals, herbalism, homoeopathy, etc. She had gone into politics after her husband suddenly died in his early 50s. Very ambitious, beautifully strong and pure in her intent. Came for homoeopathy to help with her gruelling schedule. Had been experiencing muscular tension and numbness in her legs. History of ME and back pain. To me she fitted **Sequoia** as a constitutional remedy: a "gentle giant", pure, strong, ambitious, hugely compassionate and very responsible. **Sequoia** 200c

prescribed weekly. All physical symptoms improved and she said she had felt incredibly strong and coped fabulously with her election campaign as an independent and had been re-elected.' HJ

3 'Female, 16, presented with very severely cracked feet, with deep bleeding fissures along the whole length of the soles of both feet. Naive, ambitious, gentle, very responsible, pure, bossy, strong, busy and compassionate. She was the middle of three children and not only looked after them but also both her parents! My feelings were that she had disturbed kidney/sacral energy partly due to the fact that the family had immigrated to England when she was nine which was around the time the feet had started to become a problem. My initial prescription was **Calc-carb** which did nothing for her feet. **Sequoia** 30c daily was prescribed based on her personality and the kidney relationship. The feet quickly healed.' HJ

4 'Female, 33, very severe asthma. Had previously done well with **Medorrhinum** and **Thuja**. However, after the birth of her second child the asthma was worse than it had been for years and these remedies weren't effective. She was also experiencing difficulty lactating. I remembered **Sequoia** as a remedy for this as well as for sycotic asthma. **Sequoia** 30c daily was prescribed and the asthma improved dramatically as did the breast milk.' HJ

5 'Female aged 47 years. During the consultation she complained of a pain in the centre of her diaphragm, following a cough with difficult expectoration. Breathing sounded tight and "wheezy". She described her diaphragm as being "closed in". The stomach felt tight, [she] wanted to burp but couldn't. The whole of the upper abdomen felt constricted. The patient sat hunched over, almost bent double. She said she "felt like elongating my whole body". Constriction in the stomach: better for standing and bending double.

'Based on the patient's desire to elongate I gave her **Sequoia** 30 in the consultation. Within seconds of the patient taking the remedy she described a tingling sensation in the solar plexus and a shift of energy downwards. Her voice sounded more relaxed and less tense and her breathing eased and wheeziness decreased. Over the next ten minutes she gradually straightened her body until she was almost lying in the chair leaning backwards. She commented that her whole abdomen seemed to be growing and stretching. She felt more relaxed and wanted to sleep. The tense feeling and sense of compression in her stomach had gone. The pain in the stomach/diaphragm eased.

'No other remedy was given. At the follow-up one month later the patient reported that the remedy had removed a long-standing fear of giving up smoking and she had not smoked since the previous appointment. Her chest had cleared over a couple of days and all sense of tightness, restriction and compression in the chest, diaphragm and stomach had gone. She commented that she felt taller.' **SP** (First published in *Prometheus* No. 9 December 1998.)

6 'Female, aged 50, presented with joint problems, particularly in hands, and thumbs. History of IBS and breast cancer in right breast two years prior. Client had lumpectomy but had refused chemo and wasn't on tamoxifen. There had been some query as to bone density in hips. Client had had **Causticum** in the past, along with **Phos, Rhus-tox, Aurum** and **Lycopodium** but these had never held for very long.

'Client set herself very high standards and was a very spiritual person but a bit lost as to how she should deal with this side of her character. I gave her **Sequoia** two years previously, based on the physicals of the joints and the prior cancer but moreover on the need to succeed in what she wanted to do; plus the fact that she needed grounding.

'The effect on the joints was immediate and she has remained on **Sequoia** ever since with no return of any pain; a bone density scan this year revealed the hips were normal (where they used to be at the bottom of bone density graph). The cancer remains in remission but client also remains on **Carcin**. The spiritual side of her character continues to emerge and she is in a position where she is now able to help people.' **LE**

7 'Female age 82 presented with very bad oedema of the lower legs. Both affected. No heart or kidney condition. Normal water retention remedies had little effect. **Sequoia** 30c daily enabled the body to start eliminating the excess fluid; client takes it acutely should the need arise.' **LE**

33

TIGER'S EYE

The remedy was proved by the meditation group on 14 February 1997. The remedy was later proved by the students on the Guild of Homoeopaths' postgraduate course in July 1998.

The Background

This is a quartz replacement of crocidolite (blue asbestos) or of gold asbestos. Its basic chemical composition is silicon dioxide, SiO_2 though there are impurities that complicate its structure such as sodium, magnesium and iron. Oxidation of the crocidolite fibres are transformed into limonite which are embedded in quartz. The fibres that constitute its structure are twisted and crumpled. Light is reflected by the fibres. It can appear in red, brown, gold, cream, black and blue.

According to mythology, tiger's eye is a stone of protection; it was used to ward off the evil eye and protected the wearer against spells and demoniacal energy. It achieved its reputation because the limonite fibres within the stone cause it to have the appearance of an eye; a polished example of the burnt-orange crystal makes it even more like a tiger's eye.

Keynote effects

The main effect is of creating stability in the base and sacral chakras when there has been much damage to these two centres in the history of the patient. It is best known for settling the history of abuse to the organs of the sacral centre but it does this in one who also suffers from tension and conflict held in the solar plexus manifested as liver, stomach and spleen disorder.

General symptoms

Tendency to be left-sided predominantly though symptoms may manifest on the right first and then move to the left. Tends to be at either extreme of hot or cold. General inertia and lassitude especially after an episode of extreme activity or sex. Workaholic. Nervous breakdown. Central nervous system is at the end of its tether. Suppression of developmental phases: puberty, menopause through the use of the Pill or HRT. Cancer as a result of suppression through drugs or surgical intervention especially when that is accompanied by grief (for example after an abortion, sterilization). ME. Schizophrenia. Acute hysteria. Postpuerperal insanity. Postnatal blues with confusion and unreasonable tempers like **Lachesis** but not so vicious.

Miasms

Tuberculosis, cancer, syphilis and sycosis.

Mental and emotional symptoms

Easily bewildered. Feelings as if split in two with the two halves doing different things: the will is opposed and the ego fragmented. Their fancies and desires override their common sense. Hedonistic but fully aware of the temptations and the problems inherent. Can have fits of anger and tears when conflict within reaches 'high tide'. This is often associated with menses (or suppressed menses or menopause). Feels fragmented; < from confusion about relationships where the will and ego are either suppressed or confused. Laughs in a rather manic or hysterical way. Obsessed with sexuality. Disorientation. For those who become unfocused by being bogged down in a mass of detail that clouds the real issues. Restless, fidgety hands. Anger: buried too deeply to be accessed. A sense of not being 'still' within. Can seem calm on the outside but be full of turmoil on the inside. Can be foul-mouthed. Unthinking and careless. Hysteria especially after emotional issues that include or are dominated by sexuality. Helps those who become too involved in their problems to stop navel-gazing.

Physical symptoms

Head
Frequent headaches: < going up the right side from the base of the skull. Tension in neck muscles. Left-sided sick headaches; bilious headaches with wish to lie down.

Eyes
Has an affinity for the eyes. Cataracts. Watering eyes or dry eye syndrome. Inflammation of the lower left eyelid.

Mouth
Cold sore on left lower lip.

Throat
Remedy tends to create a discharge of mucus from the throat. Foul taste.

Stomach
Nausea and retching and/or pains when overexcited or overwrought. Heartburn < being upset.

Female
Bloating and congestion in the uterine region. Symptoms of the female organs confused with those of the bowels. Ovaries feel hard as pebbles. Helps women who want to come off HRT. NBWS abortion, the coil, abdominal surgery, after delivery or miscarriage. Left ovarian problems. Cancer of the breast (left). During the proving it was received that this is a remedy, especially in low potency, to be avoided in the first three months of pregnancy.

Male
Incomplete erection; impotence. Lack of libido in aggressive or workaholic men. History of promiscuity.

Urinary organs
Pain in the right kidney. Dark urine with no smell. Split stream.

Neck and back

Stiffness and aching in the muscles at the level of the cervical spine and into the shoulders.

Extremities

Severe cramp in the left hamstring.

Considerations for the use of the remedy

Tiger's Eye is indicated in those who have experimented on and abused the sacral centre to the point of losing contact with what keeps them grounded. Gratification and sensuality have held sway over common sense too often in the past. Not only is the security of the base threatened but the solar plexus also suffers from tension and discomfort. It might also be indicated in those who are unable to find relief for their symptoms of the generative organs through other well-chosen remedies; there is a preoccupation with the distress felt in these structures which has its origins in the emotional sphere. It is as if the sacral chakra organs cannot give up their role as keepers of deep emotional turmoil. It is no surprise then that remedies such as the following need to be compared:

- **Lachesis** can have similar episodes of hysteria though it is more verbally cruel and abusive and the typical symptoms of fullness of the part with < from restriction, especially of the throat, do not appear in **Tiger's Eye**.
- **Folliculinum** has the NBWS since the Pill or HRT but it is also often indicated when there is some debate as to whether **Lachesis, Sepia** or **Pulsatilla** should be given; with **Tiger's Eye** there is no such debate.
- **Lilium Tigrinum** which is particularly left-sided and tends to be more of a 'drama queen' than overtly hysterical or, as some **Tiger's Eye** patients can be, chilled or chilling.
- **Medorrhinum Americana** can be just as violent and hysterical; just as ungrounded and disconnected; just as focused on sex and may be very hard to tell apart from **Tiger's Eye**. What can help to differentiate it is that the **Tiger's Eye** patient has a sense of needing to focus, to change and to seek balance while **Med-am** may be unaware of any such imperative.

It is worth noting that it has been said of the 200 that 'it feels like an expulsion' meaning that the remedy felt as if it was meeting a response that wanted to create a forceful expulsion of negative energy. The 1M has been described as '... this is more opening and lifting ...' as if the remedy were causing a response that was less expulsive and more relaxing and inviting of change. This may not be possible to apply to all patients as there are no rules as far as potencies are concerned but it may help to suggest one approach to prescribing in someone whose system is sensitive and reactive. (The quotes come from a cranial osteopath working closely with a patient who was taking the remedy.)

A support remedy that goes well with **Tiger's Eye** when the coil has caused any physical damage is **Avena Sativa** Ø + **Thlaspi Bursa Pastoris** 3x + **Hydrastis** 6x. This is especially true if there is a history of heavy bleeding at the period.

Esoteric therapeutics

As a healing stone it brings together the vibrations of sand and sunlight, thus it is a stone that synthesizes the energies of sun and earth. It encourages stability and peace with a greater awareness of beauty and harmony. It works, at the level of the base and sacral centres, as a disciplining force over sexuality and the emotional sphere. It is mostly for 'earthy' people. It helps to resolve internal conflicts most often felt or held in the solar plexus. It helps to soften inappropriately inflexible will in those who have become fixed in a certain attitude. It balances yin/yang energy; it balances the two sides of the brain, left and right. It helps those who find themselves feeling vulnerable to conflict. It is said to belong to the sign of Capricorn.

Tiger's Eye also provides stability to the two lower chakras. Allows for the awareness of negative states so that these lower centres can become focused and grounded. Will help to resolve conflicts originating in the solar plexus (the chakra governing ego's influence over the will) that have resulted in disharmony or illness in the lower two centres. It particularly heals the sacral chakra. Abuse of this centre from the Pill, HRT, removal of organs, sexual promiscuity and negative karma from many sexual encounters. For those whose creative energy becomes inappropriately focused in this centre so that the energy is spent and wasted rather than transformed via creative expression. Helps to calm manic creative energy when it creates problems of positive channelling; where creative energy is frustrated through excessive ambition or drive. The pivot of the action of the remedy is the solar plexus: symptoms (of presenting complaints) arising in areas influenced by the other chakras will be found to trace their origins back to the solar plexus. Symptoms (and their psychic causes) in the liver, spleen, stomach, pancreas, large and small intestines and the gall bladder may be either present as well or have a history of suppression.

It is useful to quote from *Crystal Power, Crystal Healing* by Michael Gienger (page 382) who outlines **Tiger's Eye** in the following way:

- Spiritually – Tiger's Eye helps us get through difficult phases in life without losing courage. It helps preserve that spark of trust in God that leads us on in dark moments.
- Emotionally – Tiger's Eye helps us to distance ourselves from external influences that may come storming in on us; it mitigates that influence of moods and stressful situations.
- Mentally – Tiger's Eye helps us retain an overall view in complicated, difficult situations and also helps with doubts and difficulties in making decisions.
- Physically – Tiger's Eye has a pain-alleviating effect. It slows down the flow of energy in the body and dampens over-excitation of the nerves and overstimulation of the adrenal glands.

He warns that Tiger's Eye should never be worn for more than a week.

Chakras

Crown

Disturbed dreams of violence or crime can reflect problems held in the lower centres particularly in the sacral and base. Rash reactions and behaviour with hasty decision-making all stemming from a disordered brow and solar plexus can dull the reception of inner spiritual direction. There is real disequilibrium in this remedy and madness is a feature in extreme cases. The madness is often linked to a profoundly damaged sacral centre. Both this chakra and the brow suffer irreparably from the removal of the female organs too early in life.

Brow

When troubled energy in the sacral and solar plexus chakras causes powerfully reactive responses in the brow there is little time for positive thinking or balanced decision-making. Though there is sharp perception here, a canniness that is helpful in tricky situations, there is often no time for wisdom to be brought to bear on emotional reactivity in personal relationships. The consequence of this is that the patient suffers; sometimes is in torment that is felt in the heart. Confusion and woolly-headedness are the aftermath of going with the gut reaction.

Throat
While there is a quick tongue at the service of a quick wit, this centre is often in trouble from not being able to produce the right words in a crisis. Confusion in the brow is matched by stumbling for self-expression.

Heart and thymus
There is much trauma held in this centre from a history of mistaken choices that have left the sacral plexus very damaged either energetically or sometimes physically (though see **Senecio + Tyria** as a complement). There is much blame felt in the heart and patients find it very difficult to let go of the habit of looking for causes of distress outside themselves. Often there is much to blame others for but patients cannot see that they must first change their trick of 'going for the kill' (in those with a fiery energy) or wishing ill towards others (when their energy is less reactive).

Solar plexus
This is the chakra at the core of this remedy. The liver is affected by a constant state of being in conflict; every challenge is a potential conflict where the outcome must be a clear victory over any contrary force that presents itself. The spleen suffers from overweening ambition that obscures a quieter path to a harmonious existence. The pancreas struggles with the effects of lack of peace and joy. All this is likely to stem back to difficult ancestral energy where challenge and conflict were rife.

Sacral
Hysteria in its original sense may rule this centre. Damage from physical violence, sexual perversity, surgical intervention or biochemical abuse may contribute to the problems found in this chakra. Sexual perversion may have been visited on the patient or be the result of having suffered similarly in the past. There is also the possibility of any of this stemming from previous generations in which troubled lives were never able to find any peace and resolution.

Less dramatically, this centre may well have been damaged through too much sexual activity with too many different partners early on in life. This is especially true of those who have sought to compensate for the lack of parental care through promiscuity. There is an empowering hunger for physical gratification (either now or in the past) which can profoundly affect the course of the person's life. This damages this chakra which should be yin and 'giving' in character, like the heart centre, but which becomes yang thus causing the disturbance throughout all the centres.

Base

Childhood trauma involving difficult parentage and too little compassion and love affect the development of this centre. Feeling the threat of the adult world as well as the attraction of it too early can lead to lack of caution, little respect for common-sense advice and the determination to find out for oneself what is 'out there' before having had time to learn basic survival skills. Firm foundations for life do not feature much in this remedy. Though the adrenals are of the base chakra, they are put in the service of the sacral and solar plexus chakras. If this has gone on too long then there is a profound tiredness that betrays adrenal exhaustion even to the point of chronic fatigue.

Case studies

1 'A Jewish woman with a history of dope smoking from her early teens into her 20s now had a new relationship after a broken marriage. She was obsessed with her sexual state; she was unable to experience an orgasm. She also remembered that as a child she had dreams of executing members of her family and of spiders. She had **Ayahuasca** + **Ignatia** + **Syphilinum** 200 (single collective dose). She felt that the remedy was "uncomfortable and marvellous. After taking it I was lying and crying; I had massive sobs; I felt very alone. It was as if I was carrying a heaviness. I made the decision to let it all go. I masturbated and had my first orgasm!" She was then given **Thuja** 50M with **Lac Humanum** 30 weekly (after she had mentioned things from the past). When she returned she complained of a "spinal blockage. My spine is locked in some places and it's completely flexible in others." She then had **Silver**

Fish 1M (once a week). The result was that sex was now hugely better. Shortly after this she had **Syc-co** (which brought on a profuse mucous discharge) and then **Tiger's Eye** 30 twice a week for five weeks. Her period came on time. "I really let go of something. My sacral chakra moved. I felt pain in the whole of my womb area." She felt that she had shifted her intellectual control of her sacral centre. "I let go of putting so much on the orgasm aspect of sex. I'm much lighter. I'm relaxing in that area." Now she had feelings of jealousy. She was given **Ayahuasca + Ignatia + Syphilinum** 10M with **Chalice Well** 30 weekly after which she returned wearing bright-coloured clothing (for the first time) and saying she felt remarkably well. "I have grounded."' **CG**

2 'A woman in her early 40s came for treatment having suffered from stress for a considerable time. She had a history of a variety of traumatic events any one of which would have been enough to call for deep constitutional remedies. She was not given to feeling sorry for herself; she was practical and pragmatic and though there was some bitterness at the emotional treatment she had received from boyfriends in the past and resentment towards her parents, she did not dwell on these as she told her story. She was able to cry at times and felt that this helped when it happened. She wanted to make more of her life than she had so far achieved and she said that she knew that her path had to include more spiritual work on herself. Over a number of years she came sporadically for appointments and received quite a number of deep remedies: **Nat-mur, Lachesis, Calc-carb, Lycopodium, Carcinosin, Oak, Copper Beech** among others. She felt that most, if not all of them had helped her on her journey. When she described her attraction to sadomasochistic sex and mentioned that she had been having visions of mutilated bodies she was given **Tiger's Eye** 10M, once a week for six weeks. On her return she said that she had decided that she could no longer continue with her former way of life, having difficult and sometimes cruelly violent relationships with men. She did not want to be celibate but felt that she had to trust her ability to attract the right kind of relationship in which she could feel nurtured.' **CG**

3 'A student of homoeopathy, a woman in her middle 30s who had recently had her second child, sent the following information after having been prescribed **Tiger's Eye** 30 once a week for six weeks.

"'After the second dose of the remedy I dreamt of having killed people. For my last victim I had to sneak into a house and get a plastic belt to strangle a man. I could see a woman in the next room but she couldn't see me. The wardrobe from which I took the belt was like one I had as a small child. I strangled a tall, bearded middle-aged man. When he was unconscious I stamped on his head with my boot; I could feel my heel go into the flesh of his face. I stuffed him under the desk (the one I have at home). I knew he was not dead but I didn't have time to finish the job. I don't know why I had strangled him; maybe I had been hired (to do it).

"'In the dream I heard the doorbell in the middle of the night. I was asleep in my parents' house and I could hear my mother saying, 'Yes, wait a minute.' I knew it was the police. There were three non-uniform officers and three female psychologists. My father was with them. He was very cheerful as if he had been drinking. I admitted to my mother that they had come for the right person. I told my parents that I had done something really disgusting and that I didn't know why. I told them that I'd stolen £1000 but also that I'd done something far worse and that I would go to prison. Despite protesting that I had been asleep when the crime was committed the three psychologists told me that it made no difference and that I'd have to go to hospital.

"'I was taken away and have a vague memory of security doors and buttons and that people thought that I was dangerous. I had no emotions but it dawned on me that I had no regrets. I had killed in cold blood and I knew that I had a bad side deep down inside me. I was fascinated. I came out into the street and the devil was standing there. He looked quite modern with a black and white car. 'I'll extend your contract until 2002,' he said. I replied, 'You won't get me!' He sent some dark evil spirits over to me and I protected myself with light and said, 'I send you love and light,' and made the sign of the cross. I thought I could feel a friendly angel though I also felt an angel with dark feathers like the angel of death. When I woke up I felt the dream was absolutely real. I felt these evil powers around me so I started praying for protection. I saw that everyone has a bad side which is always in us like germs in the throat. During the dream I remember wondering why I was so cruel. Somebody replied that I had taken too much **Medorrhinum** (in the past).

"'I had this dream while we were in a holiday villa in France. It was a very old house and we slept with the windows open. I felt it was very spooky in the bedroom and I lay awake in shock. I felt apprehensive about taking the third dose of **Tiger's Eye**. I dreamt that I was in bed with a child, a little girl. My mother told me it was OK and that the child had done this before. The child was naked and so was I. I bent over the child to lie on it but when my hair touched the child's body I said, 'I can't do this!' I felt that there was something terribly wrong."

'One week after taking the third dose she dreamt again. "I dreamed that I was in my car. Someone pulled out a machine gun and shot my car to pieces. I tried to hide under the seats but the shots went right through and did hurt [me]. I felt the pain in my sleep."

'The patient had complained of not feeling well since the birth. Her first period since the delivery had just occurred. She was still 'flooding'. She felt overweight though very happy about her new baby. She commented on her periods: "I always find my period is trouble; loads of blood and repression." In her letter with the dreams she also wrote down the physical and emotional reactions she had had to **Tiger's Eye**. "Uterine cramps, quite sharp, almost cutting pain. Coming and going; < in the morning after breakfast. Similar to pains I used to get. I only wanted to sit still. They lasted an hour. I had bleeding at ovulation; not actual bleeding but reddish-tinged discharge. For quite a while I had sneezing often – almost violent and very loud. The sneezing comes up after severe tingling in the nose – it's almost like an allergy. In the morning I get a lot of gelatinous discharge (nasal) and sometimes it's < when I change environment from indoors to outdoors. I didn't feel PMS while I was with my friends but very much so when I was coping with a business partner. I am very dictatorial, very critical and demanding [but he was] very condescending towards me and I felt like a little girl again and made small by my father. I had suicidal thoughts which I had not had for a long time. I know I have to take responsibility for myself and let my husband do what he wants to do. I think that I am on the right track. There was no reaction to the last two doses of the remedy, by the way."' JM

34

TUNBRIDGE WELLS WATER

The remedy was proved by two meditation groups: by the staff of the Helios Pharmacy, Tunbridge Wells, on 20 May 1995 and students of the Guild of Homoeopaths' graduate course on 15 March 1997 when the 6th potency was taken. The original idea for the remedy came from the staff at the Helios Pharmacy. They all convened at the spring in the Pantiles. They visited the local exhibition 'A Day at the Wells' to obtain a feel for the town before returning to the pharmacy. A short meditation was held to focus the minds of those involved and the remedy was potentized up to the 40th potency in small groups. Any sensations or thoughts experienced during this time and shortly afterwards were recorded and later collated to produce their remedy picture. The following is based on the article on **Tunbridge Wells Water** by Sue Palmer published in *Prometheus*, the journal of the Guild of Homoeopaths (No. 11, December 1999) and the transcript of the meditative proving by the students of the Guild course.

The Background

Tunbridge Wells is a spa town in south-east England; the waters of the spa were used from Roman times and the town was popular up until the Regency period when it began to lose favour after Brighton, on the south coast, became more fashionable. In 1606 it was recorded that Dudley, Lord North, first discovered the value of the chalybeate springs when it was reported that he had been entirely cured of 'the lingering consumptive order he laboured under'. The water then gained a considerable reputation for healing 'cold chronical distempers, weak nerves and bad digestion'. The Lord's own physician stated that the water contained 'vitriol' and that drinking it would cure 'the colic, the melancholy and the vapours; it made the lean, fat and the fat, lean; it killed flat worms in the belly, loosened the clammy humours of the body and dried the over-moist brain'. The doctor must have fancied himself something of a poet as he penned the following doggerel,

> These waters youth in age renew
> Strength to the weak and sickly add
> Give the pale cheek a rosy hue
> And cheerful spirits to the sad.

The town became a rival to Bath for a time due to the patronage of various queens of the 17th century. Lord Boyle, who visited the town in 1728, wrote, however, that most visitors were there to follow and slavishly imitate the members of the royal family who still frequented the place; he added that 'I believe these renowned wells are not of any great use. We are ordered down here commonly pour la Maladie Imaginaire, for the spirits and the melancholy to which our whole Nation are too subject. The Diversions and Amusements of the Place send us home again cheerful and the foggy Air of London with the common Disappointments of Life urge our Return the following Year. The Water has a brackish taste never palatable.'

The mineral waters are chalybeate; they are ferruginous which means that they contain salts of iron. The word 'chalybeate' is derived from the Latin for steel, '*chalybs*' which is in turn taken from the Greek, '*khalups*'; Chalybes were mythical people who lived on Mount Ida in Asia Minor who had invented methods of working with iron. Apart from iron carbonate ($FeCO_3$), the water also contains manganese carbonate ($MnCO_3$), calcium sulphate ($CaSO_4$), magnesium sulphate ($MgSO_4$), magnesium chloride ($MgCl_2$), sodium chloride (NaCl) and potassium chloride (KCl). (The proving shows that each of these chemicals has homoeo-pathic echoes in the mental and emotional aspects of the remedy.)

Thomas Sydenham, famous physician of the 18th century, prescribed chalybeate waters as a cure for hysteria. Queen Victoria, before she ascended the throne, visited Tunbridge Wells in order to imbibe the mineral waters in 1834.[50]

---

50 In our own time the water is distinctly suspect as a source of health enhancement and has anyway dwindled to a trickle partly due, probably, to the large numbers of trees that have grown up above the springs.

Keynote effects

The remedy covers the loss of power; the loss of power on the physical, mental and emotional levels all from a state of repression. The main effect is gradually to lift this pall of repression and consequent weakness when the negativity comes from social conformity and the fear of being judged; the need to join the rat race in order to achieve; the breakdown of relationships between generations; long sufferance of being servile in hopeless situations.

General symptoms

Pre-eminently a liver and spleen remedy; cleanses and balances the energies of the solar plexus. Gall stones and toxicity in the liver. Diseases of the pancreas. Bowel diseases as a consequence of liver disease: irritable bowel; Crohn's disease; pyloric stenosis; jaundice. Putrid states. Occurs in patients who have cancer or AIDS; the pains of abdominal cancer with vomiting. Intestinal worms. Very poor nutritional state: lack of assimilation and proper absorption. Excessive acidity; ulceration of the alimentary canal. Gangrene. Poor circulation with sluggish portal system; poor oxygenation. Heart pathology with palpitations and oedema; water retention. Toxicity induced by chemotherapy (and radiotherapy). Rheumatoid arthritis with distortion of joints. Allergies and candida. Skin conditions: leprosy, eczema, psoriasis, icthyosis. Tubercular conditions of the lungs: asthma and sequelae of pneumonia especially where the liver fails to cleanse the system. Lymph system is overtaxed leading to recurrent glandular fever or ME. Poor nutritional state with little assimilation. Flushes of heat with feelings of panic. Useful after traumatic accidents where the patient appears not to be fully centred back in the body; complements **Arnica**. This out-of-body state also happens after extensive allopathic treatment using drugs and surgery or after transplants.

Miasms

Cancer and syphilis.

Mental and emotional symptoms

Desolation and grief; almost without exception, the provers reported these feelings. Silent or dumb grief and sadness. Emotionally crushed. Sense of hopelessness and despair. Panic attacks: with palpitations and fear felt in the solar plexus. Fearful but finds it difficult to explain why. Feels outcast and is unable to make eye contact; ashamed of oneself. Feels separated from society or friends by the condition; feels isolated. Uncomplaining; may be unaware of how ill they really are. The more serious the condition, the less complaining they become. (Carers get the sense that the patient does not want to get better.) Patient sabotages own treatment; by antidoting or not taking the remedies or by nullifying common-sense advice on nutrition and self-help by going too far down the conventional medicine trail. Strong desire to conform to rules; fastidious in observing regulations. Feel embarrassed and uncomfortable if they are seen to be breaking the rules. Adhering to rules gives them a sense of structure they otherwise lack. Yet paradoxically may become rebellious with a strong desire to break the rules; to indulge; to have an affair; to become reckless. Promiscuity from the need to buck the family trend. They present a proper and correct mask of politeness but this can hide deceit. They conceal whatever is ugly or considered unnatural so that they are cut off from their true emotions. Self-disgust and self-loathing. Fear of intimate relationships especially between men and women. Men can feel intimidated by women's power. Refuses or avoids counselling; shies away from looking into original causes. Disease states that seem rooted in the breakdown of relationship between the child and a parent; schism between generations.

Suppressed anger especially within the sphere of relationships. Unresolved anger and bitterness between mother or father and child. Strong reluctance to speak of their own emotional issues on a deep level though there may be a compassion and understanding for others. (Of use in patients who are carers for the very ill or handicapped but whose purpose, paradoxically, is coloured by the need to be with terminally ill or hopeless and helpless people.) Prefers to be alone; does not make friends easily or does so among people who are equally emotionally handicapped. Sense of being observed. Seeks anonymity; if they cannot be alone then they prefer to be with the crowd. Apathetic and selfish; can't be bothered attitude. Nostalgic and old-fashioned. Poor concentration; mind is 'fuzzy'. Cold and unfeeling; lacks sympathy. Mood swings: wants to be full of fun and laughter but then 'dries up' and loses the will to make the effort. Complains of lack of motivation; of being stuck. Feels powerless to make positive changes. If there is an essence to the picture of TWW then it is schism or a separation which is so seemingly impossible to bridge that there is not enough will power to attempt to heal the rift, leaving the subject little apparent choice but to accept negativity and illness: it is too difficult to get better, as that would entail dealing with deep emotional issues too awful to contemplate. One has the sense that the patient has lost hope of making connections with either the past or past relationships or with present vitality.

Physical symptoms

Head

Bilious headache; < frontal region. Migraines: < forehead and into eyes with visual disturbances. Piercing pains with background dull ache with nausea and vomiting. Hair falls out; < chemo- and radiotherapy. Eruptions on the scalp: scaly and flaking with tendency to suppurate; eczema with intolerable itching = need to scratch till it bleeds. Cradle cap.

Eyes

Prefers to avoid sunlight; photophobic. Gummy eyes: thick discharge in the morning but dry eye syndrome for the rest of the time. Wants to shade the eyes as they get red and sore in the wind and bright light. (No problem with electric light.) Floaters. Cataracts. Corneal ulcers.

Ears

Eczema on the outer ear with weeping cracks: smelly, yellow exudate. Crusting in the meatus of the ear with itching and bleeding after scratching.

Nose

Acute sense of smell but pleasant things smell repulsive. Ethmoid sinus may become blocked and distort the sense of smell causing things to seem putrid.

Mouth

Bad taste with a furred tongue. Tongue is discoloured: brown or dirty green; papillae are distorted and can have the appearance of seaweed (at the back of the tongue). Dryness and thirst for water but drinks less than wants to because of water retention. Yellowish deposit on fauces. Foul breath.

Throat

Dryness with irritating cough. Unable to expectorate slimy mucus that sits in the throat pit. Claggy, yellow mucus which is thick and glutinous. Voice is easily strained.

Respiration and chest

Difficult to breathe deeply or into the abdomen. Restricted breathing due to heaviness in the chest especially around the heart area. Heart pounds with anxiety. Cardiac asthma. Angina pectoris. Thick mucous expectoration from deep in the lungs: difficult to hawk up and < cough which can be painful and which < liver and bowel symptoms. Pains under either scapula from tension in diaphragm and tight breathing and coughing. Breathing is > at night especially if bowel symptoms are < then.

Stomach

Extreme nausea with vomiting (useful during chemotherapy when **Ipecac** and **Cadmium-sulph** are insufficient). Stomach feels full and heavy; < after drinking water or taking liquid foods. Acidity: heartburn and waterbrash. Belching with burning in the oesophagus. Needs to eat little and infrequently but < hunger and << overeating. < dairy products but wants milk which <. Hot water > but only after a while. Can feel swashing in the stomach. Fear and tension felt in the stomach with pains that extend round or through to the back; pains in the cardiac sphincter area < palpitations.

Abdomen

Bloating and distension; abdomen feels unbearably heavy and loaded < a short while after a meal. Sensation of a tight band around the diaphragm with gall stones. Colic: has to bend double but pressure < so becomes restless and writhes with the pain. Feels blocked up and constipated; ileo-caecal valve becomes tender and blocked. Urge to pass stool but with no result. Foul diarrhoea passed with urgency but then followed by sense of fullness in the sigmoid flexure. Anal prolapse with waterlogged tissue of the mucous membranes. Passes blood with stools and mucus. Burning sensations in the descending colon. Constipation and diarrhoea alternate. Spleen is swollen and tender as a consequence of liver disorders. Patient tends to cradle the left side of the abdomen but is not able to bear any pressure on the right side. Always prefers loose clothing. Pot belly: she complains of feeling six-months pregnant. Jaundice: especially in small babies; become emaciated with bloated bellies. Pains: < right to left.

Female

Pains in the ovaries < Right. Abdominal symptoms all < before menses. Period pains become difficult to distinguish with bowel pains. Uterus feels swollen.

Period discharge is thick and dark and alternates with a watery leucorrhoea. Menses is clotted and can smell rotten. Herpetic eruptions in pubic area: dry and scaly with itching and soreness. Yeasty discharge: candida. Water retention < before the period; water mostly held in the abdomen but may also be in the hands and feet.

Male
Eczema of the external genitalia: sore, scaly and itching; skin becomes red and swollen. Sexual desire only felt for those beyond their reach which may encompass incestuous feelings (cf. **Nat-fluor**).

Urinary organs
Frequent urination especially at night. Bladder responds to the abdominal pressure so little is passed but urging quickly returns. Urine tests show no sign of bacterial changes. Aching in the kidneys with water retention.

Skin
Poor skin tone and discoloration: can be roughened and dry or yellowish, reddish or very sickly pale. Eczema: dry, scaly and itching with a tendency to suppurate. Ulceration with very slow healing. Ulcers suppurate with crusts that slough off revealing foul and even gangrenous-looking pus. White scales that might be seen in psoriasis or icthyosis. Heavy cradle cap that resists all other treatment. Itching but without eruption; < in liver conditions. Itching in patients who have a history of jaundice and grief (a good sign if it has occurred after other remedies). Flushes of heat with palpitations which then leave the patient cold and pale. Pustular acne and painful boils < face; neck.

Neck and back
Cannot stand or sit upright; has neither the strength nor the will power to maintain an upright posture. Neck and shoulders are stiff and achy; spine is tender and sensitive. Back feels weak and needs support yet abdominal symptoms feel > for not slouching. Pustular acne; scarring.

Extremities
Rheumatoid arthritis with distorted joints which become inflamed and painful especially < after suppressed anger from a failed relationship. Gout: < hands and feet with severe headaches; part goes deep red and has severe, sharp,

sticking pains with the swelling which may well not be of a uniformly round shape. Numbness of limbs with poor circulation.

Sleep
Frequent waking from urge to pass water or from nausea. Abdominal rumbling which prevents restful sleep. Dreams of being pursued but unable ever to see the pursuer; of fear with waking afraid; of being underground or buried alive; of arguing with someone who is breaking the rules; of anger after breaking rules; of bad weather, rioting and threatened violence. Heat in bed alternating with chilliness.

Considerations for the use of the remedy

As iron is such an important constituent of **Tunbridge Wells Water** it is worth quoting Clarke's opening words on **Ferrum Metallicum** in the *Dictionary of Materia Medica:*

> Ferrum, the Mars of the alchemists, is one of the prominent constituents of the animal body, being present in considerable quantity in the blood. It is present in many articles of daily food and, when given in excess to men or animals, its first effect is to increase the amount of iron in the blood, stimulate the appetite, augment the heart's beats and the bodily vigour. The secondary effects which ensue sooner or later if the administration of iron is continued, are those which give the indications for homoeopathic prescribing. Hahnemann describes the effects of iron on persons who habitually drink chalybeate waters: 'In such localities there are few persons who can resist the noxious influences of the continued use of such waters and remain well, each being affected according to his peculiar nature. There we find more than anywhere else, chronic affections of great gravity and peculiar character even when the regimen is otherwise faultless. Weakness almost amounting to paralysis of the whole body and of single parts, some kinds of violent limb pains, abdominal affections of various sorts, vomiting of food by day or by night, phthisical pulmonary ailments often with blood spitting, deficient vital warmth, suppression of the menses, miscarriages, impotence in both sexes, sterility, jaundice and many other rare cachexias are common occurrences.'

Clarke goes on to say that 'Iron is what may be called a "nutritive" remedy in certain defective blood conditions having an organopathic relation to the blood . . . in the anaemia of cancer and syphilis it is often of great service as an accessory and need not interfere with more specific remedies.' (That is **Ferrum** may be homoeopathic to the condition of the blood in a patient whose general condition might indicate some other similimum though Clarke warns that **Ferrum** 'is not suited to all cases of anaemia and chlorosis or even a majority of them and should never be given without discrimination and careful watching'.) Furthermore, he notes that **Ferrum** is somewhat like a cross between **Arsen-alb** and **China** in its excessive irritability of both mind and tissues which is also relevant to **Tunbridge Wells Water.**

The most obvious remedy with which to compare this one is **Berlin Wall** which is indicated in those who suffer from depression, repression, suppression and oppression. However, though both are syphilitic, **Berlin Wall** is not so noted for physical toxicity in the liver nor does it have the problem of needing to conform.

Anacardium is also worth considering as it suffers from mental conflict equally strongly as **TWW**. **Anacardium** is more to do with feeling like a square peg in a round hole and unworthy of filling the shoes of others who are admirable in some way. It is full of hidden wishful thinking not on forbidden things but on ambition; they are confused and led astray by hopes that they cannot truly fulfil. It is aware of and can appreciate qualities in others to which it aspires but has no gift to achieve. **TWW** may well be capable of achieving what it aspires to but cannot because of being hobbled by its constraints.

Arsen-alb, Calc-carb, Lyc, Nat-mur, Sepia, China, Pyrogen, Arnica, Syph, Tub-bov and **Aids Nosode** all act as intercurrents and follow well where indicated. **TWW** can be given as a liver drainage remedy in low 6x or 12x potency in support of any of the above.

Esoteric therapeutics

The brow centre is much affected in this remedy: there is a constant conflict between the inner child, the aspect of the person that never really had a chance to finish their early development, and the adult, the aspect that is ill at ease and unfit for coping with the adult world around. The struggle even seems to threaten a fear of madness.

Chakras

Crown
Disturbed sleep from difficult dreams. Spiritual awareness is made less likely by the schism felt emotionally and the disturbance to the brow centre.

Brow
This centre is disturbed by imposed moral criteria either from a parental source or as a result of restriction due to personal traumatic experience. Learned behaviour and attitude patterns restrict original thinking and cause imbalance between the ego and the intuition. Intuitive thinking may be entirely absent. Lack of freedom in the field of thought. Too much self-judgement and little mercy on oneself. Confusion leads to stomach or menstrual disorders.

Throat
Lack of self-expression from the suppression of the spontaneous. Constraint due to conforming has led to a complete lack of creativity.

Heart
Sadness and grief from imposing excessive degrees of control on the mind and emotions. Strong desire to break free and rebel which is usually kept under a tight rein. May take to drinking alcohol in excess in order not to feel the constraint in this centre.

Solar plexus
Conformity has led to suppression of the will; this causes much stress in the liver and gall bladder both of which interfere with the smooth running of this chakra. The ability to deal with challenges is complicated by the confusion in the brow centre. The lack of aspiration causes the spleen to suffer which in turn leads to stomach upsets and bowel problems. There is fearfulness in this chakra causing a tendency to feel nausea or loss of appetite.

Sacral
Generative organs are affected by loss of power over one's destiny. Any form of pathology here may be traced back to difficulties between the generations. Disgust may be a strong sense focused on this chakra.

Base

Fear and lack of security are the main impediments for solid grounding. These problems can be stronger in their influence on the organism than the grief and disappointment held in the heart. Fear is the chief factor in causing the patient to take evasive action instead of confronting problems head-on. The central nervous system may be affected by trembling or excessive reaction to being startled. The musculoskeletal system and the immune system are weakened by poor nutrition and being unfit generally.

Case studies

1   'A 30-year-old woman came to see me in 2006. Her presenting symptoms were irritability with her husband and children. Her periods had stopped. Her libido was non-existent. She said that she alternated between being depressed and angry. She said she had differences of opinion with her husband about money: he said she spent too much and she thinks that he is just "tight". She was very abrupt and during the consultation said she had had a good and happy childhood; she was the middle child from an affluent family. I felt that she was holding a lot in.

'She told me that she had had an abortion early in their marriage because at the time her husband had just found out that his father had Huntington's Chorea. Her husband was having tests done and they did not want to risk any children having it. She said she felt resentful of this especially when her husband was found to be clear of the gene.

They have two children and although she has always found it very hard to cope with being at home with them and gets very angry, shouting a lot at them, she still feels she would like another baby to replace the one she lost.

'She had various remedies over the following months which included **Sepia, Medorrhinum, Oak** and **White Chestnut.** She was eventually given **Nat-mur** and **Rose Quartz** but there was a sense that she wasn't telling the whole story and it was difficult to get to the bottom of the anger. At the consultation following the **Nat-mur** 10M she told me [something] that she had never told anyone because she was too ashamed to admit it: her mother was an alcoholic and had been ever since her younger brother had been born. This had put a lot of pressure on her during her schooldays and while growing up as she could never invite anyone home and was always making up stories to cover up. She had a reasonable relationship with her father but never felt that she was good enough or achieved enough to please him.

'I gave her **Tunbridge Wells Water** 30 and **Agnus Castus** Ø. The whole case opened up. Not only did she have her first period for over a year but she became more emotional for a while and the anger started to get a lot less. She continued to take **Tunbridge Wells Water** in ascending doses over the next few months and it turned the whole case around. She had talks with her dad and her mum; she became more accepting of her mother's alcoholism, realizing that it was not her fault. She had been able to talk to friends more and became generally much more outgoing. Since then she has worked through many more issues requiring other remedies but on occasions she has had more **TWW** when it has been necessary. I feel that **TWW** was the remedy that really made her stop having to keep up appearances and made her soften up a lot.' JL

NB When I contacted JL about the ascending potencies used in this case she sent the following email: 'The TWW case started with 30s twice weekly and went up to 10M eventually but it was interesting that it was the 30 that had such a good effect not only on her periods but mentally and emotionally, opening up a very closed case.' CG

2   'Man, 47, born in Scorpio, had had constitutional and acute treatment for psychological, heart and digestive complaints for some years. On this occasion he came having been in hospital for a kidney stone which he had managed to pass by himself after taking **Dioscorea** 200. He needed **Arnica** 1M and **Berberis** 6x on a daily basis to recover from this. He then returned to his usual theme of his bowels: he suffered from loose bowels each working day. As soon as he got halfway to work in the car he would get griping and the urge to pass a motion and be in fear that he would not reach a lavatory in time. At the weekend "everything seems to shut down". He enjoyed his employment and was good at it. What he felt anxious about in the car was getting stuck in traffic.

'He had a history of an extremely traumatic breakdown of his first marriage in which he felt devastated, humiliated and fearful. His first wife, an erstwhile patient, had had a clear picture of **Lachesis**. She had been considerably older than him and their marriage had caused a rift between him and his mother and brother. He was always excessively sensitive and fearful particularly about his health and emotional stability. When he had cleared the last of the residual symptoms in his kidney and back he took **Tunbridge Wells Water** 100: one each week for six weeks.

'On his return he said that the pattern had changed: the only day of the week on which he had a bowel problem was Monday when he would still get griping on the way to work. He had also had a severe itch that appeared without any eruption down his right flank. (The kidney pain had been on the right.) Shortly after that he broke out in eczema which has periodically flared up in acute episodes. He is far less fearful and has become more philosophical about symptoms he knows stem from his nervous disposition. What has never returned is the permanent bowel problem with the loose and explosive stools.' **CG**

3   'A physiotherapist, retired due to chronic fatigue syndrome, continued to come for treatment for her various ailments. These included persistent constipation, painful periods, thrush and cystitis and a very nervous disposition. She was in her 40th year when she began coming ten years ago. She recognized that her biggest problem was that she felt 'stuck'. She was intolerant of dairy and gluten and got typical **Lycopodium** symptoms if she indulged in these. She had to use laxatives though she preferred to rely on linseed. Her constipation was worse towards the middle of her cycle when she tended to bloat despite careful eating. She retained water and suffered bouts of colicky pains in the abdomen. Her stools were very hard when she was constipated; she had episodes of no urging whatever. She admitted to feeling melancholic and that it did not take much to make her feel sad. Even beautiful things made her feel sad. She had suffered a lot while at college and had a history of sore throats and swollen glands; a test for glandular fever had proved negative. She loved her parents but they had caused her "difficulties". Over the years she had done well on **Carcinosin**, **Pulsatilla**, **Tuberculinum**, **Lycopodium**, **Anacardium** and **Silica**. She had reacted very strongly to **Clay** but it had brightened her view of life. She felt that cranial osteopathy suited her very well and complemented the remedies. Nevertheless, the

constipation persisted. Then one day she described her concerns about her mother who was unwell. She explained that there was probably nothing much the matter with her but that she had always had a difficult time with her. Her parents matched each other well but they had argued all the time and she always felt distressed by it. She felt at odds with her parents. She was given **Tunbridge Wells Water** 30: one each week for three weeks. The result was good in that within a few days of the first dose she passed a motion consisting almost entirely of congealed and thickened mucus. "It was like mucus membrane." She now suffered far less from the constipation though "My time is mid-morning. If I miss that time then it doesn't happen in the rest of the day." Her periods were also much better with less pain and no dip in mood. She was then given **TWW** 100. When she returned she said she was doing well. She still had sluggish bowels and trapped wind but she was still eating small amounts of bread. She had far more energy and was doing more though careful to pace herself. She was getting more sinus congestion and still had water retention in her abdomen around the period. She confessed to drinking three coffees each day. She was sent off with **TWW** 100 to be taken each week for eight weeks and she promised to try and dispense with the coffee as she knew it might be affecting the remedy. Subsequently she required further remedies, the need for which was triggered by the various events and changes that continued to happen in her life including her mother's death, her husband's redundancy and whatever emotional issues became manifest after craniosacral treatment. The constipation eventually succumbed over time to the influence of **Alumina** 200, **Opium** 24 given daily for a while, **Ruby** 200 and intercurrent doses of her standby remedy, **Lycopodium**. However, it was the **Tunbridge Wells Water** that first improved her general energy levels and began the process of change in the digestive tract and to the hormones. After the first doses she never returned again to the extremity of poor energy that she suffered when the chronic fatigue was at its worst.' **CG**

35

TURQUOISE

The remedy was proved on 6 June 1997 by students on the postgraduate Guild of Homoeopaths' course.

The Background

Turquoise belongs to the phosphorus class of minerals and its chemical formula suggests just how complex a stone it is: $CuAl_6 (PO_4)_4(OH)_{8.4}H_2O$. It is hydrated phosphate of copper and aluminium. It occurs in rare crystals which are minute, cryptocrystalline masses, stalactites, veins and crusts. It varies in colour from pale blue to sky blue or greeny blue or even apple green. The masses have a waxy smooth surface. The principle places where it is mined are in Iran and in the United States. It is discovered in places where 'it has been deposited by surface waters in cracks and cavities in alumina-rich extrusive rocks in arid regions, together with phosphates, chalcedony and limonite'.[51] The hardness of turquoise varies from between 2.7 and 5 or 6 on Mohs' scale. This is due to the grain size of the crystalline aggregate.[52] It is also worth noting that turquoise as a gemstone is subject to considerable interference from traders who treat it in order to give it deeper colour. It may be impregnated with paraffin to darken it and make it easier to polish. A cherished example may turn out to be entirely synthetic; it may be made of ceramic material, glass, plastic or artificially coloured rock.

Turquoise was so named because it was in Turkey that European crusaders first set eyes on it though it was also traded by merchants of the Levant. It was known to the ancient Egyptians several thousand years before. It has long been

51 *Simon and Schuster's Guide to Gems and Precious Stones*
52 Ibid.

valued and revered in history as a stone for both healing and protection. Every previous great civilization has found in it a medicinal stone for the eyes and a charm against accidents (either to the eyes or through falls from horseback). It is first mentioned by name in the 13th century as a protector of the eyes against accidents. Middle Eastern peoples also used turquoise with their pack animals, camels, horses and mules. Any rider or driver carrying a stone would believe that it protected him from injury if an accident should befall him or his animal; the stone would absorb the physical shock and leave the master and beast free from hurt. It was also regarded as a powerful aid to the direction of the will when aiming counteroffensives against harmful forces and as a protective device against overwhelming odds. Thus, also, the American Pueblo and Apache Indians attached pieces of turquoise to their arrows to ensure accurate aim. It was claimed to heal cataracts and was particularly favoured by Arab Muslims for this purpose. Tradition tells us that the stone is able to warn the wearer of hidden danger. Turquoise was a stone protective not only of the physical body but also the spirit and it was deemed to be a guard against the 'evil eye'. It was regarded as a stone of dreams, philosophy and religion and it assisted those who underwent a spiritual journey to resist the blandishments of material life. It prevented weaknesses from becoming vices.

Judy Hall, in the *Encyclopaedia of Crystals*, says that turquoise is 'a powerful energy conduit, it releases old vows, inhibitions and prohibitions, dissolves a martyred attitude or self-sabotage and allows the soul to express itself once more. Turquoise shows how the creation of our fate depends on what we do at each moment.' Other writers have stated that it is a stone to encourage spiritual attunement; it is a healer of the spirit bringing calm and tranquillity to the mind. It is said to be associated with Sagittarius, Pisces and Scorpio.

A curious sidelight on this stone is that it has always been known to be both susceptible to the changes of weather and likely to change colour when the owner or wearer is either in danger or profoundly ill. There have been written reports of those who have died leaving a stone that has faded with the illness and demise of its owner. Turquoise should mature to its natural colour in daylight which is lighter than the blue-green that it is when it is mined from the rock.

Keynote effects

Releases pent-up emotion from the throat centre thus releasing negative energy from the heart centre. It is a remedy for enhancing the energy of the voice when there has been suppressed expression.

General symptoms

Works primarily on the throat, thymus and heart centres; secondarily on the sacral centre and on the base. Thyrotoxicosis. Globus hystericus. Multi-miasmatic but also tubercular and sycotic. Excessive production of mucus especially in the throat and upper respiratory tract. Alteration in body temperature: heat without fever. Heat in the head or in the extremities. Palpitations and panic attacks. Nervousness felt in the heart area. Hyperactivity. Swelling and pains of the extremities. Right-sided symptoms. Heat with itching. Heat with sweating. Protective of the physical body from pollution: radioactive, petro-chemical and miasmatic. Anorexia. Menopausal symptoms including fibroids and hot flushes. Tumours: brain < from radiation.

Miasms

Psora, tuberculosis, sycosis and cancer.

Mental and emotional symptoms

Strong fear of death. Panic and agitation. Deep sadness: a desire to cry with a reluctance to talk. Feels 'frightened and drowning in sadness'. Great fear of being alone. Either very loquacious or not given to talking much at all, especially about the self. If talkative then tends to be superficial or evasive, avoiding difficult emotional areas. Very busy to mask the need to talk about and resolve deep emotional issues. Skirts round controversial issues to avoid emotional conflicts. Suppressed sexual desires; lack of sexual expression. Helpful for those who have found sexual activity to be nothing much more than biology. Encourages the unifying expression of sexual love; in expressing the energy of the sacral chakra they can later release the energy of the throat centre. Feeling as if rendered speechless. Deep hurt that leaves the person feeling bereft of words. Can be tentative, timid, weak (morally) and vulnerable. The remedy encourages such positive attributes as feelings of being supported; of greater strength from replenished resources; of more intuition (wisdom); of patience and gentleness. As anxiety or grief lift these are replaced by joy and expansiveness. Has a greater sense of knowing which way to go. Has a greater sense of determination and even urgency. Is more able to finish what has been begun. Those who felt lost now feel as though they have found themselves. Changes the perspective of those who are in denial or who seem to be running away from something.

Physical symptoms

Head
Heat especially in the face.

Eyes
Heat and smarting; prickling and watering. Wants to keep eyes open to prevent pain. Cataract.

Nose
Postnasal drip.

Throat
Thyrotoxicosis. Thyroid feels swollen and heavy. Constriction around the neck. Globus hystericus. Voice control is impaired. Dysphagia. Mucous congestion.

Chest
Difficulty breathing in states of heightened emotion.

Heart
Palpitations. Nervous sensations in heart region. Panic attacks with palpitations. Sensation of a pounding heart after stress. 'Nervous' heart.

Abdomen
Sensation of emptiness in the womb of emotional origin.

Female

Loss of libido. Menopausal symptoms: hot flushes; fibroids. Sensation of emptiness in the womb. Helps to lift the physical aspect of sex onto a finer level of esoteric vibration.

Extremities

Stiffness < right side. Swelling of hands. Sensation of puffiness. Heat in the feet.

Considerations for the use of the remedy

There are a number of remedies that should be compared:

- **Ignatia** covers similar throat symptoms though it is more passionate and potentially noisier in its reactions than **Turquoise**.
- **Nat-mur** is differentiated by its modalities, taste for savoury and salt and by its more urgent thirst, none of which are particularly marked in **Turquoise** which, nevertheless, follows extremely well after this or either of the other two salt remedies.
- **Lachesis** has a strong fear of death but it is far more voluble and overtly confused than **Turquoise**. The throat symptoms are more urgent and threatening in **Lachesis** and it is far more toxic. **Turquoise** follows well in cases where **Lachesis** has not unlocked the emotional problems underlying the case.
- **Calc-carb** has just as strong a sense of death and loss, is just as much a noted remedy in thyroid pathology and as easily confused or lacking in focus as **Turquoise** but it is usually a chillier remedy. However, **Calc-carb** is very often the constitutional state that underlies a **Turquoise** state.
- **Phosphorus** is another constitution that may go into a **Turquoise** picture and the patient may have the slight and less than substantial frame and physical appearance of this remedy.
- **Peridot** is another heart-stricken remedy but it does not have the same emphasis on the throat centre as a focus for pathology and it is more threatened at the level of the wounded ego.
- **Green Jade** is decidedly a rival with **Turquoise** in the throat centre and in thyroid pathology but it is more affected by any turmoil that would upset routines, more stubborn because more strongly defended and

less sensitive to emotional pressure as it is so well defended, while **Turquoise** is generally sensitive in the manner associated with **Phosphorus**.

Turquoise has been known to be well supported by **White Chestnut Flower** in cases where there has been damage to the sacral centre. **Oak** may well be called for to follow on from **Turquoise** in a case where there are no indications for **Calc-carb** or **Phos**. Either **Blue** or **Green** are complementary when indications show similarities to one or other of these two colour remedies.

Esoteric therapeutics

It is a remedy of great peace, power and protection. It is protective of those going through any traumatic experience (and it helps to draw karmic resolution out of such experiences). It enhances the energies of the individual chakras as they are released to work on negativity whether in the form of toxicity, emotional turmoil or spiritual or psychic attack. It realigns the meridians and, like **Purple** and **Amethyst**, encourages the downward spreading flow of energy from the crown centre and subtle bodies into the lower, physical body. The stone protects the aura particularly from the damage caused by drugs (either recreational or allopathic) and from radioactivity. It can awaken a person to the danger they place themselves in by using such substances. It is useful in those patients who have any underlying fear or fears that would, if released, feel as if they might be destructive. The remedy lets the fear rise to the surface safely to be expressed harmlessly but curatively from the throat centre. So it is regarded as a vital remedy for those who hold deeply entrenched fear. (Consider it for those who cannot sing or who choke easily or in those old **Nat-mur** cases which seem never to budge.) This remedy deals more effectively than **Nat-mur** does with cases of suppressed shock to the heart and throat centres. It allows the expression of the hurt to come out without anger or resentment but with clarity of understanding and acceptance. This remedy is excellent for the communication of the truth. Promotes moral and spiritual courage. It is useful for public speakers as it enhances fluency and clarity of expression as well as protection of the throat centre which can quickly become exhausted with overuse of the voice. This stone can also awaken the thymus centre to healing energies but in a safe mode. (Hence, **Turquoise** can be a complementary support to remedies such as **Berlin Wall**, **Chalice Well**, **Jet**, **Thymus Gland**

and **Syphilinum.**) Also helps to foster intuition. Clarifies those cases where there is lack of direction or even of any movement at all due to mixed miasmatic inheritance. Works well in support of the nosodes especially **Tuberculinum**. A remedy to consider for the passage through birth and death.

As a homoeopathic influence on the patient it is a remedy for the voicing of the heart and mind. It is often needed in those who have something very decisive and decided to say about emotional issues that for one reason or another have never found any expression. With this lack of vocalizing of what lies in the chakras above and below the throat, there grows a latent fear that is to do with a fundamental lack of security. The patient feels unsafe to use the voice for what he or she has to say. It is also a remedy that provides a degree of protection to those who are going through any form of long-drawn-out trauma especially one during which little is voiced but much is stored up in the mind and the heart.

Chakras

Crown
The remedy is one to foster truthful receiving of spiritual guidance. A sense of clarity and tranquillity settles into this chakra.

Brow
Truth is the keynote in this centre. For a long time the patient may have held back from saying what needs to be said for fear that the truth would be painful and damaging. Intuition is enhanced so that there is a better awareness of how and when what needs to be said, should be delivered to those who need to hear it.

Throat
Much trauma and grief is prevented from being expressed properly through this centre because of fear. It is of great value in those who have often needed **Ignatia** in acute prescribing or **Nat-mur** for constitutional reasons but where the results have had only partial success. The same can also be true of those who have needed **Lachesis**; these are the **Lachesis** cases of people who do not fit the typically venomous constitutional picture but who have attributes of **Lachesis** that leave room for considering other remedies.

Heart

Deep grief suffuses the aura of the heart especially when it is associated with fear of hurting others that would cause a sense of loss. 'Loss' is a strong theme in this centre especially in those who have Scorpio strongly in their astrological chart. The fear of death is also concerned with 'loss'. When the throat is finally able to voice the trauma it is done without anger or resentment.

Solar plexus

The remedy aids stomach qi as it assists discrimination in the brow centre. When descending qi is faulty due to 'swallowed' emotions and especially when there is rising fire in the form of acidity, **Turquoise** will ease trouble in this chakra if there are other indications for it.

Sacral

Confusion and congestion occupy this centre especially when the cause for needing the remedy lies in love relationships. As a sycotic remedy, mucus congestion, thickening of tissue and water retention may well be part of the overall picture.

Base

Poor grounding as distress in the heart, throat and head contribute to lack of awareness about what is real or unreal, what should be revealed and what may be kept back or ought to be kept back and what would be of benefit to others and what would be a release for the self. Fear, too, causes great stress to this centre; hypochondriasis. May be of help in those cases where it is not certain whether the tubercular or sycotic miasm is uppermost; after **Turquoise** this may become evident. Assists the patient to become much clearer about their own position, condition, situation by relieving them of the tendency to be negatively introspective.

Case studies

1 'Woman in her early 60s who had been thoroughly browbeaten by her first husband came for treatment because of difficulty with her throat. She found it difficult to swallow, often had to clear her throat of phlegm

and felt a sense of constriction. Despite being a quietly spoken and thoughtful person who was rather timid, she had been given **Lachesis** on previous occasions which had helped rather than not though had not cleared the condition. She was not overtly afraid of anything though she gave off a sense of anxiety; this being despite the fact that she had recently married for a second time and was very content. She frowned frequently and seemed often to be at a loss for words. She was given **Turquoise** 1M. Shortly afterwards she rang the clinic to complain of an acute sore throat in which all the physical symptoms seemed so much worse. She was content to be reassured that the remedy was causing an aggravation and said that she would see it through. When she returned for her follow-up appointment she felt much better. She had been able to tell a relative who had been troubling her exactly what she had needed to say for a long while.' CG

2 'Woman in her mid 60s, a regular patient, needed help to go through a stressful crisis in her marriage. She liked to use **Ignatia** 10M: "It gives me some control over my emotions when I need to keep things together." However, her husband was "giving me hell" by being unpredictable in his attitude, behaviour and temper. She felt silenced by him. She was given **Turquoise** 200 once a week. She said that she loved the remedy as it made her feel so relaxed in the throat. Though her husband went on to find other ways to aggravate her and caused her further trauma by going off on holiday without her, she remembered the calming effect of the remedy.' JM

3 'A very old lady who was a medium by profession came complaining that her mediumistic powers had gone. She was alarmed by this and saddened. Her chakras were not in alignment and her aura showed that she was blocked at the throat and the brow. It does sometimes happen that mediums lose their gift before they come to the end of their lives. She was given **Turquoise** 30c. When she returned she had recovered all her abilities and was very content.

  'I often use **Turquoise** as an auric protection remedy when the throat chakra is weak. I also find it useful to encourage patients to tell the unvarnished truth. [See also **Purple** and **Moldavite**.] In such cases I give the 30th potency daily for four weeks. A dose of the 30th potency just before hands-on healing to align the chakras is very effective. **Turquoise** is also helpful when the thymus gland is blocked and inaccessible to other indicated remedies [see **Thymus Gland** in *Volume I*]. I have also noted that **Turquoise** is very useful to support **Conium** in cases of cataract.' JM

36

YELLOW

The remedy was proved by both meditation groups of the Guild; the first session was on 19 September 1997 and the second, one month later.

When ordering this remedy from the pharmacy, it is helpful to differentiate it by asking for **Yellow (Guild)**.

The Background

Pictorially, yellow is one of the colours of light (gold and silver being others). It is associated with the sun (golden yellow light) and thus with the heart centre (yellow and blue mix to make green, the traditional colour of the heart chakra) and earth.

Biologically, yellow is the colour of warning especially when it appears in stripes with black or dark brown. Warnings alter our perception instantly; whatever we may be doing, if a natural sign of warning is present then our primitive reflexes react immediately. This suggests that yellow, sometimes in combination with other colours, affects the thalamus and hypothalamus, endocrine glands that are part of the primitive brain and that regulate the functions of reaction. One of the consequences of becoming alert to potential danger is that we start to pump adrenalin, flooding the system with accessible energy in order to fight or flee (see below in 'General symptoms').

Yellow is also associated with the liver as the traditional colour of both bile (though it can be brownish or green) and of several remedies that treat the liver: **Chelidonium, Lycopodium, Taraxacum, Hydrastis, Sulphur** and **Achillea Millefolium** as well as **Turmeric**.

While blue is often associated with a calming, yin influence and red is associated with fire and anger and is predominantly yang, yellow is often associated with spiritual energy; the energy that returns that which has crystallized into matter, back into ether. However, colour therapists regard yellow as a stimulating colour, particularly of the intellect as it is capable of speeding up the mental processes of creative thought. Practitioners use it to clear a foggy brain. Overstimulation with yellow can lead to the opposite: exhaustion and depression. Yellow is also used in colour therapy to foster healing of skin conditions.

Keynote effects

Yellow should encourage elimination through the activity of the lymphatic system (sweat) and the bowels. It lightens the toxic burden and enlightens the mind and spirit. It galvanizes the earth element when that threatens stagnation.

General symptoms

A remedy that initiates transformation and regeneration. Useful in all systems of the body especially the lymphatics, the liver, the bowels and the skin. Also on the emotional body after trauma. Has a calming effect on those who have lived through a series of traumas or who are perpetually agitated for some reason that is not evident; has an enlivening effect on those who are suppressed or torpid due to loss of perspective or even identity. Useful where emotional problems are beginning to impede the physical processes of the body; so, often called for in draining potential pathology from the system. Close to this are symptoms that arise through changing states which may be developmental ones or due to force of circumstance. Where there is a process of metamorphosis going on which brings on symptoms that arise from the threat to the status quo. Nausea, sensations of emptiness, anxiety in the heart area, loss of energy can all arise from this. Pains are burning and stinging; feelings of being scalded. Hypersensitivity to extraneous sounds. It is seen as one of the great cleansing remedies and it has a great affinity for and works well with **Sulphur.** For those who have excessive amounts of adrenalin in their systems, **Yellow** may become an important remedy to drain resulting toxicity: this is typically seen in children with learning difficulties whose infantile startle reflex is still in play and interfering with the developing autonomic nervous system. (Children with attention deficit and hyperactive disorder come into this category.) Releases pent up energy that has been unable to find any expression because of suppression or emotional abuse.

Miasms

Psora, tuberculosis, sycosis, radiation and leprosy.

Mental and emotional symptoms

Feelings of not being grounded. A sense of not wanting to be here. Feeling cut off and unconnected. Wanting to retreat in the face of the sense that there is a major change looming. Difficulty in expressing exactly how they feel; throat chakra is seized up. Confusion and muddle; **Yellow** can bring peace of mind, stillness and calm; restores clarity of thought. One of the remedies to consider where there is a deep history of trauma which the patient is reluctant to let go of or is unaware of holding on to. Quietens the mind and engenders a state of relaxation. Lack of confidence from years of being cowed (especially by parents). Creative energies are locked away and need to be released. Patient can be leading a very narrow, conventional existence. A remedy for fear and terror; < after experiencing a frightful event or for those who feel fear for no apparent reason. Perhaps there is in this aspect of the remedy a connection with yellow being the traditional colour of cowardice; not cowardice in the face of physical danger but in the pursuit of anything that would encourage expansion and growth. Useful where fears prevent moving forward developmentally. Deep distrust of life. Disbelief in their own abilities. Encourages the expansion of the patient's horizons. Helpful for those who have done a lot of heart-searching to no great effect; who have been to counselling for years but not achieved much change. Patient may come in a crisis with the feeling that they just can't take any more – yet this is revealed as their usual pattern. Allows people to surrender to the inevitable. Negative Leo states: laziness; can't be bothered but remedy can restore the opposite. Great anxiety.

Physical symptoms

Head
A feeling of confusion with a tight head. Unable to hold head up with the neck; too heavy.

Eyes
Burning and stinging. A feeling as if there is smoke in the eyes. Tightness.

Mouth and Throat

Dryness. (Burning sensation with sore tongue.) Restriction in throat. Tickling < right side. Thyroid underactivity.

Chest

Constriction and oppression. Feeling heavy in the heart area or empty. Wheezy breathing.

Heart

Palpitations due to overstimulation (which is possibly due to hyperthyroidism). A physical sense of the burden of grief. Irregular heartbeats.

Abdomen

Congested liver and spleen. Constipation (or chronic diarrhoea). Burning sensations especially with sense of being bunged up. Nausea and empty feelings.

Female

Any condition may need **Yellow** where there is a process of change struggling to go on (puberty, menopause) but that becomes stuck. Menstrual irregularities; endometriosis. Flushes of heat, even inflammations of the internal organs. Helps to ease the restriction of the womb during pregnancy and delivery.

Urinary organs

Flow of urine increased.

Skin

Eczema. Skin is flaky and itchy, red and sore. Threatens suppuration as there is liver toxicity. Scar tissue that remains irritating.

Back

It is said to assist the Kundalini energy especially where this has been damaged by adverse experiences in the past. Will assist other spinal remedies in their work of healing injuries or blocked energy due to musculoskeletal distortion.

Extremities

Pains in limbs with stiffness and some swelling (left side: knee and neck).

Considerations for the use of the remedy

Yellow can be usefully compared with several other remedies:

- **Calendula** which has great potential when given to one who is unable to let go of the trauma of an accident.
- **Sulphur** which is often used either as an opening remedy in much suppressed cases or as an intercurrent in those who have had acutes suppressed for which **Yellow** may also be considered.
- **Green**, made by mixing blue and yellow, is also a transformative and regenerative remedy though, on the physical level, it is more to do with the physical structure of bones, joints and ligamentous tissue.
- **Tuberculinum** which shares the desire to seek outside themselves for something different, something new though it is usually more restless physically than **Yellow** and has more of an explosive temperament.

Yellow is important in healing the lymph system, the liver and the spleen. It works well (perhaps best) when used in lower potencies in combination with other related remedies. It has a natural affinity for the organ remedies: **Liver, Ovary, Lung, Kidney** and **Thymus Gland**. It is, when put into combinations, the ingredient that makes such triple remedies into extremely effective drainage remedies.

Many of the symptoms of **Yellow** are accompanied by a certain amount of anxiety. This is in some measure due to the adrenal drive that is part of the **Yellow** picture. Unfortunately the adrenal flow is inappropriately directed so that the patient cannot channel it and use it purposefully. The use of **Yellow** in combination (or on its own) can help to restore a balanced adrenal flow. One of the first symptom changes to notice is likely to be a considerable degree of calmness and even contentment at feeling more settled.

Suggested combinations (though intuition and a thorough knowledge of remedy relationships are indispensable in selecting remedies for combining):

- **Yellow + Carduus Marianus + Chelidonium**: this is one of the most satisfactory combinations for the drainage of the liver and gall bladder. It works on the organs themselves and on the associated meridians.

- **Yellow + Clay + Wheat** (or **Gluten**): cleanses the bowels, the liver and the small intestine when these are torpid and sluggish; when there is candida and allergies; when there is eczema with a weak immune system (frequent colds and coughs). It can be used in the 6x, 12x, 6c or 30c potencies on a daily basis after an indicated dose of **Okubaka** in a high potency. It will also work to complement a high dose of **Sulphur** when that is indicated.
- **Yellow + Okubaka + Wheat** (or **Gluten**): useful as a drainage remedy in irritable bowel syndrome to support **Lycopodium** or **Nat-sulph**.
- **Yellow + Thuja + Arsen-alb** (or **Arsen-iod**): it will treat the blood and lymph as well as balance the flow of energy that is thoroughly disturbed by any suppressive treatment that may have been given already. This will work particularly well after indicated doses of the nosodes – though **Sulphur** instead of **Arsenicum** may well be better suited to follow **Psorinum** especially in eczema. This is a combination (using the **Arsen-iod**) that can be thought of in leukaemia.
- **Yellow + Liver + Lycopodium** (or **Chelidonium**): this combination in 12x will act as both a liver cleanse as well as a tonic. It can be given in warm water for speedier results. It will support the action of constitutional remedies that are indicated.
- **Yellow + Kidney + Urtica Urens**: strengthens and cleanses the kidneys and bladder. Can increase the flow of urine and support a change of diet intended to lower the acid levels in the body. May help to promote the break-up of stones and gravel.
- **Yellow + Lung + Tuberculinum**: this can cleanse and strengthen lungs after acute infections or after years of chronic lung trouble. Helps to drain the bronchioles and the bronchi and free the alveoli of clogging mucus so the exchange of gases improves. This works well after **Phos, Nat-sulph, Arsen-alb, Stannum, Puls, Kali-carb, Ant-tart, Lyc, Med-am**. This combination has been used successfully in encouraging the lungs of smokers to drain stagnant, toxic mucus from their base.
- **Yellow + Thuja + Oak** (or **Ayahuasca**): this combination is for intractable cases of back injuries. It helps maintain the flow of Kundalini energy going up and down the spine while the site of the injury heals itself.
- **Yellow + Pineal + Thuja**: is of use in children of precocious maturity who become easily exhausted. They lack concentration yet are bright;

they are inclined to internalize everything and tend to self-reference anything that occurs around them. Their anxieties are often irrational or concerned with their performance. This combination can support both **Phosphorus** and **Lycopodium** well.

- **Yellow** + **Pituitary** + **Calc-carb** (or **Baryta-carb**): this is a combination for slow development either in physical or mental maturity (or both) when indicated remedies have not effected any change.

Esoteric therapeutics

Yellow holds the essence of both yin and yang. It is the colour of the earth (yin) as well as of the light from above (yang); **Yellow**, the remedy, has an influence on the drawing down of yang energy into the system to mix with the earth yin. This process is associated with the esoteric activity of the stomach and its relationship with the kidneys and spleen: the forging of creative, aspirational, upward surging energy and with the intestines: the downward, eliminating energy of the waste system. **Yellow** is a remedy of the stomach meridian; when this meridian is seen to be out of sync in the body then this remedy should be considered.

Yellow is said to assist the mind in changing states of consciousness: when a patient is ready to allow personal developmental growth to occur, **Yellow** eases the passage. As part of this, it also heals the 'soil' in which trauma takes root thus it is a remedy to consider in those who find it so hard to let go of the vestiges of tragedy and accident. It is a remedy of new beginnings, of awakenings; it is useful in those who need to start again from square one in order to set out on a new path of discovery. This would be true even in those who are struggling with serious pathology. It is a remedy that reminds us that it is never too late.

Chakras

Crown

A remedy to encourage the patient back to a spiritual path; as they heal their physical pathology or emotional turmoil, **Yellow** fosters the link with the spiritual source. Helps people to rise above the hurly-burly of the world; to remain rooted in the base but relieved of the adrenal driven rush of modern life. Particularly useful in those who face burnout.

Brow

Blankness of the mind: patients feel that they need peace and quiet in which to think. Neither the intellect nor the intuition is able to operate effectively; both are compromised by poor drainage of the lymphatic system, by radiation or by toxicity in the system. Difficult to see what needs to be done for feeling of being cut-off or of confusion or from a mixture of churning mind and lack of self-belief. Encourages clarity of vision and thought.

Throat

The throat centre feels blocked and may be affected by excessive radiation: from air travel or from X-rays and other sources of radiation toxicity. Despite clear hearing, unable to hear what is said to one. Despite intelligence, unable to say what one truly means.

Heart

Yellow covers the connection between the heart centre and the spinal column. In cases where there is heart centre trouble as well as chronic spinal symptoms, this remedy is called for. It is indicated in those who have blocked energy in the spine at the level of the heart. (This is often manifest in those who have different symptoms below the level of the diaphragm and above it: cold lower extremities and hot torso; weakness in the arms and torso but strength in the legs, etc.)

Solar plexus

Detoxifies the liver and intestines. Affects the gall bladder and liver meridians profoundly as well as the stomach and large intestine meridians. Restores integrity to the lymphatic system and its reservoir, the *cisterna chyle*. Helps patients deal with challenges that would otherwise be maintaining causes that would dissipate the energies of other, perhaps more obviously indicated remedies.

Sacral

A continuing struggle to make sense of the world when there is a fundamental difficulty in making any shift in consciousness that would require expansion and greater independence and stretching beyond the safe haven of the base centre. This centre may never have been fully awakened from fear of full expression of sensuality.

Base

A remedy of the base centre to bring into focus that which needs to be done before there is any moving on to new growth or development. A remedy for new beginnings but only once old difficulties that have contributed to a general holding back have been resolved or, at least, once a start has been made to resolve them. **Yellow** is an uncompromising remedy and will often work to ensure that the patient's innate self-healing process starts to process negative energy through physical eliminative measures.

Practitioners' comments

Comments from practitioners include the following, recorded at a regular monthly gathering of homoeopaths in Sussex where they study new remedies in particular:

- 'I use it a lot with **Thymus Gland** to support eczema cases. I use it in "x" potencies or in 30 and 1M.'
- 'I've used it to treat great toxicity in a very large patient with so much grief and oedema. It's fantastic for lymph drainage and water retention or lymph, bowel and skin conditions.'
- 'It's great for grounding in cases where there's toxicity. A radiation case given **Yellow** 12x, **Zinc** and **MRPG** gently opened the doors . . . no aggravations using it.'
- 'In combination, **Lung** + **Yellow** + **Tub** is great for chronic lung problems. (It worked well when I) gave it to a patient who had double pneumonia.'
- '. . . given to a patient who "felt like a child peeping over the blankets" . . . they needed to move on, make decisions and take more responsibility. I've found that it works well with **Nat-mur**.'

An accidental proving

'A woman who had been coming to the clinic for many years but who only ever seemed to respond to remedies given in acute crises, was the subject of some despair. She was a very willing patient but also very blocked emotionally. (She refused to believe that there was any such thing as 'stress'.) She suffered from irritable bowel, bouts of excruciating proctitis, arthritic pains in all the joints of her extremities (though the focus of pain shifted from one site to another), severe skin rashes with histamine reactions, lichen planus, chronic vaginitis, acne rosacea and bouts of deathly exhaustion (which surprised no one as she was always throwing herself into a wall of work). She had had innumerable remedies for her chronic complaints that seemed to be well indicated and she had also had regular sessions of cranial osteopathy, shiatsu, acupuncture and naturopathic treatment. All her practitioners came to the same conclusion (which made them feel better in their collective impotence to help her): she was an intractable case. She came one day complaining more of her liver and her digestion than usual. She was given **Yellow** 30 to be taken one a day for ten days.

After a few days, when she came down to breakfast, her husband looked at her and exclaimed, "You're yellow!" When her son came in he said, "You're yellow!" and this was enough for her to look in the mirror and call an ambulance. She was indeed yellow from head to foot. She was taken into hospital and subjected to tests, no one thinking to ask her how she felt. (They did not even ask her if she was feverish, itching or nauseous.) The tests proved "inconclusive"; the doctors were stumped. When it was apparent that she was not suffering more than her usual symptoms, she was allowed home. It took five weeks for the yellow colour to clear, the last place affected being the palms of her hands. At the end of this time, it was apparent that she was no longer complaining of her liver symptoms and she has never returned to complain about irritable bowel symptoms since that date. What subsequently developed, however, was what doctors told her was a chronic viral problem that was characterized by periodic bouts of severe urticarial rashes over her neck and face; the chief symptom of this was the vivid redness of the condition. Doctors ruled out Lupus. Perhaps what had been brewing in her solar plexus had now found an external expression.

Case studies

(See also **Silverfish** in *Volume I*, where the first case features **Yellow**.)

1 'HS (two years and eleven months). At 13 months HS sustained severe scarring over his right arm from boiling water. He was hospitalized and left with deep scarring and red skin for which he has been wearing a

pressure bandage. HS has been treated for a wide range of conditions arising from birth trauma, vaccination and a traumatic circumcision. Sometimes the work has been complemented by cranial osteopathy. He has had trauma remedies including **Buddleia**, **Syphilinum** and **Arnica**. Treatment is ongoing.

In April 2003 there was the opportunity to prescribe a remedy specifically for the scald scarring which HS was picking at and aggravating. **Yellow** 9x b.d. was given. In October HS's mother reported that the scald scar was very much improved, the skin was much smoother and less red. HS has not been bothering about it for some time.' **TH**

2   'A young lady in her thirties came to see me some six years ago. She had been brought up in a remote part of Africa as a child, the eldest of three, along with her two younger brothers. Her mother was very domineering but found life very hard in Africa and could not cope with the three children especially when her husband had to travel a lot with his job. My patient became responsible for the parenting, care and discipline of her younger brothers when her mother couldn't cope. She found the African tribal folk both fascinating and intimidating. Her father was very preoccupied with his job and rather distant and she found the only way to get his attention was by doing well with her education. She was often very frightened and felt emotionally inadequate to deal with all the problems.

'The family came back to England and she went to university, where she got a degree and went on to do her master's degree. She also excelled at playing the violin but outside this she could not cope with life. When she came to me she described herself as a child hiding under the blankets peeping over the edge afraid to come out. She had just finished her master's and needed to find somewhere to live and a job and was terrified. She was also seeing a counsellor on a weekly basis who suggested she should have homoeopathy. Since this time she has moved a long way. She had increasing doses at various times of **Carcinosin** and **Lycopodium** and **Nat-mur**, **Calc** and **Yellow**. She cut the ties with her mother for a while and learned to stand on her own two feet, but now has a good balanced relationship with all her family including her mother.

'She now lives away from London and has a very full life working as a university lecturer and examiner and as a trainer for Volunteer Services Overseas. She also plays in an orchestra and has a full intellectual life. She bought a house and has furnished and decorated it without allowing her mum to tell her how and what to do. This was a huge achievement. During the years she has had **Yellow** sometimes on its own and sometimes in addition to another remedy. She is always analysing things in her head and I have found it helps her to contact her heart and feelings to decide emotionally and spiritually what is right for her. It always seems to help her to find that inner peace and groundedness that she craved so much.' JL

3   'Female, 56, with autoimmune thyroid condition, seemingly triggered by a session with a reflexologist. She felt frightened by the experience and felt attacked by the therapist. My sense was that there was some sort of past-life relationship here. I had not treated this patient before and do not normally perceive past life on the first meeting. However, during my studies at the Guild I had learnt to give **Yellow** as a remedy to release fear from past life. So I gave it as a single dose of **Yellow** 10M to which we had almost immediate relief of the overactive thyroid symptoms. Instead, the patient developed bright red marks on her feet and calves that resembled burns. She dreamt she had been burnt as a witch. I had just been on a course with Ian White on Australian Bush Flower Essences. Ian has produced a remedy for burns and for those who had been burnt as witches in past life: Mulla Mulla. I gave this and the "burns" disappeared. The thyroid remains normal.' HJ

4   'Female, 52, diagnosed with fatty liver. No symptoms except for abnormal liver enzymes on blood tests. She was **Phosphorus** constitutionally. However, this produced no change in the liver enzyme readings until **Yellow** 30c given daily. I chose **Yellow** as the fatty liver had occurred during menopause and the patient had lots of menopausal symptoms which were not responding well to treatment: flushes, anger, night sweats and flooding menses. I felt that the menopausal process was not an easy transition. The underlying fear was of growing old (**Phosphorus**) but the **Yellow** also reduced the menopausal symptoms considerably.' HJ

5 'Female, 66, diagnosed with chronic lymphocytic leukaemia (C.L.L.). I prescribed **Arsenicum Album** 200c which I alternated with **Carcinosin** 200c using Dr Ramakrishnan's plussing method. Although the leukaemia remained under control with this combination, the blood readings were not improving. I decided to add in **Yellow** 30c daily as a medicine simply to work on the lymphatic system. Ever since, the blood tests have improved. The patient has now had C.L.L. for six years but has not needed any chemotherapy. Originally she was told she would probably need it within two years. The white blood cell count is very gradually improving.' **HJ**

6 'A boy aged two came having bad dreams. He had always been a poor sleeper but now would stand in his cot at night, red-faced, screaming and inconsolable. A new baby had been born in the family which was upsetting him even more. His only vaccinations had been for tetanus and polio at 12 months. **Tub-bov**, **Belladonna**, **Puls** and **Blue** did nothing. His mother commented that he loved colours and knew the names of all of them, his favourite being yellow. A quick reference to the notes followed and he was given **Yellow** 30 for three successive nights. He slept peacefully after the first dose and has continued to do so since.' **ME** (First published in *Prometheus* No. 12 June 2000.)

7 'Female, age 48, presented with pain in liver region; felt as if she were filled with water; digestive system a mess. Emotionally, history of multiple grief: alcoholic father who was verbally abusive; was very hard on herself and a people-pleaser; attracted emotionally unavailable people in her life. Initially remedies such as **Carc**, **Nat-mur**, **Causticum** were prescribed but had little effect.

'In the third consultation client suspected many traumas were also coming from past lives. On the basis of this, the fact that the solar plexus area was completely congested and her upbringing with her father, I prescribed **Yellow 30c**.

The effect was immediate and huge: produced an "angry" headache, the sinuses became congested but felt that she was starting to "let go". A termination previously avoided surfaced and the start of many dreams and images from previous lives. Three years on the client is still shifting stuff, her digestion is virtually there, peace has been made with her dad and many tears have been shed.

'I still use **Yellow** in increasing doses should the solar plexus area become congested or in her words "toxic". **Yellow** will always start the clearing process and enable her to move on with whatever emotion has become lodged in that area.' LE

8   'Female, 55, had previously brought her daughter to see me because her father had died three years previously. She decided to make an appointment for herself. She presented with horrific sinus congestion, upper and lower sinuses, stomach bloated, constipated and no energy for life at all. Emotionally, was still grieving sudden death of husband but history revealed that her father had died when she was aged seven, grandmother when she was ten and there was the loss of family pets.

'**Nat-mur** was effective at starting to work on the grief and by the second consultation she was in better spirits, particularly as the constipation was easing. Over the following six months, many things improved except for the sinus congestion: thick yellowy discharge, fairly constant, and slight constipation; awful headaches. I combined **Yellow 6c + Clay 6x + Thuja 6c** to try to encourage the sinuses to start draining and clear out all the muck. This worked well and she obtained much relief from this combination.

'**Yellow** at this potency cleared all the constipation, and worked brilliantly as an aid to sinus congestion.' LE

PART III

Appendix I Radiation Pollution

Radiation is a medical hazard of our time. For all the necessity of its various uses, there is risk to humanity from its effects. Some people are more affected by radiation toxicity than others.[53] While the minute, measurable amounts of radiation involved in, say, a radioactive dye test may well not be harmful to the majority, there can be no doubt that there are sensitive individuals who need both protection and medication because of being exposed to even such minimal radiation.

Radiation takes different forms. We commonly think of X-rays as the most usual source of risk but many are convinced that working in or living near power stations is detrimental to health.[54] Patients who have undergone necessary tests such as barium enemas, have subsequently complained of symptoms that are relieved by such remedies as **Baryta-carb** and **Baryta-iod** or combination remedies such as **X-ray + Baryta-carb + Pyrogen + Rad-brom** 6x.[55]

Radiation pollution is a problem even when it is not injected into our bodies for medical reasons. Travellers are exposed to radiation in the atmosphere; it is one of the causes of severe jet lag in those who are susceptible. It is apparent that there are jet lag 'black spots': flying over areas of America or over the southern Pacific where nuclear tests have been carried out, for example.[56]

53 One patient, who was an inspector for nuclear power plants and claimed to have been exposed to more than 50 times the safe limit of radiation, was constitutionally well and had no reaction whatever to any radiation remedies.

54 One such patient who worked at a nuclear power plant on the south coast of England complained of constant tiredness and had a worryingly dark grey complexion, both of which symptoms are consequences of radiation toxicity.

55 This combination remedy has been used successfully in patients who have had a barium enema as part of the investigation of irritable bowel syndrome where there is a history of compacted faeces in the large intestine that has led to chronic, continual absorption of toxicity.

56 One patient, a retired commercial pilot whose face and body were covered in skin cancers, claimed it was common knowledge that the Geiger counters in the planes' cockpits would go over into the red zone when flying over certain areas where nuclear tests had been carried out and even over nuclear power plants.

(It is, perhaps, not surprising that **Arnica** has been used successfully for jet lag on numerous occasions as this remedy is known for its ability to remove radiation toxicity from the body.)

However, microwave technology has introduced another radiation threat which is far less controlled as it is abroad in the environment pervasively and in closer proximity. Both mobile phones and the masts that emit the signals by which they operate are sources of insidious danger that it would be a mistake to dismiss; even while the majority of us make use of them. What is interesting is that the effects on the human body of both forms of radiation are similar, with the characteristic deathly tiredness, inability to coordinate the mind either in thought or in relation to physical movement and weakness being the most obvious early signs. All radiation remedies have these symptoms in common to some degree.

Radiation is not only a toxic threat; it is also a miasm. At least, it is a miasm by default, so to speak; it can behave like one even though it is not an inheritable disease state in the same class as the well-known miasms. Changes wrought on the tissues of a parent through radiation pollution may affect the child. We should be in no doubt that radiation of any sort is capable of making genetic alterations in those who are susceptible and in those who inherit genes from them. After all, science acknowledges the dangers: doctors advise radiotherapy patients not to go near their relatives for a substantial period of time after their treatment.

The part of the body most vulnerable to radiation is the thyroid gland. It is the organ of the body involved in iodine metabolism and it is iodine that is most attractive to radiation. It is no accident that so many of the remedies associated with iodine are listed as remedies for pathology of this gland. This includes the sea remedies as the oceans hold so much iodine.

Those who are able to see the aura of someone affected significantly by radiation tell us that damage occurs first in the auric field. They report that radiation 'tears holes in the aura and the areas affected become grey and otherwise colourless'. From such 'holes', energy leaks away somewhat as if a plug had been taken out of a basin. A common place for such an energy leak is at the base of the spine; it is a direct assault on the base chakra. This is a cause of the exhaustion felt by all those who suffer from this peculiar form of toxicity.

Radiation also has another characteristic habit: it migrates from one part of the body to another, often to distant parts. It can travel round the body either through the blood, the lymph or via the meridians, those subtle energy channels of the body. Yet it may do its most obvious damage on the skin where it can cause symptoms that look like anything between eczema and cancerous ulceration. What is certain is that radiation toxicity is syphilitic in its sinister insidiousness, carcinogenic in its potential and psoric in its protean range of symptomatology. It is sometimes a hidden maintaining cause that it takes a long while to see.

Sources of potential radiation toxicity in patients

Power stations, X-rays, barium meals and radioactive dye tests, Wi-Fi computers, microwave ovens, CD players, mobile-phone masts and mobile phones. Some practitioners would include the sun in this list. (Laser treatments do not cause radiation toxicity though lasers are harmful to the tissues of the body. Patients need to be protected against the effects of this form of treatment; **Ruby** is one remedy that will afford such protection.)

Remedies from radioactive sources

Plutonium, Radium Bromide, Radium Iodatum, Caesium, Cobalt, Baryta Carbonicum and Baryta Iodatum, X-ray, Strontium Carbonicum, Sol, Microwave Radiation Pulsed G3, Japanese White Oleander.

New remedies that may positively affect radiation toxicity in the body

Ayahuasca, Clay, Emerald, Goldfish, Green, Japanese White Oleander, Moldavite, Moonstone, Plutonium, Purple, Rainbow, Rose Quartz, Ruby, Sea Holly, Winchelsea Sea Salt, Sequoia, Yellow.

New remedies that may help to lift the radiation miasm

Emerald, Jet, Moldavite, Plutonium, Rainbow, Ruby, Yellow.

Parts of the body most affected by radiation

Thyroid, thymus gland, **lymphatic system**, the central nervous system, **skin**, bone, blood, liver, kidneys and **sex organs**.

Effects of radiation on the body

Alters endocrine function and metabolism; interferes with the glandular organism; burns, ulceration and necrosis; deformities of the body's structure; disease of the heart and circulation, of elimination; alteration of the body's temperature control; weakness, debility and emaciation. It may be a hidden or additional feature to take into consideration in cases of chronic fatigue syndrome, ME and certain kinds of cancer especially those involving the lymph glands or blood.

Effects of radiation toxicity on the mind

Confusion and disorientation; memory loss, increasing symptoms of senility and mental degeneration; inability to register things; mental stagnation; difficulty in communication; difficulty in using language; tendency to be easily distracted; easily deluded about one's condition and about external circumstances. Also hyperactivity of mind with mental restlessness. Radiation engenders fearfulness and anticipatory feelings.

Effects of radiation toxicity on the emotions

Lack of emotion; desire to curl up and shut out the world; feelings of inadequacy; depression; being detached; emotional exhaustion; ultrasensitivity but also violent thoughts and reactions.

Appendix II Remedies That Have a Reputation for Grief

'Ailments from Grief' is a very familiar rubric, possibly the most well known, commonly looked-up and probably the most easily abused. In this volume more remedies have potentially been added to that rubric which cannot make the prescriber's task any easier.

The rubric is a problem because it has too few remedies in it to encompass all forms of grief and because the old favourites of **Nat-mur**, **Staphysagria**, **Causticum**, **Pulsatilla**, **Carcinosin**, **Aurum** and **Ignatia** are so readily resorted to without sufficient differentiation; it is so easy to identify their footprints in so many cases. It is so often said that this or that patient is 'a typical **Nat-mur**' or 'an obvious **Staphysagria**' or 'a classic **Pulsatilla**'; we take it for granted these remedies will perform the miracle of helping a patient to shed their grief with a dose of one or another of them. It is not reasonable to expect that these old favourites constitute the limits of our experience of grief and we misunderstand the nature and energy of grief if we do expect them to.

Grief is often multifaceted and multilayered even in the one patient. Grief may be the result of a traumatic emotional event, a series of events, a traumatic accident, a long period of emotional stress or a difficult birth or even a conception stigmatized by negativity. Grief can be complicated by and interwoven with layers of other life events such as surgery and anaesthetics, medical drugging, physical accident, sudden changes of fortune and miasmatic susceptibility. Grief can also be 'inherited' from previous generations. From those of our forebears who have been unable to resolve their own conflicting emotions and have passed on their susceptibility, we may rerun patterns of behaviour that lead us to experience emotions that could be found in past history. The very source of grief may be the ongoing turmoil caused by an unstable and ever-changing relationship between one generation and another. This can all be incremental through several generations. To risk sanction from those who would deny that homoeopathy has any place in such areas, for those who believe in past lives, grief can be of a karmic origin which requires some form of expiation or resolution and which will throw up in the present life opportunities for this. It is not infrequently that we come across patients who have a range of several of these different grief origins in their history and to imagine that only one remedy will do the job is wishful thinking.

So protean is grief in the variety of effects it has on an individual's energy that it is not good enough to assume that grief and withheld tears, strong thirst and a liking for salt are sufficient indication for a dose of **Nat-mur** to expunge the well of unhappiness that has been so buried in the heart centre of a patient. So often it *is* enough to prescribe **Nat-mur** and expect a positive result but not one that will necessarily afford the patient lasting wellness; it will only manage one step of the patient's journey. In any **Nat-mur** there is always more to unearth. In so many cases today it is true that the more a patient works on him- or herself, the more there is to uncover. This is where many of the new remedies and the controversial ways of prescribing them can be invaluable. To use them means that we not only have to know their materia medica but also their relationships with others including those that are useful for organ drainage.

It is common enough that a patient with a grief-laden heart centre also suffers from trouble in other parts of their system; trouble that is physical and potentially threatening to the physical constitution when the emotions are opened up. This is more true of remedies such as **Lachesis** and **Aurum** than, say, **Ignatia** or Nat-mur (even if these latter may be of value in cases of physical pathology). One of the reasons for this is that in many remedies grief is not confined to the heart centre. **Lachesis** invests grief in the throat and generative organs. **Ruby**'s grief may seem to be more centred on the solar plexus. There is a whole list of new and old remedies that covers grief hidden in the thymus gland. In these and other cases it may be important to make sure the elimination system is working efficiently first by prescribing drainage remedies. 'Yes, but if the indications are there for **Nat-mur** or **Causticum**, we should give that first as the centre of any case is the emotions,' is the rebuttal.

Sometimes it is gentler and swifter in the long run to ensure that the bowel, kidney, bladder and perhaps the skin are able to eliminate well before encouraging a patient to dig deep into an area of their lives that has been so repressed that it will require a considerable amount of energy to achieve resolution. If we can minimize aggravations before giving a remedy that might provoke a physical eliminative reaction then we should. This is most especially true of those who are suffering from physical pathology as well as grief. A patient will trust the process of healing more if the journey is taken in carefully managed stages.

The following thumbnail comparison of the new and old grief remedies is a guide to differentiation.

Himalayan Crystal Salt

- Grief is deeply rooted in family history, like **Aquamarine**, and may have a dark energy.
- Patient feels more challenged by the prospect of change than **Winchelsea Sea Salt** and is less able to adapt quickly.
- The route to pathology is towards the heart while in **WSS** it may be towards carcinogenic changes.
- It is less resentful and brittle than **Nat-mur** having a more unconditional sense of compassion.
- There is a great need for the outdoors; even more than with **WSS** which has a passion for the sea or **Nat-mur** which may be averse to the sea and the sun.

Winchelsea Sea Salt

- It has all the same modalities as **Nat-mur** but it is more restless and less cynical.
- It is less reserved than **Nat-mur** in relation to other people; may seek out the opinion of others or hang on their words as it gives them a sense of gained strength.
- Emotions may be just as deeply felt and held as in the other salts but can appear to be 'drowning'.
- It is far more likely to have a deep longing to be by the sea while **Nat-mur** may have an aversion to it.

Eryngium Maritimum

- It is even drier than the salts; drier in heart, body and mind.
- The personality is more threatened with desiccation.
- It is more sceptical (though not cynical), brusque and even apparently rude.
- It tends to form calculi and stones.
- It is a very psoric and carcinogenic remedy.

- It is extremely tenacious, stoic and is defensive of the deeply hidden story of grief.

Aquamarine

- This shares a deep karmic load with the salt remedies.
- The grief in this remedy stems further back in history than in any other remedy even in cases where the patient is unaware of its origins.
- This has a sense of destructive desolation and despair which brings it into comparison with **Buddleia.**

Buddleia

- There is always the element of deep shock with the grief.
- They feel very detached from the 'now' in their state of grief and desolation.
- They feel bowed down and depressive and may not be very communicative.
- They suffer from emotional paralysis like **Conium, Purple** and **Phos-ac,** though are usually more demonstrative of grief than these.

Japanese White Oleander

- It is more mentally absent than **Buddleia** though on a par with **Phos-ac.**
- The sense of being overwhelmed is in the nervous system of **JWO** but in the emotional body of **Buddleia** and the salts.
- There is more silent dread in **JWO** rather than **Buddleia's** 'How can this have happened?'
- It is more likely to be surly than **Buddleia;** can be torpid one moment and angry and even aggressive the next.

Emerald

- Grief is much to do with hurt to the ego.
- Inhibitions remind us of **Nat-mur** though it is less chronically embittered and warmer-hearted; less communicative than **WSS.**
- It can be full of righteous anger which lifts it to a level above the suppressed grief of the other salts, **Purple, Conium** and **Eryngium,** etc.
- The origins of the grief may stem from parental control or abuse.

Conium

- Grief is more about the loss of what once was than of having been subjected to the negative energy of another person.
- It follows or precedes **Nat-mur** well.

Aurum Metallicum

- Grief is much about the loss of status, money and ambition.
- It is followed well by **WSS** or **Emerald.**

Lycopodium

- Grief is about the failure to achieve and fulfil potential.

Chalice Well

- This is one of the most useful remedies for acute or ongoing situations full of grief; helps in letting go of interfering emotions.
- There is more self-searching than in other grief remedies: 'Am I doing the right thing?'
- Oppression is strong in the present while other remedies feel the oppression from the past.
- This helps to prevent a person from developing a deep state of **Nat-mur.**

Ruby

- While **CW** cannot let go in a general sense, **Ruby** cannot let go of a specific old relationship.
- It can be vehement and intolerant but this comes from a passionate nature while **CW** is often less focused and more vulnerable.
- It stores its grief in the solar plexus rather than the heart centre.

Rhodochrosite

- It feels the lack of nurture most strongly.
- It can resemble **Nat-mur** in its brittle and embittered attitude though is more demonstrative and hopeful of emotional reciprocation.

Rose Quartz

- Grief is centred on 'home'; there is always an aspect of needing to be at home either geographically or within the heart of another.

Green Jade

- Strongly defended against the world it can be hard-hearted and cynical.
- It shuts out the world of emotions and is deaf to emotional problems.
- They feel that there is an emotional traffic jam going on around them.
- It puts pathology into the throat and thyroid.
- It is like a cross between **Nat-mur** and **Sepia**.

Cardamom

- Like **White Chestnut Flower**, it is a chronic of **Staphysagria** and like WCF it has a pacifying or calming influence unlike **Staphysagria** which can sometimes foster anger and righteous justification for perpetual revenge.
- Stoic like **Oak** it is impatient and irritable like **Nat-mur** but lacks courage unlike the other two.
- It tends to lead a life of 'nose to the grindstone' and without much recognition which is craved but with a longing for peace and quiet.
- It craves balance in life above all else.

Bluebell

- There is an acute crisis of grief with lack of confidence and fearfulness; akin to **Chalice Well**.
- There are strong feelings of grief over the father figure.
- It is easily distracted and full of phobias.

Plutonium

- It has much to do with grief hidden deep in past or family history.
- The process of unearthing the grief is deeply transformative if cathartic.
- It is often characterized by a sense of fragmentation in the personality.
- It works well with **Thymus Gland** to unlock the forgotten past.

Appendix III New Remedies and the Energy Centres of the Body

The following is a guide to the 72 plus remedies appearing in *Volumes 1* and *2* of *The New Materia Medica* and their affinity for and influence on the chakras. Those in bold type are not necessarily deeper-acting; simply more often indicated when that chakra is struggling. The lists of well-known remedies that follow in parentheses are not exhaustive; the remedies mentioned are those which have an affinity for the associated chakra. There are inevitably names missing from the lists but this is only from want of experience to date.

Crown
Amethyst, Ayahuasca, Birdsong (Blackbird), Blackberry, Black Obsidian, **Buddleia,** Dolphin Sonar (Song), Hornbeam, Hyacinthoides Non-Scripta, Japanese White Oleander, Lumbricus, Moldavite, **Moonstone,** Plutonium, **Purple,** Rainbow, **Rosebay Willowherb,** Sandalwood, Statice, Stonehenge, Thymus Gland, Viscum Album

(*Arg-met,* ***Cann-ind,*** *Carcin, Iridium,* ***Luna, Opium, Thuja,*** *Viscum-alb*)

Brow
Ash, Amethyst, Blackberry, Chalice Well, Copper Beech, Cotton Wool, **Goldfish,** Green, **Lapis Lazuli,** MRPG, **Moldavite,** Oak, Okubaka, **Orange,** Pluto, Pomegranate, **Rainbow,** Rhodochrosite, Ruby, Salix Fragilis, Sandalwood, Sequoia, Silverfish, Silver Birch, Stonehenge, **Sycamore Seed,** Turmeric, Viscum Album

(*Aeth, Agar, Ailan, Anac,* ***Arg-met,*** *Arsen-alb, Arsen-iod,* ***Baryta-carb,*** *Bell,* ***Calc-carb, Calc-iod,*** *China, China-sulph, Cimic, Coff, Ham, Hell, Hyos, Hyper, Lyc, Mang,* ***Merc-sol*** *[Viv], Nat-sulph, Nit-ac, Phos-ac, Plat, Plum, Proteus, Psor, Silica, Stram, Sulph, Sulph-iod, Syphilinum, Thuja, Tub, Verat-alb*)

Parathyroid

Blue, Ivy Berry, Moonstone, Oak, Rhodochrosite, **Rose Quartz**

(Arnica, Belladonna, Calc-carb, Hypericum, Ledum, Lyc, Pall, Plantago, Puls, Tub)

Throat

Blue, Emerald, Hazel, Goldfish, **Ivy Berry**, Moonstone, MRPG, Pluto, Rainbow, **Rhodochrosite**, Rose Quartz, Rutilated Smoky Quartz, **Sea Salt**, Tunbridge Wells Water, **Turquoise**, Viscum Album

(Arg-met, Caust, Ign, Iod, Kali-bich, Kali-iod, Kali-mur, Kali-sulph, Lac-can, Lach, Lyc, Nat-mur, Puls, Rad-brom, Spon)

Thymus

Aquamarine, Ayahuasca, Berlin Wall, Black Obsidian, Buddleia, **Chalice Well**, Eryn-mar, **Goldfish, Hornbeam**, Jade, Japanese White Oleander, **Jet**, Latrodectus, Lotus, Lumbricus, Moldavite, Oak, Olive, Peridot, **Pluto**, Rainbow, **Rhodochrosite**, Rose Quartz, Sandalwood, Statice, **Thymus Gland**, Turquoise, Winchelsea Sea Salt

(Arsen-alb, Baryta-carb, Carcin, DPT, Ign, Lac-hum, Staphys, Syphilinum, Thuja, Tub)

Heart

Amethyst, Aquamarine, Ayahuasca, Berlin Wall, Blackberry, **Buddleia, Cardamom**, Chalice Well, **Emerald, Golden Beryl, Goldfish, Green**, Hazel, **Himalayan Crystal Salt**, Hornbeam, Ilex Aquifolium, Jade, Japanese White Oleander, Jet, **Latrodectus**, Lotus, Moldavite, Neem, **Oak**, Olive, Peridot, Rainbow, **Rhodochrosite, Rose Quartz**, Ruby, Salix Fragilis, Silver Birch, Statice, Tunbridge Wells Water, **Winchelsea Sea Salt**, White Chestnut Flower

*(Ambra, Ammon-mur, Anac, Ant-crud, Arsen-alb, **Aurum**, Calc-mur, **Carcin**, Caust, Crat, Cycl, **Ign**, **Lac-hum**, Lach, Mag-mur, **Nat-mur**, Phos-ac, Proteus, Puls, Staphys, Tub)*

Solar plexus

Berlin Wall, **Blackberry, Black Obsidian**, Black Tourmaline, Cardamom, Clay, Copper Beech, **Golden Beryl**, Green Tourmaline, Hazel, Ilex Aquifolium, Ivy Berry, Jet, Lotus, **Lumbricus**, Oak, **Okubaka**, Organic Brown Rice, Pomegranate, **Red, Ruby**, Rutilated Smoky Quartz, **Sodium Bicarbonate**, Tunbridge Wells

Water, **Turmeric**, Viscum Album, White Chestnut Flower, Winchelsea Sea Salt, Yellow

(Ailan, Aloe-soc, Ambra, Ant-crud, Bell, Bellis, Bryonia, Calc-sulph, Card-mar, Cham, Chel, China, Coloc, Dys-co, Ferr, Gaertner, Ham, Hepar, Hydras, Kali-ars, Lach, Lyc, Mag-carb, Mag-mur, Morgan, Morgan-Gaertner, Nat-phos, Nat-sulph, Nux-vom, Phos, Pyro, Sulph, Thuja, Tub, Verat-alb)

Sacral

Ash, **Blue**, Cardamom, Clay, **Copper Beech**, **Golden Beryl**, Goldfish, Hazel, Hyacinthoides, Ilex Aquifolium, **Pomegranate**, **Red Chestnut Flower**, Rhodochrosite, Rutilated Smoky Quartz, Salix Fragilis, Sandalwood, **Senecio + Tyria Jacobaea**, Sequoia, Silver Birch, Tiger's Eye, Viscum Album, **White Chestnut Flower**

*(Ambra, Apis, Arg-nit, Benz-ac, **Berb-vul**, Cann-sat, Canth, Cimic, **Follic**, Kreos, **Lach**, Lil-tig, Lyc, Med, **Med-am**, Nat-sulph, Nit-ac, Plat, **Puls**, Sabal, Sabina, **Sepia**, Sycotic-co, Syphilinum, **Thuja**)*

Base

Amethyst, Ash, **Ayahuasca**, Blackberry, **Black Obsidian**, **Black Tourmaline**, **Buddleia**, Cardamom, Chalcancite, **Clay**, **Clear Quartz**, Copper Beech, Cotton Wool, Dolphin Sonar, Emerald, **Golden Beryl**, Goldfish, Green, **Green Beech**, Hazel, Hornbeam, Hyacinthoides Non-Scripta, Ilex Aquifolium, Jade, **Jet**, **Lotus**, **Lumbricus**, MRPG, **Malus Domestica**, **Moldavite**, Neem, **Oak**, Olive, Peridot, Pomegranate, Plutonium, Rhodochrosite, **Rosebay Willowherb**, Rose Quartz, Rutilated Smoky Quartz, Salix Fragilis, **Sequoia**, Silverfish, Silver Birch, Sodium Bicarbonate, Viscum Album, White Chestnut Flower, **Yellow**

*(Acon, Aesc-hip, Alum, **Arsen-alb**, Ammon-carb, Ant-tart, Arg-met, **Arnica**, **Baryta-carb**, Bellis, Borax, Bryonia, **Calc-carb**, Calc-fluor, Calc-phos, Calc-sil, Calc-sulph, Calen, Carb-an, **Carb-veg**, **Carcin**, Caust, **Conium**, Cuprum, Ferr, Fluor-ac, Graph, Ham, Iridium, Kali-bich, Kali-carb, Kali-phos, Kali-sulph, Kreos, Leprosinum, **Lyc**, Mag-carb, Mag-phos, Mag-sulph, Mang, Med, **Med-am**, Morgan, Nat-carb, Nat-phos, Nat-sulph, **Nux-vom**, **Opium**, Petr, Phos-ac, **Phos**, Plum, **Psor**, Puls, Rad-brom, Rhus-tox, **Silica**, Stannum, **Sulphur**, Syphilinum, **Thuja**, Tub, Zinc)*

Appendix IV Leprosy, Its Miasm and Its Nosode, Leprosinum[57]

Leprosy is a progressive, chronic disease of low infectivity. *Mycobacterium leprae* spreads through the body rather like dry rot creeps through the wooden structure of a house. It causes changes to skin, bone, glands and the soft organs; particularly the liver and spleen. It has a long period of incubation, sometimes of many years. It especially affects 10- to 20-year-olds and boys more than girls. It can take up to 40 years to manifest. Its chronic course begins with the development of lesions on the skin and damage to the peripheral nerves; tumorous growths form in the skin, nerves and membranes. It has a particular propensity for affecting the bones of the face, the nasal cavities, the palate and the phalanges of the feet and hands.

Leprosy cannot be cultured in vitro; it needs living tissue on which to form. Infection has been thought to be through skin lesions or via mucous membranes; it is believed that it is contracted during childhood. Other theories as to its origins in the body include that of the bacterium being inhaled on dust particles into the respiratory system. Offspring of lepers are more likely to develop the disease than others.

There are two forms of leprosy: lepromatous and tubercular. In the former, skin lesions are painless macules that are freely disseminated across the body; they are rosy or shiny. The skin of the face and ear lobes are the most affected parts though the onset is very gradual. There are also episodes of fever and pain in the peripheral nerves. Gradually the skin becomes thickened and corrugated with a tendency to oedema. The loss of the eyebrows is characteristic as are painless lumpy nodules like ganglia. Internally there is a gradual breakdown

57 We are greatly indebted to Prakash Vakil, a homoeopath in Mumbai, who studied and treated leprosy for some while, for his insight into the disease and his development of the nosode. His painstaking work was published by the International Foundation for Homoeopathy in their publication *Proceedings of the 1991 Professional Case Conference (Small remedies and interesting cases III)*. For a full description of the history of leprosy see this author's *The Companion to Homoeopathy*.

of the mucous membranes which eventually leads to ulceration. Deformity of the nasopharyngeal mucosa and the nasal cavity develops; iritis and blindness often follow.

Tubercular leprosy has scanty dissemination of the macules though there are well-defined patches of lesions with raised edges and a pebbly surface. The skin becomes dry and hairless, scaly and depigmented. Lesions most often appear on the legs, especially on the shins where they are erythematous. Peripheral nerves become thickened and palpable; neuritis occurs at the extremities. Sensory and motor nerves are damaged while there is surface anaesthesia. The skin becomes cold, inelastic and shiny with an absence of sweat. Muscles become fibrotic and contracted. There is facial palsy. The sinuses are chronically active. Perforating ulcers appear at points of pressure. Tuberculoid tumours form along nerve lines and these become caseated; they form cold abscesses that develop without inflammation and are filled with white pustular matter.

From this description it is possible to see parallels with other miasms, most especially syphilis, psora, tuberculosis and cancer. In cases where patients manifest pathology that is similar to the leprous state, it is reasonable to consider the use of **Leprosinum**, the nosode, when indicated remedies fail to achieve positive changes. (Obvious examples include ringworm, vitiligo, some varieties of eczema, erythema nodosum, ganglia, Bell's palsy, iritis and ozaena.) **Leprosinum** was proved in India where the disease is still prevalent. In order for us to see how **Leprosinum** might be appropriately used in western Europe we need to exercise a certain amount of intuition. As a 'picture' the remedy may seem to be remote from people born in Britain but if we view it as a remedy for the removal of a block to cure then it becomes of more than passing interest. We need to bear in mind that the energy of this miasm lies dormant and has not been obviously manifest for many generations. It is often difficult to see the miasm for all that goes on in complex cases, and the use of the nosode is commonly neglected; it may appear as a last resort. Results may at first seem frustrating as it is a remedy that may require frequent repetition till any shift is observable; perhaps this is a reflection of the remote depth of history within the patient.

General symptoms

Deformities, especially minor ones such as 'rat-bitten' ears though there can be the foreshortening of limbs or missing digits. Nodules and lumps under the skin; wrinkling of the skin. Loss of hair especially of the face. Oily or waxy skin though there is a general lack of sweat. Neuropathy and neuritis. Oedema especially of the feet and ankles. Pains in the joints. Numbness and tingling; pins and needles especially accompanied by icy coldness of the part affected. Osteoarthritis. Psoriasis, icthyosis, scleroderma. Dryness of the whole body; pruritis. Tendency to ulceration and suppuration. Aggravation from the sun or radiating heat. Amelioration from rest and gentle motion.

Mental and emotional symptoms

Attribute their condition to fate and believe that medicine will not achieve a cure. May feel that no one should ever suffer like this yet may also be hopeful of recovery. There is a strong sympathy for others (even overweening) especially those in a similar plight. Wants sympathy but hides the need. Cannot bear the idea that others might learn of their condition as they feel shame strongly. Become thoroughly dejected and isolated; seek solace in religion especially among minority denominations. Strong desire for company but only with like-minded people in order to avoid rejection. A deep sense of rejection. Mildness of character; tend to be unnaturally accepting of whatever befalls them. Despite what may appear as a victim mentality, they can be irritable especially when shown too much sympathy or charity. Defensive of others who might be at a disadvantage.

Patients who are likely to show signs of the leprosy miasm are:

- those who belong to minority groups
- those who seek consolation, security and support in nonconformist faiths
- children who are subjected to bullying: dyslexics and others with medium or severe learning disabilities
- those who have been subjected to prolonged emotional stress and feel ostracized
- patients who have all other typical signs of the tubercular miasm but lack the excessive sensitivity, mood swings and fiery nature
- those who live or work without prospects within a large institution through no choice of their own
- those who have a victim mentality

• those who are subject to the powerful influence of others especially if these others are parents, spouses or managers who are tubercular or syphilitic in nature.

The new remedies associated with the leprosy miasm

Aquamarine, Berlin Wall, Curcuma Longa, Dolphin Sonar, Goldfish, Hazel, Himalayan Crystal Salt, Jet, Malus Domestica, Moldavite, Oryza Sativa, Senecio + Tyria, Statice, White Chestnut Flower.

Familiar remedies that are complementary to the nosode

Anac, Arsen-alb, Calc-carb, Carb-ac, Carb-an, Carbo-veg, Causticum, Graphites, Iris-vers, Kali-iod, Lach, Mephitis, Nat-carb, Nat-mur, Phos, Psor, Sec, Sepia, Silica, Tub.

Bibliography

Agrawal, Dr YR, *A Treatise on Bowel Nosodes*, Vijay Publications, 1981

Berkow, Beers, Bogin, Fletcher, *The Merck Manual of Medical Information* (Home Edition), Merck & Co, Inc., 1997

Boericke, Oscar, MD, *Homoeopathic Materia Medica with Repertory*, Boericke & Runyon, 1906

Chancellor, Philip M, *Illustrated Handbook of the Bach Flower Remedies*, The CW Daniel Co Ltd, 1971

Clark, Andrew, *Minerals* (Hamlyn Nature Guides), Hamlyn, 1979

Clarke, JH, MD: *A Dictionary of Practical Materia Medica*, Homoeopathic Publishing Co, 1903

Culpeper, N, *Culpeper's Complete Herbal*, Wordsworth Editions, 2007

Gienger, Michael, *Crystal Power, Crystal Healing, The Complete Handbook*, Cassell, 1998

Grieve, Mrs M, *A Modern Herbal*, Harcourt, Brace & Co, 1931

Griffith, Colin, MCH RS Hom, *The Companion to Homoeopathy*, Watkins, 2005
— *The Practical Handbook of Homoeopathy*, Watkins, 2006
— *The New Materia Medica Volume I*, Watkins, 2007

Hamaker-Zondag, Karen, *Tarot as a Way of Life*, Samuel Weiser, Inc., 1997

Hall, Judy, *The Encyclopaedia of Crystals*, Godsfield Press, 2007

Harper-Shove, Lt Col F, *Prescriber and Clinical Repertory of Medicinal Herbs*, The CW Daniel Co Ltd, 1938

Hsueh-Lien, Tsao & Thornton, Bruce, *Meridians*, Astrolog Publishing House, 2004

Julian, OA, MD, *Materia Medica of New Homoeopathic Remedies*, Beaconsfield Publishers, 1979

Kaptchuk, TJ, *The Web that has No Weaver*, Congdon & Weed, 1983

Keble Martin, W, *The Concise British Flora in Colour*, Ebury Press & Michael Joseph 1965

Kozminsky, Isidore, *The Magic and Science of Jewels and Stones*, Cassandra Press, 1988

Lad, Dr Vasant, *Ayurveda, The Science of Self-Healing*, Lotus Press, 1984

Lessell, Dr Colin B, *The Biochemic Handbook*, Thorsons, 1984

Lyman, Kennie (editor), *Simon and Schuster's Guide to Gems and Precious Stones*, Simon and Schuster, 1989

Melody, *Love is in the Earth, A Kaleidoscope of Crystals*, Earth-Love Publishing House, 1991

More, D & White, J, *The Illustrated Encyclopaedia of Trees*, Timber Press, 2002

Murphy, Robin, *The Homoeopathic Medical Repertory*, Hahnemann Academy of North America, 1993

Orion, Rae, *Astrology for Dummies*, Wiley Publishing, Inc., 1999

Oken, Alan, *Complete Astrology, A Modern Guide to Astrological Awareness*, Bantam Books, 1973

Page, Dr Christine R, *Frontiers of Health*, The CW Daniel Co Ltd, 1992

Paterson, Jacqueline Memory, *Tree Wisdom (The Definitive Guidebook to the Myth, Folklore and Healing Power of Trees)*, Thorsons, 1996

Quelch, MT, *Herbal Remedies and Recipes and Some Others*, Faber & Faber, 1945

Rehman, Abdur, (editor), *The Encyclopaedia of Remedy Relationships in Homoeopathy*, Thieme Verlag, 2005

Scholten, Jan, *Homoeopathy and Minerals*, Stiching Alonnissos, 1993

Sherr, Jeremy, *The Homoeopathic Proving of Plutonium Nitricum*, Narayana Publishers, 1999

Smits, Tinus, MD, *Autism, Beyond Despair*, Emryss Publishers, 2010

Stuckenschmidt, HH, *Twentieth Century Music* (World University Library), Weidenfeld & Nicolson, 1969

Vermeulen, Frans, *The Synoptic Materia Medica*, Merlijn Publishers, 1992

Weiss, Rudolf Fritz, MD, *Herbal Medicine*, Beaconsfield Publishers, 1988

Winston, Julian, *The Heritage of Homoeopathic Literature*, Great Auk Publishing, 2001

Wren, RC, FLS, *Potter's New Cyclopaedia of Botanical Drugs and Preparations*, (revised Williamson and Evans), The CW Daniel Co Ltd, 1988

INDEX